Male Sexual Dysfunction

Male Sexual Dysfunction

EDITED BY

Robert J. Krane, M. D.

*Professor and Chairman, Department of Urology,
Boston University School of Medicine; Urologist in
Chief, University Hospital, Boston*

Mike B. Siroky, M. D.

*Associate Professor of Urology, Boston University
School of Medicine; Attending Surgeon and Director,
Neuro-Urology Laboratory, University Hospital, Boston*

Irwin Goldstein, M. D.

*Assistant Professor of Urology, Boston University
School of Medicine; Director, Division of Urology,
Boston City Hospital, Boston*

LITTLE, BROWN AND COMPANY
BOSTON/TORONTO

1983

Contents

Contributing Authors

George S. Benson, M. D.
Associate Professor of Surgery (Urology), The University of Texas Medical School at Houston; Active Staff, Department of Urology, The Hermann Hospital, Houston
CHAPTER 3

Jerry G. Blaivas, M. D.
Associate Professor of Urology and Director of Neurourology, Columbia University College of Physicians and Surgeons; Attending Urologist, Presbyterian Hospital, New York
CHAPTER 24

Roy P. Finney, M. D.
Professor of Surgery (Urology), University of South Florida College of Medicine; Chief, Section of Urology, James A. Haley Hospital, Tampa
CHAPTER 21

Steven C. Fischer, Psy. D.
Assistant Professor, Division of Psychiatry, Boston University; Associate Director, Behavior Therapy Unit, Boston University Medical Center, Boston
CHAPTERS 15, 19

Irwin Goldstein, M. D.
Assistant Professor of Urology, Boston University School of Medicine; Director, Division of Urology, Boston City Hospital, Boston
CHAPTERS 7, 11, 16

John G. Gregory, M. D.
Professor of Urology, Saint Louis University School of Medicine; Director of the Program in Urology, St. Louis University Group of Hospitals, St. Louis
CHAPTER 25

Ibrahim S. Hawatmeh, M. D.
Clinical Assistant Professor, Saint Louis University School of Medicine; Attending Surgeon, Genitourinary Surgery, St. Louis University Group of Hospitals, St. Louis
CHAPTER 25

Erik Houttuin, Ph. D., M. D.
Assistant Professor, Department of Surgery (Urology), Saint Louis University School of Medicine; Attending Surgeon, St. Louis University Group of Hospitals, St. Louis
CHAPTER 25

Milorad J. Jevtich, M. D.
Attending Urologist and Vice-Chairman, Department of Urology, Washington Hospital Center, Washington, D. C.
CHAPTERS 13, 14

Udo Jonas, M. D.
Chairman, Department of Urology, University of Leiden; Chairman, Department of Urology, Academisch Ziekenhuis, Leiden, The Netherlands
CHAPTERS 2, 3

Kailash R. Kedia, M. D.
Assistant Professor of Urology, Case Western Reserve University School of Medicine; Chief of Urology, Division of Urology, Metropolitan General Hospital, Cleveland
CHAPTER 4

Robert J. Krane, M. D.
Professor and Chairman, Department of Urology, Boston University School of Medicine; Urologist in Chief, University Hospital, Boston
CHAPTERS 2, 7, 11, 12, 18

Gary Leach, M. D.
Assistant Clinical Professor of Urology, University of California, Los Angeles, School of Medicine; Staff Urologist and Director of Urodynamics Laboratory, Kaiser Foundation Hospital, Los Angeles
CHAPTER 20

Robert M. Levin, M. D.
Assistant Research Professor of Urology and Director of Urologic Research, The University of Pennsylvania School of Medicine, Philadelphia
CHAPTER 3

Terrence R. Malloy, M. D.
Associate Professor of Urology, The University of Pennsylvania School of Medicine; Chief of Urology, Pennsylvania Hospital, Philadelphia
CHAPTER 17

Daniel D. Maxwell, M. D.
Attending Radiologist, Radiology Department, Washington Hospital Center, Washington, D. C.
CHAPTER 14

JoAnn McConnell, Ph. D.
Assistant Professor of Neurobiology and Anatomy, The University of Texas Medical School at Houston, Houston
CHAPTER 3

Arnold Melman, M. D.
Associate Professor, Mount Sinai School of Medicine of the City University of New York; Associate Director, Department of Urology, Beth Israel Medical Center, New York
CHAPTER 3

Harris M. Nagler, M. D.
Assistant Professor of Urology, Columbia University College of Physicians and Surgeons; Assistant Attending Urologist, Presbyterian Hospital in the City of New York, New York

CHAPTERS 9, 10

Herbert F. Newman, M. D.
Lecturer in Surgery, Mount Sinai School of Medicine of the City University of New York, New York

CHAPTER 1

Pat O'Donnell, M. D.
Assistant Professor, Department of Urology, University of Arkansas College of Medicine; Chief, Urology Section, Veterans Administration Medical Center, Little Rock

CHAPTER 20

Carl A. Olsson, M. D.
Professor and Chairman, Department of Urology, Columbia University College of Physicians and Surgeons; Director of Urology, Presbyterian Hospital, New York

CHAPTER 10

Leonard M. Pogach, M. D.
Assistant Professor of Medicine, College of Medicine and Dentistry of New Jersey, Newark; Attending Physician, Endocrinology, Veterans Administration Medical Center, East Orange

CHAPTER 6

Michaela H. Purcell, R.N., M.S.N.
Nurse Clinician, Department of Urology, Saint Louis University School of Medicine; Nurse Clinician, St. Louis University Group of Hospitals, St. Louis

CHAPTER 25

Shlomo Raz, M. D.
Associate Professor of Surgery/Urology, University of California, Los Angeles, School of Medicine; Attending Surgeon, Department of Urology, UCLA Medical Center, Los Angeles

CHAPTER 20

Mike B. Siroky, M. D.
Associate Professor of Urology, Boston University School of Medicine; Attending Surgeon and Director, Neuro-Urology Laboratory, University Hospital, Boston

CHAPTERS 2, 7, 11, 12, 18

Michael P. Small, M. D.
Clinical Professor of Urology, University of Miami School of Medicine, Miami
CHAPTER 22

Alma Dell Smith, Ph. D.
Assistant Professor of Psychiatry (Psychology), Boston University School of Medicine; Staff Psychologist, University Hospital, Boston
CHAPTERS 15, 19

Michael J. Torrens, M. Phil., Ch. M., F. R. C. S.
Clinical Tutor, University of Bristol; Consultant Neurosurgeon, Frenchay Hospital, Bristol, Great Britain
CHAPTER 5

Judith L. Vaitukaitis, M. D.
Professor of Medicine and Physiology, Boston University School of Medicine; Head, Section of Endocrinology and Metabolism, Boston City Hospital, Boston
CHAPTER 6

Keith Van Arsdalen, M. D.
Fellow in Urological Research, The University of Pennsylvania School of Medicine, Philadelphia
CHAPTERS 3, 17

Alan J. Wein, M. D.
Chairman, Division of Urology, The University of Pennsylvania School of Medicine; Hospital of the University of Pennsylvania, Philadelphia
CHAPTERS 3, 17

Ralph deVere White, F. R. C. S.-Ed.
Associate Professor of Urology, Columbia University College of Physicians and Surgeons; Attending Urologist, Presbyterian Hospital, New York
CHAPTER 9

Max K. Willscher, M. D.
Assistant Clinical Professor of Urology, Boston University School of Medicine, Boston; Urologist, Elliott Hospital and Catholic Medical Center, Manchester, New Hampshire
CHAPTER 8

Preface

G. F. Lydston, one of the early pioneers in the treatment of male sexual dysfunction, observed in 1908 that the impotent patient does not seek the cause of his problem, only relief from his predicament, which Lydston described as "a flaccid penis in a physiological emergency." Nearly 70 years passed before therapeutics advanced to the point that it can provide a reasonable hope of relief for the great majority of patients with sexual dysfunction. Because sexual dysfunction has many possible etiologies, treatment has often been fractionated in the past between psychiatry, endocrinology, neurology, physical medicine, and urology. This chaotic state of affairs produced, on a research level, relatively slow progress in understanding the mechanisms of sexual dysfunction and, on a clinical level, relatively ineffective patient treatment.

Two trends have become apparent in the last decade that are rapidly changing the approach to male sexual dysfunction. One is the establishment of multidisciplinary clinics designed to focus the efforts of specialists in the various fields that impact on the problem of sexual dysfunction. The organization of such clinics is designed to promote a cooperative effort in the evaluation and treatment of patients. As one example, patients diagnosed to have organic impotence are nevertheless evaluated psychologically to resolve issues of fear and anxiety about surgical therapy. Postoperatively, if further psychologic counseling or therapy is required, the already established relationship with the psychologist or psychiatrist is easily resumed. Conversely, patients with psychogenic impotence who have failed psychologic sex therapy can more easily be considered for surgical therapy in such a setting. The multidisciplinary approach thus offers the patient a treatment program that ultimately should prove more successful in alleviating sexual dysfunction.

The second trend is the emergence of the urologist as the primary coordinator of care for the patient with sexual dysfunction, whether the cause of that dysfunction is an organic, a psychogenic, or as sometimes occurs, a combined one. In one sense, this is merely a reaffirmation of the historical role of the urologist as a specialist in diseases of the male genital tract. In another sense, it recognizes the importance that prosthetic surgery has recently assumed in the treatment of impotence.

We have attempted in this book to collate the knowledge gained from our experience and that of our contributors in evaluating and treating the male patient with sexual dysfunction. Such knowledge has accumulated exponentially in recent years. Some diagnostic techniques, such as sacral evoked response studies, now increasingly routine, did not exist 10 years ago while others, such as measurement of penile blood pressures and nocturnal penile tumescence examinations, were in their infancy. Therapeutic techniques have also advanced rapidly, particularly with respect to prosthetic implantation and microvascular bypass surgery. With this increased experience has come the realization that physical mechanisms play a much greater role in male sexual dysfunction than previously believed.

The purpose of this text is to provide a comprehensive background for physicians, psychologists, nurses, and allied health professionals concerned with male sexual dysfunction. The trend toward the multidisciplinary approach is reflected in contributions from sex therapy, psychology, endocrinology, physical medicine, neurosurgery, and urology. The first several chapters are concerned with basic neurovascular physiology and methods of assessment. Following this, the various treatment modalities are discussed in detail by individuals experienced in each particular technique.

We wish to acknowledge our debt to the contributing authors without whose expert and timely efforts this endeavor could not have been completed. We also are very grateful to Ms. Karen E. Cooper and Ms. Lorelei Satariano, our secretaries, for their administrative skill and devotion to duty.

R. J. K.
M. B. S.
I. G.

Male Sexual Dysfunction

Physiology of Erection: Anatomic Considerations

HERBERT F. NEWMAN

In the human, the criterion for full penile erection is the assumption of a straight line between the mobile, pendulous portion of the penis and its root, fixed to the ischiopubic ramus. These two components communicate freely with each other, and the flooding of their potential spaces while they are contained in a firm envelope converts them into a single, rigid organ. Erection is the function of the corpora cavernosa, whereas the corpus spongiosum is concerned with ejaculation. The latter will maintain a length pari passu with the corpora cavernosa and will attain slight turgescence, but never significant rigidity. Necessarily, their architectures differ.

The *corpora cavernosa* consist of an irregular, interconnecting network of spaces produced by *trabeculae* made up of collagenous, elastic, and smooth muscle fibers. Each corpus is surrounded by the *tunica albuginea,* a dense, fibrous layer with little elastic or smooth muscle tissue. It is continued between the two corpora as an incomplete septum with multiple openings permitting free communication between the two. In the flaccid penis, the tunica is 2.0 mm thick, decreasing to about 0.5 mm when the organ becomes erect. It is only slightly extensile but can experience enormous pressures without bursting. The tunica about the spongiosum is much thinner, contains considerable elastic tissue, and stretches easily.

The *pudendal arteries* furnish the entire blood supply to the corpora. Their extrapenile anatomy and that of the terminal aorta, with its pelvic branches, are of importance to the vascular surgeon treating impotence. The monograph of Ginestie and Romieu [12] describing normal and aberrant anatomy of the pudendal arteries should be consulted by the angiographer. On reaching the perineum, each pudendal artery sends out a fine perineal branch as well as two branches to the corpus spongiosum, the *bulbar* and *urethral arteries.* It continues as the *artery of the penis,* dividing just outside the crus into two terminal branches. One, the *dorsal artery* of the penis, goes anterior to the crus and corpus cavernosum, to leave the pelvis under the arcuate ligament. The other, the *deep artery* of

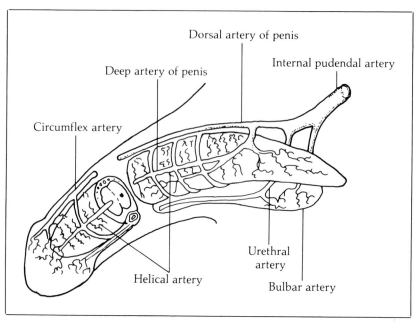

Figure 1-1. The arterial supply to the penis.

the penis (artery of the corpus cavernosum), enters the crus and traverses the entire length of the corpus cavernosum in an axial position (Fig. 1-1). There are extensive anastomoses between all the arteries of the penis, and ligation of one pudendal artery will not cause penile gangrene and may not result in impotence unless other vessels are compromised. Within the corpora cavernosa, branches of the deep artery of the penis furnish end vessels, the helicine arteries and the nutrient vessels to the trabeculae and tunica albuginea. The *helicine arteries* are sinuous vessels directed toward the tunica and glans in an arborizing manner; they are most prominent in the proximal part of the corpora. They enter the trabeculae and finally open into the cavernous spaces.

Erection is produced by the shunting of arterial blood into the cavernous spaces through arteriovenous (AV) *anastomoses.* Müller's study [19] of the penis in 1835 initiated the concept of a vessel's joining an artery to a vein without an interposing capillary network. Since then, an enormous literature on the subject of anastomoses has developed, and an excellent summary was done by Clara in 1939 [4]. Particular attention to their presence in the penis has been made by Vastarini-Cresi [27] and Stieve [23].

In his important article, Conti [5] described three types of AV anastomoses in the penis:

1. The variety found in the dartos tunic resembles the classic glomerular digital AV anastomosis. There is a coiled afferent artery, an intermediate segment, and a coiled afferent vein with meager mural musculature. The intermediate part is characterized by an endothelium that often is lined with cuboidal cells, the absence of an internal elastic lamina, a media marked by epithelioid cells, and poor separation between the replaced longitudinal and circular muscle fibers.

2. A rare variety described by Stieve with the anastomotic segment (a thin-walled vessel arising from short, straight branches of the deep artery and opening directly into the cavernous spaces).

3. The helicine arteries themselves act as the major source of shunting. Their terminal branches represent the intermediate segment with a thick wall containing epithelioid cells and devoid of an internal elastic lamella. They open into the cavernous spaces that, lined by endothelium, act as the afferent venous component of the AV anastomosis. The size of the anas-

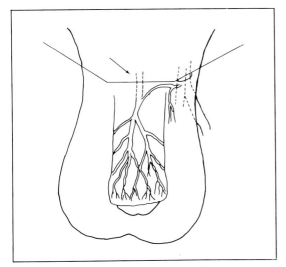

Figure 1-2. Superficial dorsal vein of the penis, emptying into the left saphenous vein. *Arrow* indicates an anastomosis with the deep dorsal vein of the penis.

tomotic lumen is controlled by the epithelioid cells in some as yet unclear manner. On the basis of electron microscopy, Fujimoto and Takeshige [11] did not believe they were degenerated or undifferentiated smooth muscle cells.

PENILE CIRCULATION

There are three major sets of veins composing the venous outflow of the penis; they are the superficial, intermediate, and deep, and there are multiple unnamed communicating vessels.

1. The *superficial dorsal vein* of the penis may be single, multiple, or forked. Draining a subcutaneous network of veins from the prepuce to the symphysis, it opens into one saphenous vein or, less frequently, into both or directly into the femoral (Fig. 1-2).

2. The *deep dorsal vein* (dorsal profunda) is the intermediate vein of the penis. Arising from a plexus in the glans, it travels in a sulcus between the two corpora, deep to Buck's fascia, to enter the pelvis under the arcuate ligament. Although usually single, it may be branched or multiple. Thin-

walled *venae comitantes* often accompany the dorsal arteries of the penis.

3. The *deep* or *profunda veins* of the penis are one or more vessels draining each corpus cavernosum. They leave the crus in an area uncovered by the ischiocavernosus muscle to enter the prostatic plexus. The corpus spongiosum similarly empties into the bulbar veins.

4. Communicating veins. *Emissary veins* are short channels that arise in the corpora and penetrate the tunica albuginea. Superior emissary veins leave the cavernosa to enter the deep dorsal vein directly, whereas the inferior vessels join similar branches from the spongiosum to form the *circumflex veins*. These, arising on both sides in the sulcus between the corpus spongiosum and the cavernosa, course transversely outside the tunica albuginea but go deep to Buck's fascia to enter the deep dorsal vein (Fig. 1-3). Some posterior branches leave the spongiosum to join the bulbar veins.

Anastomotic channels join the superficial dorsal vein to the deep dorsal vein, behind the coronal sulcus and in front of the symphysis. Multiple deep channels join the glans to the corpus spongiosum.

Within the pelvis, the deep dorsal vein and branches from the superficial dorsal veins enter the prostatic plexus, whereas the deep veins of the penis and bulbar veins join the internal pudendal vein, which communicates not only with the prostatic plexus but also the hypogastric veins. Valves have been described in the superficial dorsal, deep dorsal, circumflex, and pelvic veins that have been considered by Fitzpatrick [9] important for "sustained" erection.

Disagreements between anatomists as to the exact drainage of each component of the penis have been largely resolved by cavernosography. The prepuce and tissues superficial to Buck's fascia drain into the superficial dorsal veins. The proximal portions of the corpora cavernosa and spongiosum empty through the deep veins of the penis. The glans and pendulous part of the corpus spongiosum drain into the deep dorsal vein

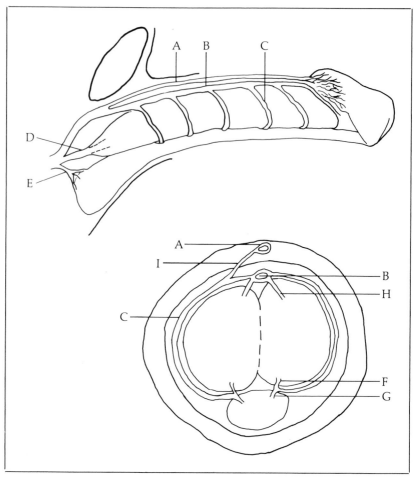

Figure 1-3. Penile veins. A. Superficial dorsal vein. B. Deep (profunda) dorsal vein. C. Circumflex vein. D. Deep (profunda) vein of the penis. E. Bulbar vein. F. Inferior emissary vein from corpus cavernosum. G. Superior emissary vein from corpus spongiosum. H. Superior emissary vein from corpus cavernosum. I. Anastomosis between superficial and deep dorsal veins.

of the penis. The pendulous segment of the corpus cavernosum empties predominantly into the deep veins of the penis and, to a lesser degree, through the deep dorsal vein. If fluid is injected under pressure into the cavernosal spaces, all three sets of veins fill [30]. These common drainage patterns may be altered in such pathologic states as priapism and impotence.

POLSTERS—DO THEY EXIST?

Intravascular protrusions in the penile vessels were described first by Ercolani [8] in 1869, but they are generally called *von Ebner polsters* or *cushions* in the urologic literature. They are characterized by a split in the internal elastic lamella, and the intervening space is filled with longitudinal smooth muscle and con-

nective tissue fibers (Fig. 1-4). Multiple cushions may appear within the same circumference, and there is great variability in the degree to which they may encroach on the lumen. Their length and proximity to each other vary from microns to millimeters.

Deysach [6] denied their existence, and Benson [1] could not find penile cushions in males undergoing a sex transference operation. Newman [20] reported their presence in about one-third of the muscular arteries or

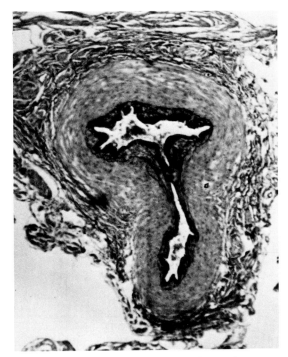

Figure 1-4. Polster at point of branching of a helicine artery.

veins seen in the average cross section at the base of the adult pendulous portion, but none were seen in the penis of a newborn. Polsters have been found in pudendal vessels outside the penis and in other muscular vessels, e.g., lingual, carotid, occipital, vertebral, axillary, subclavian, radial, palmar, brachial, femoral, peroneal, tibial, hepatic, renal, gastric, mesenteric, ovarian, temporal, and coronary arteries (Lie [17], Kiss [15]). Conti [5] attributed considerable importance to their role in the mechanism of erection. He believed relaxation of the polsters in the penile arteries together with active contraction of those in the veins induced erection; he believed that the reverse causes detumescence.

What do the polsters represent? Many theories have been offered:

1. That they represent centers of growth was suggested by Wright [29] because they are more common in the lower extremity, as compared to the upper, and are more frequent in the first two decades of life. There is no evidence of cellular activity in the cushions, and the concept of a soft-tissue growth center comparable to an epiphysis is highly speculative.

2. Hirsch [14] believed that they are inflammatory reactions in the penis because, he claimed, he always found signs of inflammation in the genital tract. However, their presence extragenitally, even in the fetus, precludes this possibility.

3. Conti [5] believed that they are anatomic structures with physiologic function. This notion is sheer teleology, arguing function from appearance. They are not present in the newborn penis. Conti admitted that contraction of arterial polsters in the relaxed penis was an exception to their behavior elsewhere in the body. They demonstrate a great diversity in appearance and occur so close to each other that they probably furnish passive resistance to flow, rather than selective diversion.

4. Robertson [21] advanced the theory that they represent a response to stress and aging. This is the most attractive hypothesis because the polsters are likely to be present at points of branching, tapering, curvature, or external attachment of vessels. Texon [25] demonstrated that these are the very places where a decrease in lateral pressure exerts traction on the intima. Lie and Brown [17] felt that pulsatile stress at these points was significant. Linear stress was held responsible by Dock [7], on the basis of finding polsters in the beating epicardial vessels of the fetus but not in the fingers or flexure levels of the popliteal arteries. His notion that the increase in length in systole produces linear stress is easily applicable to the human penis.

The relationship between the polsters and arteriosclerosis is obscure and warrants investigation. Their locations are similar to those of the early lesions in arteriosclerosis, and the histologic distinction between the two is blurred. In the older patient, they are early sites for frank atherosclerotic changes (Ruzbarsky [22]). Their absence in Benson's cases who were on massive doses of estrogen [1] is highly significant.

Many investigators who consider a restricted venous outflow as essential to the induction or maintenance of erection have sought anatomic support:

1. Penile venous sphincters. Haines [13] described a smooth muscle sphincter in the wall of the deep dorsal vein of the penis where it passes under the arcuate ligament. This has not been confirmed, and his illustration suggests a polster.
2. Striated muscle action. Müller [19] postulated that contraction of the ischiocavernosi muscles constricted the deep veins of the penis, and, as late as 1962, Lindner [18] claimed they aided erection by compressing the crura against the pubic bone. Testut [24] attributed to the muscles of Houston and Müller, slips from the cavernosae muscles, a slinglike action on the deep dorsal vein. Cadiat [3] has demonstrated anatomically that these muscles could not compress the deep veins of the penis; Kollberg and co-workers [16] found them quiescent by electromyography during erection; and, in Bors's review [2], flaccid paralysis did not preclude reflex erection.
3. Smooth muscle action. Valentin [26] suggested that contraction of the trabecular smooth muscle would restrict venous outflow, and Testut [24] claimed a similar effect on the superficial veins by the smooth muscle fibers in the dartos tunic.
4. Sluices in the wall of the deep vein of the penis described by Deysach [6] have not been confirmed.
5. Venous compression by rising intracorporeal pressure. Conti [5] suggested that the shunting of arterial blood into the corporeal spaces could compress the thin-walled veins at the periphery. Similarly, Fitzpatrick [9] claimed that the expanding shaft compressed the circumflex veins between the tunica albuginea and Buck's fascia.

REFERENCES

1. Benson, G. S., et al. Neuromorphology and neuropharmacology of the human penis. *J. Clin. Invest.* 65:506, 1980.
2. Bors, E., and Comarr, A. E. Neurological disturbances of sexual function, with special reference to 529 patients with spinal cord injury. *Urol. Surv.* 10:191, 1960.
3. Cadiat, M. Étude sur les muscles de perinée. *J. de l'Anat.* 1877.
4. Clara, M. Die arteri-venöse anastomosen. *J. Barth Leipzig,* 1939.
5. Conti, G. L'erection du penis humain et ses bases morphologico-vasculaires. *Acta Anat.* 14:217, 1952.
6. Deysach, L. J. The comparative morphology of the erectile tissue of the penis with especial emphasis on the probable mechanism of erection. *Am. J. Anat.* 64:111, 1939.
7. Dock, W. F. The predilection of arteriosclerosis for the coronary arteries. *J.A.M.A.* 131:875, 1946.
8. Ercolani, J. B. Des tissus des organes erectiles. *J. de l' Anat.* 1869.
9. Fitzpatrick, T. J. Venography of the deep dorsal venous and valvular system. *J. Urol.* 111:518, 1974.
10. Fitzpatrick, T. J., and Cooper, J. F. A cavernosogram study on the valvular competence of the human deep dorsal vein. *J. Urol.* 113:1479, 1975.
11. Fujimoto, S., and Takeshige, Y. The wall structure of the arteries in the corpora cavernosa of the penis of rabbits: Light and electron microscopy. *Anat. Rec.* 181:641, 1975.
12. Ginestie, J. F., and Romieu, A. *Arteriography of Internal Pudendal Artery.* The Hague; Mijoff, 1978.
13. Haines, R. W. An unstriped sphincter of the dorsal vein of the penis. *J. Anat.* 107:385, 1970.
14. Hirsch, E. W. The so-called arterial valves in the penile arteries. *J. Urol.* 25:61, 1931.
15. Kiss, F. Anatomisch-histologische untersuchungen über die erektion. *Ztsch. f. Anat.* 61:455, 1921.
16. Kollberg, S., Petersen, I., and Stener, I. Preliminary results of an electromyographic study of ejaculation. *Acta Chir. Scand.* 123:478, 1962.
17. Lie, J. T., and Brown, A. Normal Structure of the Vascular System and General Reactive Changes of the Arteries. In J. L. Fairbairn, L. I. Juergens, and J. A. Spittell, Jr. (eds.), *Peripheral Vascular Diseases* (4th ed.). Philadelphia: Saunders, 1972.
18. Lindner, H. H., and Feldman, S. E. Surgical anatomy of the perineum. *Surg. Clin. North Am.* 42:877, 1962.

19. Müller, J. Entdeckung der bei der erektion des männlichen gliedes wirksamen Arterien bei dem menschen und dem thieren. *Arch. Anat. Physiol. u. Wiss. Med.* 202, 1835.
20. Newman, H. F., and Tschertkoff, V. Penile vascular cushions and erection. *Invest. Urol.* In press.
21. Robertson, J. H. Influence of mechanical factors on the structure of the peripheral arteries and the localization of arteriosclerosis. *J. Clin. Pathol.* 13:199, 1960.
22. Ruzbarsky, V., and Michal, V. Morphological changes in the arterial bed of the penis with aging: Relationship to the pathogenesis of impotence. *Invest. Urol.* 15:194, 1977.
23. Stieve, H. *Harn und geschlechts-apparat (Zweiter Teil): Siebenter Bar. Handb. d. mikr. anat. d. menschen.*, Berlin: *J. Springer*, 1930.
24. Testut, L., and Latarjet, A. *Appareil Urogenital* (vol. 5). *Traité d' Anatomie Humaine* (8th ed.). Paris: Doin, 1930.
25. Texon, J. Mechanical Factors Involved in Atherosclerosis. In A. W. Brest and J. H. Mayer (eds.), *Atherosclerotic Vascular Disease.* New York: Appleton-Century-Crofts, 1967.
26. Valentin, G. Uber den verlauf der blütgefasse im dem penis des menschen und einiger saugetiere. *Arch. Anat. Physiol. u. Wiss, Med.* 1838.
27. Vastarini-Cresi, G. Communicazioni dirette tra le arterie e le vene (anastomosi arterio-venose) nei mammiferi. *Mon. Zool. Ital.* 13:136, 1902.
28. Von Ebner, V. Uber klappenärtige vorrichtungen in den arterien der schwellkörper. *Anat. Anz.* 18:79, 1900.
29. Wright, I. The microscopical appearances of human peripheral arteries during growth and aging. *J. Clin. Pathol.* 16:499, 1963.
30. Wrobel, S. Zylne krazenie oboczne pracia w obrazie radiologicznym. *Pol. Przegl. Chir.* 45:849, 1973.

2

Neurophysiology of Erection

MIKE B. SIROKY
ROBERT J. KRANE

The mechanism of penile erection until recently has received scant research attention since Conti's classic description [8] in 1952. Recent research has focused on the neural innervation of the penis as well as on control of the penile vasculature. This chapter deals with the neurovascular physiology of erectile function and reviews recent research results when they are appropriate to the discussion.

OVERVIEW

All levels of the central and peripheral venous system participate in the neural mechanism of erection. Because of the dominance of the cerebral cortex, the processing of sexual stimuli is much more complex in humans than in lower animals. Nevertheless, the preoptic hypothalamic region appears to be an important center controlling heterosexual behavior in most species. The efferent pathway from the hypothalamus proceeds along the medial forebrain bundle, through the substantia nigra of the midbrain, and into the ventrolateral pons. In the spinal cord, the efferent tracts are probably within the lateral columns, but this is unclear. The efferent impulses exit the spinal cord through the thoracolumbar and sacral autonomic nerves.

The penis is innervated by both divisions of the autonomic nervous system as well as by somatic sensory nerves. The sacral parasympathetic nerves, when stimulated, cause penile erection, but these nerves are almost certainly preganglionic in nature. The thoracolumbar nerves, when stimulated, cause detumescence of the erect penis, although they appear also to control tumescence of the corpus spongiosum. The corpora cavernosa have a very significant adrenergic innervation. Clarification of the neural mechanism by which the penile vasculature is controlled during erection and detumescence will require further research.

INNERVATION OF THE PENIS

Sensory

As is shown in Figure 2-1, somatic innervation of the penis is provided by the pudendal nerves, which arise from sacral segments

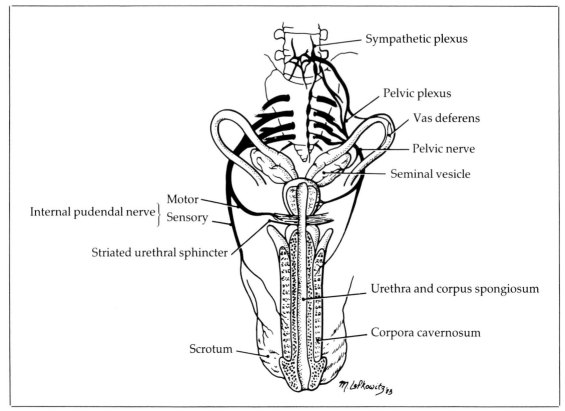

Figure 2-1. Autonomic and somatic innervation of the male internal genitalia. Details of peripheral neuronal organization are not included.

S2 to S4. The *pudendal nerve* is a mixed motor-sensory nerve that provides motor supply to the perineal striated muscles as well as sensory supply to the penile skin [54]. Sensory receptors in the glans penis and penile skin are described as nonspecific, free, and spray-like nerve endings [36]. In the deeper layers of the skin, pacinian corpuscles may be found.

It is of interest that receptors in the glans penis of certain species (e.g., the cat) have been shown to be androgen dependent [9]. The function of these receptors is indicated by the fact that anesthetization of the glans penis [9] or section of the dorsal penile nerves [22] impairs the ability of the animal to achieve intromission, although penile erection itself remains unchanged.

The functions of the pudendal nerve and its central afferent pathway have been studied with electrophysiologic techniques. Although both the pudendal and the tibial nerves are mixed motor-sensory nerves, the conduction velocity in the pudendal nerve is significantly slower [38]. Futhermore, conduction velocities in the afferent tracts of the spinal cord subserving the pudendal nerve were also much slower when compared to stimulation of other peripheral nerves.

In our own clinical work, we have been able to determine the latency of response in the appropriate area of the cerebral cortex after pudendal nerve stimulation. The response has been termed the *genitocerebral evoked response* (GCER). The central conduction time of the GCER is approximately 28 msec, also significantly slower than the central conduction time for the posterior tibial nerve (see Chap. 16).

Motor
The corpora cavernosa and corpus spongiosum receive motor innervation from the pelvic nerves, which arise from sacral cord

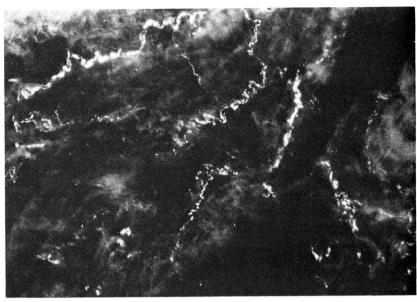

Figure 2-2. Fluorescence photomicrograph of human corpus cavernosum using glyoxylic acid method. (Photo courtesy of JoAnn McConnell, Ph.D.)

segments S2 to S4 (see Fig. 2-1). The pelvic nerves constitute the major motor input to the penis. However, sympathetic fibers from the thoracolumbar spinal cord also supply the penile vasculature, particularly the corpus spongiosum.

The report by Baumgarten and co-workers [3] in 1969 concerning adrenergic fibers in the corpus cavernosum provided considerable impetus to further research on the motor innervation of the penis. They found abundant adrenergic fibers in the corpus cavernosum of the cat and monkey, but a less prominent adrenergic nerve supply to the corpus spongiosum. Other investigators, however, reported conflicting results, finding a predominance of cholinergic over adrenergic fibers [26, 47].

Baumgarten's findings have been confirmed by investigators using the recently developed glyoxylic acid histofluorescence technique. Benson and McConnell [4, 37] have demonstrated marked histofluorescence (specific for catecholamines) in the corpus cavernosum of rat, rabbit, cat, monkey, and human (Fig. 2-2). The histofluorescence was evenly distributed throughout the corpus cavernosum, without regional variation. The corpus spongiosum contained far less histofluorescence. In contrast, acetylcholinesterase-positive fibers were scant in human corpus cavernosum.

The significance of these findings is still unclear. Do the adrenergic fibers arise from thoracolumbar sympathetic nerves (long adrenergic nerves) or from postganglionic adrenergic nerves in the penis (short adrenergic neurons)? Whereas Benson and McConnell did not demonstrate catecholamine-containing cell bodies in their material, Dail and Evan [10] found short adrenergic neurons in the rat penis [10]. Furthermore, what is the role of these adrenergic nerves in the mechanism of penile erection? In vitro experiments have shown that norepinephrine causes an alpha-adrenergic-receptor–mediated contraction of the corporal smooth muscle, whereas acetylcholine has no effect [4, 27, 37]; this suggests an active, rather than passive, role for the corpora, one mediated by adrenergic mechanisms.

NEUROPHYSIOLOGIC OBSERVATIONS
The neurogenic mechanism of penile erection was first demonstrated by Eckhardt [13] in

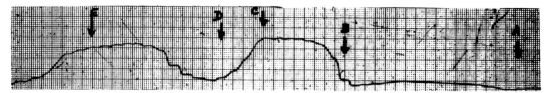

Figure 2-3. Recording of canine intracorporeal pressure during various nerve-stimulation experiments. A. Pelvic nerves (PN) and hypogastric nerves (HG) were stimulated simultaneously, producing low-level pressure increase. B and D. HG stimulation stopped. C and E. Stimulation restarted. Stimulation parameters 4 V, 1 msec duration, 20 Hz. Calibration: 1 box vertical = 20 cm H_2O. 1 box horizontal = 5 sec.

1863 when he reported that electrical stimulation of the sacral parasympathetic nerves produced penile erection in dogs [13]. He termed these nerves *nervi erigentes*. After Eckhardt's report, Gaskell [16] found that the nervi erigentes exit from the spinal cord by the anterior nerve roots S2, S3, and S4. This basic schema has been corroborated many times by subsequent investigators [11, 21].

Cholinergic Mechanisms

Attempts to elucidate the pharmacologic mechanism of erection soon followed Eckhardt's report. With one exception [40], most investigators found that atropine had little or no effect on nerve-induced penile erection in dogs [11, 21, 31]. Direct arterial injection of acetylcholine produces little or no change in vascular tone in the corpus cavernosum [11, 41]. It has long been known, however, that nicotine [30] as well as other ganglionic blocking agents [5] can block completely penile erection induced by pelvic nerve stimulation. Thus, pharmacologic studies of penile erection demonstrate that acetylcholine is almost certainly not the neurotransmitter finally responsible for vascular engorgement of the penis. The evidence is most consistent with the view that the pelvic nerves are preganglionic and synapse with more distal neurons, whose transmitter is unknown.

Adrenergic Mechanisms

Early work on hypogastric (sympathetic) nerve stimulation led to contradictory results. Partial penile erection was observed in dogs by Bacq after hypogastric nerve stimulation [2]. In contrast, Langley and Anderson [30] observed only vasoconstriction in the external male genitalia of various experimental species. Furthermore, surgical extirpation of both sympathetic chains below the diaphragm does not interfere with erection in the otherwise intact cat [46]. Stimulation of the sympathetic trunk or hypogastric nerves causes detumescence of pelvic nerve–induced erection in the cat [46] as well as in the dog [5] (Fig. 2-3).

Neuropharmacologic studies of the response of penile vessels to adrenergic agents were first reported by Elliott in 1905 [14]; he found that epinephrine caused the penile arteries of the dog to contract. This has been confirmed by recent studies involving the penile vessels [41] as well as the corporal smooth muscle [4]. These effects are blocked by pretreatment with an alpha-blocking agent such as phentolamine. However, Dorr and Brody [11] could not produce erection in dogs by intraarterial injection of norepinephrine.

Our own studies [51] have demonstrated that direct arterial injection of isoproterenol, a beta agonist, can induce partial penile tumescence in the dog (Fig. 2-4). It seems increasingly clear that adrenergic mechanisms play an important role in penile erection. Whether other neuroactive agents such as prostaglandins, vasoactive intestinal polypeptide (VIP) [43], substance P, and adenosine triphosphate (ATP) play a role remains to be determined.

Somatic Mechanisms

The *pudendal nerve* is a mixed motor-sensory nerve that provides somatic afferent innervation (dorsal nerve of the penis) as well as

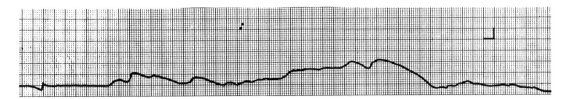

Figure 2-4. Change in canine intracorporal pressure secondary to intraarterial injection of 5 mg terbutaline sulfate, a beta agonist. Injection occurred at start of long arrow beneath recording. Calibration is same as in Figure 2-3. Note that the response is considerably less than that obtained by pelvic nerve stimulation. (Reprinted from R. J. Krane and M. B. Siroky, Neurophysiology of erection. *Urol. Clin. North Am.* 8:1, 1981. With permission of W. B. Saunders Co.)

efferent innervation to the perineal striated musculature. In rhesus monkeys, section of the dorsal penile nerve resulted in less frequent attempts at intercourse [22]. In cats, this procedure largely prevented successful intromission [9, 46]. In dogs, contraction of the perineal striated muscles produces more rapid tumescence, but erection still occurs in the absence of perineal muscle activity [19]. The perineal striated muscles appear to play an auxiliary role in humans as well [29].

CENTRAL CONTROL MECHANISMS
Spinal Cord
The classic experiments of Root and Bard [44] provide insight into the complementary roles of the thoracolumbar (sympathetic) and sacral (parasympathetic) outflows from the spinal cord. These investigators showed that, after ablation of the entire sacral spinal cord, male cats attained full erection in the presence of estrous females. If the spinal cord was transected above the sympathetic outflow, however, erections were abolished. These results demonstrate that at least a portion of the erectile response is mediated by the thoracolumbar outflow in some animals.

The clinical correlate of this experiment is traumatic spinal cord injury. After complete sacral cord lesions, up to one-fourth of patients may demonstrate potency [5], although the quality of their erections was not described. In these patients, only psychogenic stimuli lead to erections. With lesions above T8, psychogenic stimuli are no longer effective, but local stimuli become increasingly effective (reflex erection). With cervical cord injuries, nearly all patients experience reflex erections.

More light has been shed on this phenomenon by a recent study of erectile function in spinal cord injury [7]. The majority (82%) of patients with complete lesions above the thoracolumbar outflow (T12) had reflex erections involving the corpora cavernosa as well as the corpus spongiosum. In contrast, only 35 percent of patients with lesions below T12 had such erections, the majority having erections involving only the corpora cavernosa. Thus, the spinal cord segments controlling the corpus spongiosum appear to have their outflow at T11-T12 (Fig. 2-5).

Higher Centers
The cerebral cortex and subcortical structures control penile erection as well as sexual behavior in general. The role of the temporal lobes in sexual function was demonstrated by the classic studies of Kluver and Bucy [28]. After bilateral temporal lobectomy, rhesus monkeys demonstrated increased heterosexual, homosexual, and autosexual behavior. Similar results have been reported in cats [48]. MacLean's experiments in the monkey have demonstrated positive loci for erection in the gyrus rectus of the cerebral cortex, the angulate gyrus, the paraventricular nucleus of the hypothalamus, and the mamillary bodies [12, 34, 35]. Electroencephalographic studies have shown that the hippocampus also plays a role in penile erection. The hippocampus and cingulate gyrus constitute important centers in the *lumbic lobe of Broca*, which has been called the emotive or visceral brain [33] and which has extensive connec-

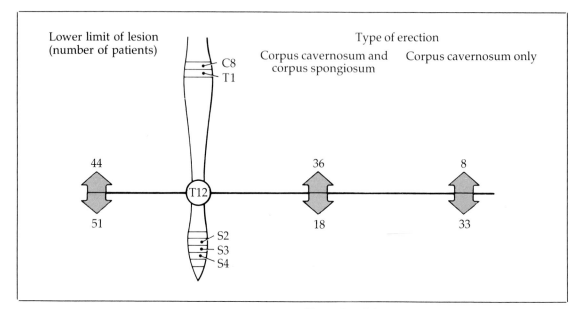

Figure 2-5. Schematic drawing to demonstrate that erections of corpora cavernosa and corpus spongiosum are controlled by different spinal cord segments. (Based on data of P. A. Chapelle, J. Durand, and P. Lacert, Penile erection following complete spinal cord injury in man. *Br. J. Urol.* 52:216, 1980.)

tions with the thalamus and hypothalamus (Fig. 2-6).

The efferent pathway from the hypothalamus appears to be through the medial forebrain bundle. More caudally, the outflow proceeds through the substantia nigra in the midbrain and then descends into the ventrolateral pons.

The mamillary bodies and cingulate gyrus are concerned with processing visual stimuli, whereas the gyrus rectus receives olfactory stimuli. The finding of positive loci for erection in the visual system in primates suggests an evolutionary progression from the primacy of olfactory stimuli in lower species to inclusion of visual stimuli in higher species.

Certain subcortical structures have been shown to influence the level of sexual activity. Lesions in the medial preoptic region of the hypothalamus abolish sexual activity in experimental animals [52] (Fig. 2-7). Conversely, electrical stimulation of this region of the hypothalamus facilitates mating activity in male rats [56]. In monkeys, stimulation of nearby structures such as the dorsomedial nucleus of the hypothalamus results in increased sexual activity [42].

Thus, in lower animals as well as in primates, the preoptic–anterior hypothalamic region is an important center for determining heterosexual behavior. It is of interest that only heterosexual activity is abolished by lesions in this region, whereas autosexual behavior is unaffected. Furthermore, these effects are not mediated by changes in testosterone metabolism, which remains unchanged.

Neuroendocrine Factors
Our knowledge of central neurotransmitter mechanisms is still rudimentary. There is evidence, however, that brain serotonin levels may play a role in neural control of sexual activity. For example, parachlorophenylalanine (PCPA), which is known to decrease brain serotonin synthesis, will enhance testosterone-induced sexual activity in various experimental animals [15]. Another central neurotransmitter, dopamine, also has been shown to play a role in male sexual behavior. Administration of L-dopa to male rats increases sexual activity, whereas dopamine receptor blockade with haloperidol blocks this effect [55]. These results suggest that male sexual activity is inhibited by central

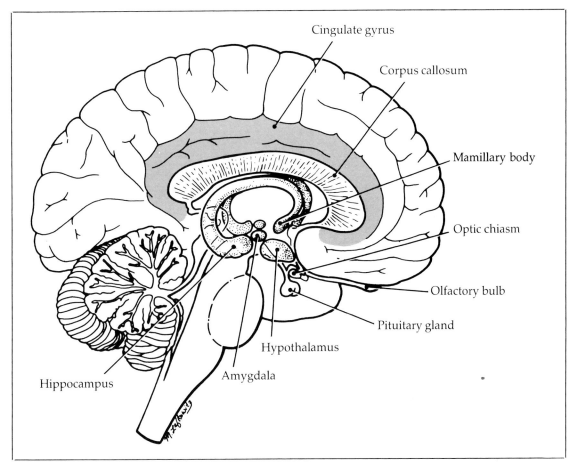

Figure 2-6. Component parts of the limbic lobe of the brain (visceral brain).

serotoninergic mechanisms and stimulated by dopaminergic mechanisms [18].

HEMODYNAMICS OF ERECTION

The internal pudendal arteries, branches of the anterior hypogastric arteries, provide blood supply to the corpora cavernosa, the corpus spongiosum, and the superficial perineal tissues. The internal pudendal arteries have four terminal branches, i. e., the superficial perineal (scrotal), the artery of the bulb, the deep penile, and the dorsal penile. On entering the corpus cavernosum, the deep penile artery divides into multiple, markedly tortuous branches (helicine arteries). More distally these become the vascular spaces of the corporal tissue, with free anastamoses between the two corpora [1].

Henderson and Roepke [21] demonstrated that pressure within the corpora cavernosa rises during erection in the dog until it approaches that in the aorta. At the same time, venous outflow from the penis is increased considerably. Angiography of the internal pudendal artery demonstrates little or no filling of the corpora at rest, but a twofold increase in flow through the pudendal artery during erection (Fig. 2-8). Whether venoconstriction plays any role remains controversial.

The microvascular anatomy of the penis was carefully studied by Conti [8] in 1952. Because he found muscular polsters, or cushions, in the penile vessels, Conti proposed the following mechanism for penile erection (Fig. 2-9): (1) arteriovenous shunts are closed, resulting in shunting of arterial blood into the

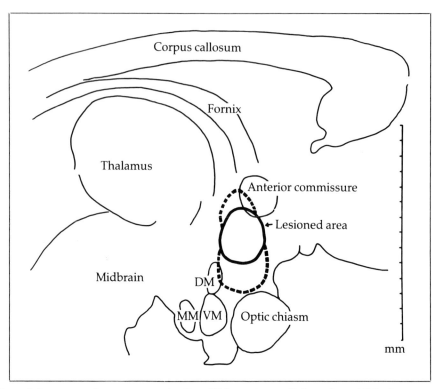

Figure 2-7. Sagittal section of rhesus monkey brain, 1.5 mm lateral to midline. Solid line: sexual activity regularly abolished. Dotted line: variability of lesions. Symbols: MM: mamillary bodies; VM: ventromedial nucleus; DM: dorsomedial nucleus. (Reprinted from J. C. Slimp, B. L. Hart, and R. W. Goy [52]. With permission of Elsevier Scientific Publishing.)

Figure 2-8. Pelvic nerve–induced erection in the dog. Stimulation on and off is indicated by small deflections in line above aortic blood pressure. Notice that marked increase in internal iliac artery flow access occurs within 2 sec of onset of nerve stimulation, whereas corporal pressure begins to rise 12 sec later even if nerve stimulation is stopped.

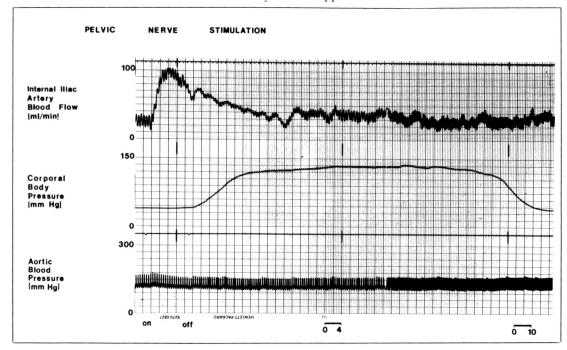

Time [sec]

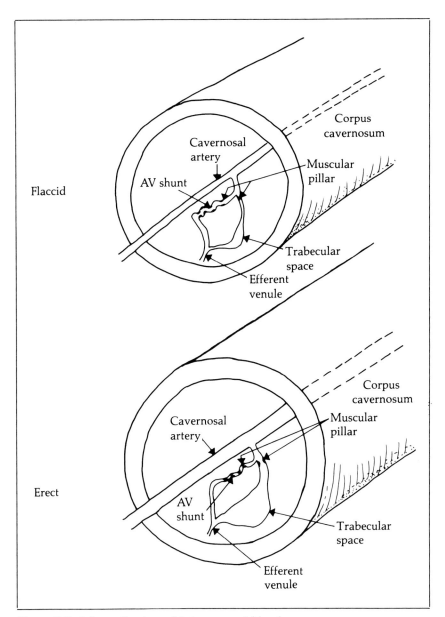

Figure 2-9. Schematic view of intracorporal blood flow regulation based on G. Conti, L'erection du penis humain et ses bases morphologio vascularis. *Acta Anat. (Basel)* 14:17, 1952.

cavernous spaces; (2) the deep efferent veins are occluded; and (3) blood flow to the superficial penile tissues is decreased.

Although it is clear that an active mechanism is responsible for rediverting arterial blood into the corporal spaces, the role of Conti's polsters (previously described by von Ebner) is unclear. Many investigators have been unable to find polsters in the corpus cavernosum of human [4] and rat [32]. However,

myoendothelial cells are known to proliferate after injury to the vessel [6] or with arteriosclerosis [20]. Thus, Conti's "polsters" may simply represent age-related degenerative changes in the penile vessels rather than physiologic structures.

CLINICAL CORRELATION
The role of the parasympathetic and sympathetic nerves in penile erection has been discussed above. Thus, it is not surprising that traumatic and metabolic lesions of the peripheral nerves lead to erectile impotence.

For example, the incidence of impotence in diabetic men is 2 to 5 times that in age-matched controls, ultimately affecting 50 percent of the diabetic population [14]. It has been shown that impotence and somatic or autonomic neuropathy coexist in 82 percent of cases [24, 45]. Therefore, clinical studies appear to indicate that peripheral neuropathy plays an important role in the sexual dysfunction of diabetic men, although angiopathy increasingly is being recognized as an etiologic factor.

Traumatic spinal cord lesions are well known to alter sexual function, as has been discussed above. About one-fourth of men with multiple sclerosis are impotent [23] and generally have a diminished or absent bulbocavernosus reflex [57]. Idiopathic degeneration of the lumbosacral sympathetic neurons also has been related to impotence, loss of sweating, and orthostatic hypotension [25]. Other spinal cord disorders that may cause impotence are syringomyelia, spinal cord tumor, tabes dorsalis, and arachnoiditis.

Supraspinal lesions and diseases also are known to influence sexual function. It has been reported, for example, that two-thirds of patients with *temporal lobe epilepsy* suffer impotence; this is in contrast to relatively few patients with other types of epilepsy [17]. Head injuries may result in impotence, despite otherwise complete recovery [53]. Impotence also has resulted from neurosurgical procedures intended to relieve myoclonus [39]. The surgical lesions include the septum pellucidum, an area known to contain positive loci for erection.

Patients with Parkinson's disease may have impotence that is not entirely explained by their motor disability. A prominent feature of this disease is degeneration of the substantia nigra, an area of the midbrain that serves as an efferent pathway for penile erection. The Shy-Drager syndrome also has been associated with impotence and loss of libido. Autopsy studies of this disorder have demonstrated degeneration of the substantia nigra [49].

REFERENCES

1. Alvarez-Morujo, A. Terminal arteries of the penis. *Acta Anat. (Basel)* 67:387, 1967.
2. Bacq, Z. M. Recherches sur la physiologie et la pharmacologie du systeme nerveux anatonome: XII. Nature cholinergique et adrenergique des diverses innervations vasomotrices du penis chez le chien. *Arch. Int. Physiol. Biochim.* 11:311, 1935.
3. Baumgarten, H. G., Falck, B., and Lange, W. Adrenergic nerves in the corpora cavernosa penis of some mammals. *Z. Mikrosk. Anat. Forsch.* 95:58, 1969.
4. Benson, G. S., et al. Neuromorphology and neuropharmacology of the human penis. *J. Clin. Invest.* 65:506, 1980.
5. Bors, E., and Comarr, E. A. Neurological disturbances of sexual function with special reference to 529 patients with spinal cord injury. *Urol. Surv.* 10:191, 1960.
6. Borst, H., and Enderlen, V. Die transplantation von Gefassen und ganzer organen. *Dtsch. Z. Chir.* 99:54, 1909.
7. Chapelle, P. A., Durand, J., and Lacert, P. Penile erection following complete spinal cord injury in man. *Br. J. Urol.* 52:216, 1980.
8. Conti, G. L'erection du penis humain et ses bases morphologio vascularis. *Acta Anat. (Basel)* 14:17, 1952.
9. Cooper, M. L., and Aronson, L. R. Behavioral implications of a histological study of the sensory innervation of the penis of intact and castrated cats. *Am. Zool.* 9:570, 1969.
10. Dail, E. G., and Evan, A. P. Experimental evidence indicating that the penis of the rat is innervated by short adrenergic neurons. *Am. J. Anat.* 141:205, 1974.
11. Dorr, L. D., and Brody, M. J. Hemodynamic mechanism of erection in the canine penis. *Am. J. Physiol.* 213:1526, 1967.
12. Dua, S., and MacLean, P. D. Localization for penile erection in medial frontal lobe. *Am. J. Physiol.* 207:1425, 1964.
13. Eckhardt, C. Untersuchungen uber die Erection des Penis beim Hund. *Beitr. Anat. Physiol.* 3:123, 1863.
14. Elliott, T. R. The action of adrenaline. *J. Physiol. (Lond.)* 32:401, 1905.
15. Ferguson, J., et al. Hypersexuality and behavioral changes in cats caused by administration of *p*-chlorophenylalanine. *Science* 168:499, 1970.
16. Gaskell, W. H. Preliminary communication to the Physiologic Society of London on the structure, distribution and function of the nerves which innervate the visceral and vascular systems. *J. Physiol.* 7:1, 1886.

17. Gastaut, H., and Collomb, H. Etude du comportement sexuel chez les epileptiques psychomoteurs. *Ann. Med. Psychol.* 2:657, 1954.

18. Gessa, G. L., and Tagliamonte, A. Role of brain monoamines in male sexual behavior. *Life Sci.* 14:425, 1974.

19. Hart, B. L., and Kitchell, R. L. Penile erection and contraction of penile muscles in the spinal and intact dog. *Am. J. Physiol.* 210:257, 1966.

20. Haust, M. D., More, R. H., and Movat, H. Z. The role of smooth muscle cells in the fibrinogenesis of arteriosclerosis. *Am. J. Pathol.* 37:377, 1960.

21. Henderson, V. E., and Roepke, M. H. On the mechanism of erection. *Am. J. Physiol.* 106:441, 1933.

22. Herbert, J. The role of the dorsal nerves of the penis in the sexual behavior of the male rhesus monkey. *Physiol. Behav.* 10:293, 1973.

23. Ivers, R. R., and Goldstein, M. P. Multiple sclerosis: A current appraisal of symptoms and signs. *Mayo Clin. Proc.* 38:457, 1963.

24. Jimenez, J. F., et al. Impotence and diabetes mellitus. *Eur. Urol.* 3:78, 1977.

25. Johnson, R. H., et al. Autonomic failure with orthostatic hypotension due to intermediolateral column degeneration. *Q. J. Med.* 35:276, 1966.

26. Klinge, E., and Penttila, O. Distribution of noradrenaline and acetylcholinesterase in bull and rabbit penile erectile tissue. *Ann. Med. Exp. Biol. Fenn.* 47:17, 1969.

27. Klinge, E., and Sjostrand, N. O. Contraction and relaxation of the retractor penis muscle and the penile artery of the bull. *Acta Physiol. Scand.* [Suppl.]:420, 1974.

28. Kluver, H., and Bucy, P. C. Psychic blindness and other symptoms following bilateral temporal lobectomy in rhesus monkeys. *Am. J. Physiol.* 119:352, 1937.

29. Kollberg, S., Petersen, J., and Stener, I. Preliminary results of an electromyographic study of ejaculation. *Acta Chir. Scand.* 123:478, 1962.

30. Langley, J. N., and Anderson, H. K. The innervation of the pelvic and adjoining viscera: III. The external generative organs. *J. Physiol.* 19:85, 1895–1896.

31. Langley, J. N., and Anderson, H. K. The innervation of the pelvic viscera and adjoining viscera: IV. The internal generative organs. *J. Physiol.* 19:122, 1895–1896.

32. Leeson, T. S., and Leeson, C. R. The fine structure of cavernous tissue in the adult rat penis. *Invest. Urol.* 3:144, 1965.

33. MacLean, P. D. The lumbic system ("visceral brain") in relation to central gray and reticulum of the brainstem. *Psychosom. Med.* 17:355, 1955.

34. MacLean, P. D., Denniston, R. H., and Dua, S. Further studies on cerebral representation of penile erection: Caudal thalamus, midbrain and the pons. *J. Neurophysiol.* 26:273, 1963.

35. MacLean, P. D., and Ploog, D. W. Cerebral representation of penile erection. *J. Neurophysiol.* 25:29, 1962.

36. Malinovsky, L., and Sammerova, J. Sensory innervation of the clitoris and penis in the macaque. *Folia Morphol.* 20:192, 1972.

37. McConnell, J., Benson, G. S., and Wood, J. Autonomic innervation of the penis: A histochemical and physiological study. *J. Neural Transm.* 45:227, 1979.

38. Meyer, M., LaPlante, E. S., and Campbell, B. Ascending sensory pathways from the genitalia of the cat. *Exp. Neurol.* 2:186, 1960.

39. Meyers, R. Three cases of myoclonus alleviated by bilateral ansotomy, with a note on postoperative alibido and impotence. *J. Neurosurg.* 19:71, 1962.

40. Nikolsky, W. Ein Beitrag zur Physiologie der nervi erigentes. *Arch. Anat. Physiol. (Lpz.) Jahrgang.* 209, 1879.

41. Penttila, O. Acetylcholine, biogenic amines, and enzymes involved in their metabolism in penile erectile tissue. *Ann. Med. Exp. Biol. Fenn.* [Suppl.] 44:9, 1966.

42. Perachio, A. A., Alexander, M., and Marr, L. D. Hormonal and social factors affecting evoked sexual behavior in rhesus monkeys. *Am. J. Phys. Anthropol.* 38:227, 1973.

43. Polack, J. M. Vipergic nerves in the penis. *Lancet* 2:217, 1981.

44. Root, W. S., and Bard, P. The mediation of feline erection through sympathetic pathways with some remarks on sexual behavior after deafferentation of the genitalia. *Am. J. Physiol.* 150:80, 1947.

45. Rubin, A., and Babbott, D. Impotence and diabetes mellitus. *J.A.M.A.* 168:498, 1958.

46. Semans, J. H., and Langworthy, O. R. Observations on the neurophysiology of sexual function in the male cat. *J. Urol.* 40:836, 1938.

47. Shirai, M. Studies on the male sexual impotence: IV. On peripheral nerves controlling erection. *Jpn. J. Urol.* 64:1, 1973.

48. Shreiner, L., and Kling, A. Behavioral changes following rhinencephalon injury in cat. *J. Neurophysiol.* 16:643, 1953.

49. Shy, G. M., and Drager, G. A. A neurological syndrome associated with orthostatic hypotension. *Arch. Neurol.* 2:511, 1960.

50. Siroky, M. B., and Krane, R. J. The mechanism of penile erection: A neuropharmacologic study. *Surg. Forum* 30:545, 1979.

51. Siroky, M. B., and Krane, R. J. Unpublished studies, 1979.

52. Slimp, J. C., Hart, B. L., and Goy, R. W. Heterosexual, autosexual, and social behavior of adult male rhesus monkeys with medial preoptic anterior hypothalamic lesions. *Brain Res.* 142:105, 1978.

53. Stier, E. Disturbances of sexual functions through head trauma. *J. Nerv. Ment. Dis.* 88:714, 1938.

54. Sugita, A. Experimental studies on the neurogenic bladder report: VI. Experimental and histological studies of the pudendal nerve. *Jpn. J. Urol.* 55:423, 1964.

55. Tagliamonte, A., et al. Evidence that brain dopamine stimulates copulatory behavior in male rats. *Rev. Farm. Terap.* 4:177, 1973.

56. Van dis, H., and Larsson, K. Induction of sexual arousal in the castrated male rat by intracranial stimulation. *Physiol. Behav.* 6:85, 1971.

57. Vas, C. J. Sexual impotence and some autonomic disturbances in men with multiple sclerosis. *Acta Neurol. Scand.* 45:166, 1969.

3

Erectile Physiology

Adrenergic Innervation of the Human Penis: In Vitro Studies

GEORGE S. BENSON
JOANN MCCONNELL

Penile erection has been classically considered to be a parasympathetically mediated event. For over 30 years, however, both clinical [15] and laboratory [13] evidence has accumulated that demonstrates that penile erection also may be controlled by the sympathetic nervous system.

In the experiments described below, we have attempted to answer four questions concerning the adrenergic innervation of the human penis:

1. Are penile "polsters" innervated by adrenergic neurons?
2. Are penile blood vessels and/or the erectile tissue of the corpus cavernosum itself innervated by adrenergic neurons?
3. Can adrenergic nerves in the penis be demonstrated at the ultrastructural level?
4. What is the response of penile erectile tissue to in vitro adrenergic stimulation?

ARE PENILE POLSTERS INNERVATED BY ADRENERGIC NEURONS?

The distribution of blood flow within the penis during erection and detumescence is thought to be controlled by smooth muscle columns (*polsters*) within the vascular intima. Although these structures were first described by von Ebner in 1900, Conti [4] popularized the importance of these structures in penile arteries and veins. On the basis of morphologic evidence in cadavers, he hypothesized that contraction and relaxation of these structures could determine the magnitude and direction of penile blood flow. If Conti's hypothesis is indeed correct, the smooth muscle in the polsters should receive autonomic innervation.

Penile tissues from three groups of patients (male transsexuals undergoing gender reassignment operations, men undergoing penectomy for cancer, and children undergoing

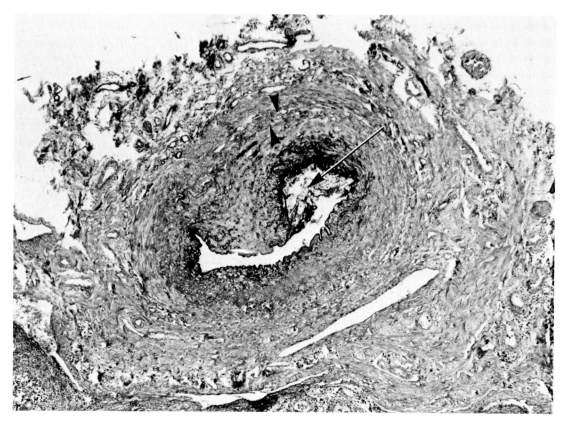

Figure 3-1. Cross section of a human penile artery showing an atherosclerotic plaque with characteristics suggestive of a "polster." Note the thickened intima and duplicated internal elastic lamina (*arrowheads*). Note also the subendothelial deposition of fibrin, which is characteristic of atherosclerosis (*arrow*). (Magnification before reduction: x200)

excision of penile chordee) have been studied to assess the morphologic appearance and frequency of polsters. Tissue obtained from transsexual patients demonstrated a few polsters within veins of the corpus spongiosum (CS), but none were seen in the corpus cavernosum (CC) [1]. The ages of these transsexuals were 24 to 35 years, and all had been treated with oral estrogens for at least 1 year prior to surgery. No structures resembling polsters were seen in penile tissue obtained from children. In a detailed study of tissue obtained from men (aged 49–62) undergoing penectomy for cancer, no incontrovertible evidence of polsters as described by Conti was found [4], although similar structures occasionally were encountered. These were nevertheless, identified as either branching points of vessels, intimal smooth muscle cell cushions, or atherosclerotic lesions in various stages of development (Fig. 3-1).

The significance of intimal smooth muscle cushions and their relationship to athero-

sclerosis is somewhat controversial. Cushions are found in humans in early childhood, usually at branch points of vessels, and have been demonstrated to increase with age [11]. At least some of these cushions appear to be related to the formation of atherosclerotic plaques. It is interesting that Conti described duplication of the internal elastic lamina as well as longitudinal smooth muscle columns as characteristics of polsters. We now recognize that these morphologic findings are characteristic of atherosclerosis.

All of the tissue that we examined, except that obtained from the transsexuals, was from specimens that had been processed previously. Since histofluorescent techniques to identify adrenergic nerves require fresh tissue, we were not able to evaluate every polster for adrenergic innervation. The material obtained from the transsexuals demonstrated a few polsterlike structures, but these polsters had no demonstrable innervation.

We therefore offer an alternative explanation of the significance of polsters. First, the smaller structures represent irregularities of the vascular wall associated with branching vessels. Their appearance depends on obtaining fortuitous sections in the appropriate plane. We recognize that at least some of these cushions may represent early atherosclerotic lesions. Second, the larger vascular wall irregularities represent various stages in the development of atherosclerotic lesions. Such lesions typically arise at branching points of vessels, may be found in the first and second decades of life, and increase in severity, if not in number, with increasing age. It is not surprising, therefore, that any one section, especially of young penile tissue, may be devoid of polsters. One would not expect such structures to be innervated, and we have not been able to demonstrate any innervation to these structures. To our knowledge, no evidence exists that demonstrates an adrenergic innervation to polsters, and, furthermore, no evidence supports the hypothesis that polsters normally control regional penile blood flow.

ARE PENILE BLOOD VESSELS AND/OR THE ERECTILE TISSUE OF THE CORPUS CAVERNOSUM ITSELF INNERVATED BY ADRENERGIC NEURONS?

Through light microscopy, we have examined penile tissue obtained from male transsexual patients treated with ethinyl estradiol for 1 year prior to their operative procedure and tissue from adult males undergoing various urologic procedures. With hematoxylin and eosin and smooth muscle stains, the CC and CS are shown to consist of numerous cavernous spaces partitioned by trabeculae, which are composed of bundles of collagen, elastic fibers, fibroblasts, and groups of smooth muscle cells. The CS has smaller trabeculae with few smooth muscle cells and larger veinlike cavernous spaces.

Tissue from the transsexuals was also studied for adrenergic localization by using the glyoxylic acid histofluorescence technique [5]. Catecholaminergic glyoxylic acid–fluorescent fibers and terminals can be seen in both CC and CS. In CC, numerous glyoxylic acid–fluorescent fibers wind through the trabeculae and approach the walls of the cavernous spaces (Fig. 3-2). Very few histofluorescent fibers occur in CS, but the blood vessels of both corpora often demonstrate adrenergic varicosities in their outer tunic.

Acetylcholinesterase (AChE) localization was utilized to identify presumptive cholinergic nerves [8]. AChE-positive fibers are seen infrequently in human CC and CS. A small number of these fibers can be demonstrated in the CC, but they are sparse or lacking in the CS. The fibers often are arranged in small bundles and may appear near arterioles. Most arterioles demonstrate such AChE-positive structures in the tunica adventitia.

It appears, therefore, that the smooth muscle of the spongy tissue of CC receives dual autonomic innervation and that the adrenergic innervation is denser than the cholinergic innervation. The blood vessels of the penis are also supplied by both adrenergic and cholinergic nerves.

CAN ADRENERGIC NERVES IN THE PENIS BE DEMONSTRATED AT THE ULTRASTRUCTURAL LEVEL?

With the electron microscope (EM), human erectile tissue demonstrates cavernous spaces and trabeculae of varying sizes. The cavernous spaces are lined by endothelial cells (similar to those found in blood vessels), and the trabeculae are composed of varying amounts of smooth muscle, fibroblasts, elastic fibers, collagen, capillaries, and nerves. The trabeculae in CS are smaller and contain few smooth muscle cells and nerve fibers; they are composed primarily of connective tissue elements.

Neural elements are not seen with any frequency in human erectile tissue. Occa-

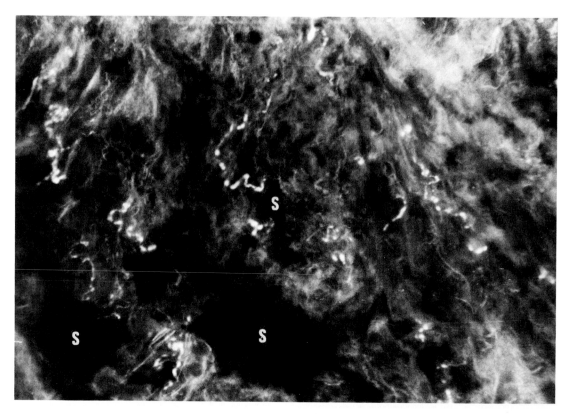

Figure 3-2. Fluorescence photomicrograph of human corpus cavernosum after treatment with glyoxylic acid. The tortuous and brilliant adrenergic fibers stand out against the duller background of autofluorescent connective tissue. Some fibers approach the cavernous spaces (S). (Magnification before reduction: x100)

sionally, profiles of small, unmyelinated nerve bundles containing two to six fibers and/or varicosities are seen, but single fibers or terminals are rare. Vesicles within these varicosities are diverse, but most are small (400–600 Å in diameter), opaque, and granular vesicles without an electron-lucent halo at the periphery. Other varicosities contain large (600–1800 Å in diameter) granular and opaque vesicles that are often elongated and lack a halo. A similar type seen in conjunction with small vesicles tends to be spherical and to have an electron-lucent halo. Large clear vesicles (600–900 Å in diameter) are also seen occasionally.

For more precise EM information, we have fixed tissue with glutaraldehyde-dichromate (G-DC), which allows for specific identification and localization of catecholamines. Under the specific conditions employed, electron-dense chromium is deposited on vesicles containing norepinephrine and dopamine. Tissue fixed in G-DC demonstrates some small, highly electron-dense vesicles, which are considered to be chrome-positive and therefore to contain norepinephrine (Fig. 3-3). Some of the small opaque or granular vesicles, however, are similar in both the control and G-DC–treated material. Neither the glutaraldehyde nor the G-DC–fixed tissue demonstrates small clear vesicles of the type considered to be cholinergic. Varicosities in large clear vesicles have been hypothesized to be sensory, whereas those with large opaque vesicles fit the descriptions for purinergic or peptidergic nerve fibers [3].

At an ultrastructural level, therefore, adrenergic nerves can be identified within CC. The G-DC technique confirms that at least some of the small vesicles in nerve varicosities contain catecholamine.

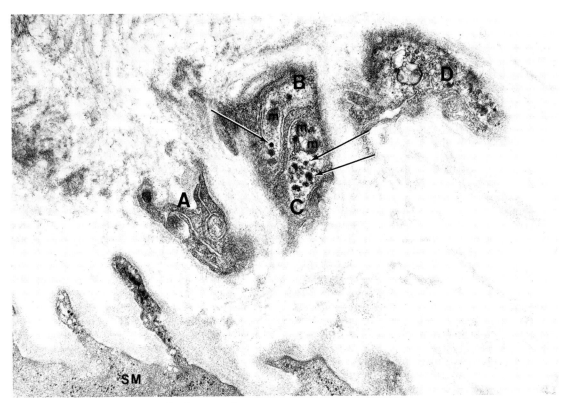

Figure 3-3. Electron micrograph of a smooth muscle cell (*SM*) and adjacent nerve fibers in the human penis. Extremely electron-dense, chromium-positive vesicles can be seen in the varicosities labeled *B* and *C* (*arrows*). Other cellular organelles shown well are mitochondria (*m*), small opaque vesicles, and small and large dense-core vesicles. Nerve bundle *A* contains only indistinct nerve fibers, and *D* indicates a varicosity with a large population of small opaque and dense core vesicles. (Magnification before reduction: x25,000)

WHAT IS THE RESPONSE OF PENILE ERECTILE TISSUE TO IN VITRO ADRENERGIC STIMULATION?

In in invitro muscle-bath chambers, strips of human CC obtained from transsexuals contract when exposed to norepinephrine. This contraction is blocked by pretreating the tissue with phentolamine, and the contraction is unaffected by pretreatment with propranolol. This contractile response is therefore thought to be secondary to alpha-adrenergic receptor stimulation. In high concentration, acetylcholine occasionally produces a minimal contraction that is blocked by atropine.

All of our transsexual patients had been treated long-term with oral estrogen. Hormonal manipulation has been reported to alter responses of other tissues to adrenergic stimulation [7, 14]. The responses obtained in CC of estrogen-treated humans are qualitatively identical, however, to those seen in CC of nonhormonally treated monkeys [10]. It would appear, therefore, that the primary response of human penile erectile tissue to pharmacologic stimulation is alpha-adrenergic receptor–mediated contraction.

COMMENT

The experiments described above demonstrate that the human penis is innervated by adrenergic nerves and that the primary response of the erectile tissue of the corpus cavernosum to pharmacologic stimulation is an alpha-adrenergic receptor–mediated contraction. The significance of this adrenergic innervation and its importance in normal penile physiology, however, are not known.

Increased arterial inflow into the penis appears to be the primary physiologic event that leads to erection [12]. Since Eckhardt's demonstration in 1863 that stimulation of the sacral parasympathetic nerves in the dog results in penile erection, it has been thought that parasympathetic cholinergic nerves either dilate penile arteries or cause shunting of penile blood flow through so-called polsters. As was said above, we do not think that the polster hypothesis is tenable. Furthermore, evidence has accumulated that refutes the concept that erection is controlled exclusively by parasympathetic nerves acting through cholinergic receptors. Data that implicate adrenergic innervation as well as speculation that implicates peptidergic and purinergic nerves in the erectile process have been presented [6, 9]. It should be emphasized, however, that all of these pharmacologic data have been obtained from animal models; no direct pharmacologic evidence for the neurotransmitter responsible for erection is available in humans.

We have demonstrated that the erectile tissue of CC as well as the penile vasculature is innervated by adrenergic nerves. At present, the erectile tissue of CC serves no known function other than to act as a reservoir for increased blood volume during erection. One can speculate that the adrenergically innervated smooth muscle of the erectile tissue does perform a physiologic function. An attractive hypothesis is that, with sympathetic discharge at the time of seminal fluid emission, adrenergic stimulation causes the erectile tissue to contract, further entrap blood within the cavernous spaces, and cause the already erect penis to become even more turgid.

The functional significance of the adrenergic innervation of the penile vasculature is also unknown. Does adrenergic stimulation cause penile blood vessels to constrict or to dilate? With the burst of sympathetic activity during seminal fluid emission, one could hypothesize that adrenergic stimulation results in vasoconstriction, thereby decreasing blood flow and causing penile detumesence. Recent animal data, on the other hand, suggest that adrenergic, particularly beta-2, agonists may actually cause penile erection [6].

Both anatomic and pharmacologic studies demonstrate that the human penis is adrenergically innervated. The influence of this innervation on the penile erectile tissue and blood vessels is not known. The relative importance of adrenergic and cholinergic, as well as possibly nonadrenergic, noncholinergic nerves, in the control of penile erection and detumesence remains to be elucidated.

REFERENCES

1. Benson, G. S., et al. Neuromorphology and neuropharmacology of the human penis. *J. Clin. Invest.* 65:506, 1980.
2. Benson, G. S., McConnell, J. A., and Schmidt, W. A. Penile "polsters": Functional structures or artherosclerotic changes? *J. Urol.* 125:800, 1981.
3. Burnstock, G. Purinergic nerves. *Pharmacol. Rev.* 24:509, 1972.
4. Conti, G. L'erection du penis humain et ses bases morphologicovasculaires. *Acta Anat.* 14:217, 1952.
5. de la Torre, J. C., and Surgeon, J. W. A methodological approach to rapid and sensitive monoamine histofluorescence using a modified glyoxylic acid technique: The SPG method. *Histochemistry* 49:81, 1976.
6. Domer, F. R., et al. Involvement of the sympathetic nervous system in the urinary bladder internal sphincter and in penile erection in the anesthetized cat. *Invest. Urol.* 15:404, 1978.
7. Hodgson, B. J., et al. Effect of estrogen on sensitivity of rabbit bladder and urethra to phenylephrine. *Invest. Urol.* 16:67, 1978.
8. Karnovsky, M. J., and Roots, L. A "direct coloring" thiocholine method for cholinesterases. *J. Histochem. Cytochem.* 12:219, 1964.
9. Klinge, E., and Sjostrand, N. O. Contraction and relaxation of the retractor penis muscle and the penile artery of the bull. *Acta Physiol. Scand.* [Suppl.] 420:1, 1974.
10. McConnell, J. A., Benson, G. S., and Wood, J. Autonomic innervation of the mammalian penis: A histochemical and physiological study. *J. Neural Transm.* 45:227, 1979.
11. Neufeld, H. N., Wagenvoort, C. A., and Edwards, J. E. Coronary arteries in fetuses, infants, juveniles, and young adults. *Lab. Invest.* 11:837, 1962.
12. Newman, H. F., Northup, J. D., and Devlin, J. Mechanism of human penile erection. *Invest. Urol.* 1:350, 1963.
13. Root, W. S., and Bard, P. The mediation of feline erection through sympathetic pathways with some remarks on sexual behavior after deafferentiation of the genitalia. *Am. J. Physiol.* 151:80, 1947.

14. Schreiter, F., Fuchs, P., and Stockamp, K. Estrogenic sensitivity of alpha-receptors in the urethra musculature. *Urol. Int.* 31:13, 1976.
15. Whitelaw, G. P., and Smithwick, R. H. Some secondary effects of sympathectomy with particular reference to disturbance of sexual function. *N. Engl. J. Med.* 245:121, 1951.
16. Wood, J. Electron microscopic localization of amines in the central nervous system. *Nature (London)* 209:1131, 1966.

Catecholamine Levels in Penile Corpora
ARNOLD MELMAN

The rapidity with which penile erection occurs after psychic or physical stimulation suggests that penile tumescence is a neurovascular event. In a classic experiment reported by Eckhard 120 years ago, he claimed that the path to erection in the dog was through the sacral parasympathetic nerves that he termed the *nervi erigentes* [4]. Although parasympathetic control of erection has been generally accepted since Eckhard's report, both modern experimental evidence and clinical experience suggest that adrenergic neurons may be responsible for penile tumescence. This adrenergic control is probably mediated at the intracorporal level through the vascular and smooth muscle network of the erectile tissue. The clinical evidence supporting adrenergic control is the presence of a high incidence of erectile dysfunction accompanying the use of antihypertensive medication possessing adrenergic-blocking activity. There is no similar evidence of erectile failure accompanying the widespread use of anticholinergic drugs. Experimental support for the role of adrenergic neurons mediating penile erection is the subject of this section.

SYMPATHETIC FUNCTION
Measurement of adrenergic nerve function, particularly in organs located below skin level, is technically difficult and must be done indirectly. The response of humans to a shift in posture from supine to upright is mediated through vasoconstrictor adrenergic sympathetic nerves. The measurement of blood pressure, pulse, and plasma norepinephrine during postural changes is used as a general index of alterations of sympathetic nerve function [6]. If a tissue biopsy is available, direct measurement of the tissue content of norepinephrine, the principal transmitter of the sympathetic neurons, can be used as an index of sympathetic neuronal activity [1].

The histologic appearance of adrenergic nerves of smooth muscle is unlike that of the better known cholinergic nerve endings of the peripheral nervous system. Therefore, a description of the basic structure of adrenergic nerves will be presented in an overview of the synthesis, storage, and release of norepinephrine. In addition, the measurement of norepinephrine content of human erectile tissue and of experimental rat corpora will be given.

STRUCTURE

The sympathetic nerves control vascular smooth muscle throughout the body [7]. Vanhoutte [13] and Weiner [15] in recent excellent reviews have carefully emphasized that adrenergic nerve endings, which are the final link of the vasomotor sympathetic centers in the brain, are influenced by many local factors, including physical, chemical, and pharmacologic events. Innervation of all vascular smooth muscle is by postganglionic sympathetic nerves. The cell bodies of these nerves are located in the retroperitoneal ganglia. The density of innervation of the muscle cells by sympathetic nerves varies from organ to organ. For example, both the iris and vas deferens are particularly rich in adrenergic nerves.

The nerve endings of each sympathetic axon form a terminal ground plexus over the receptor cells (Fig. 3-4). The *plexus* may be thought of as a network of axons coursing over, along, and around smooth muscle cells. The endings contain *varicosities;* these nonmyelinated swellings on the axon are approximately 10 nm apart and overlie the receptor cells. Each cell may be covered by several varicosities. *Junctional clefts,* the space between the smooth muscle cells and the terminal varicosities, may vary from actual contact to a distance of 4 nm. Each varicosity contains nearly 1500 storage vesicles, or membrane-covered packets, of norepinephrine. The total content of norepinephrine in each vesicle [3] is $4\text{--}6 \times 10^{-3}$ pg.

SYNTHESIS OF CATECHOLAMINE

Norepinephrine is synthesized in the axoplasm of postganglionic neurons. The initial,

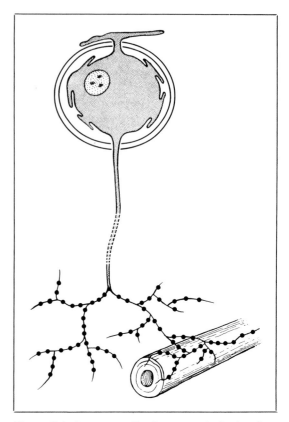

Figure 3-4. A postganglionic neuron is depicted. The terminal axon branches many times and contains vesicles of norepinephrine. The axon branches lie in the outer third of blood vessel walls or lie over the surface of the smooth muscle cells of the penile corpora.

slowest, and therefore the rate-limiting, step is the conversion of the amino acid L-tyrosine, obtained from plasma, to L-dopa by the enzyme tyrosine hydroxylase. L-Dopa is decarboxylated to dopamine in the axoplasm. The dopamine then taken up by the storage vesicles is converted to norepinephrine by the enzyme, dopamine β-hydroxylase (Fig. 3-5). The antihypertensive drugs reserpine and guanethidine inhibit the uptake of dopamine into the vesicles. Regulation of norepinephrine synthesis occurs through alteration of tyrosine hydroxylase activity. Increased norepinephrine concentration in the tissue cytosol results in a negative-feedback effect of tyrosine hydroxylase activity and a change in both enzyme kinetics and production of end product. The converse is similarly true, in

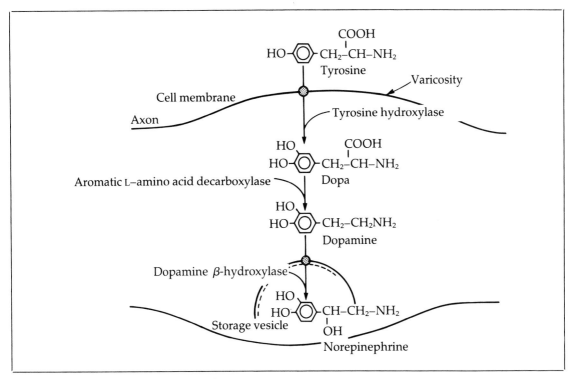

Figure 3-5. Schematic representation of a sympathetic vesicle and norepinephrine production.

that tyrosine hydroxylase activity and synthesis are increased after repeated nerve stimulation, which causes depletion of tissue norepinephrine content.

STORAGE AND RELEASE OF CATECHOLAMINES

The vesicular membrane protects norepinephrine from degradation by cytoplasmic monoamine oxidase. Other substances that are also present in storage vesicles include the enzyme dopamine β-hydroxylase and chromogranins. Nerve stimulation triggers the release of norepinephrine and the other components of the storage vesicle. The release is accomplished by a process of exocytosis. That process is dependent on the influx of calcium into the vesicular membrane. At present, it is believed that the neurotransmitter is released directly into the intracellular space. It is not known whether each nerve impulse causes a specific number of vesicles to release their entire content or whether a number of vesicles simultaneously release some fraction of their total content into the space (junctional cleft). Norepinephrine released after neural stimulation may have one of several fates. The majority of the substance is picked up by its receptor on the smooth muscle cells. Alternatively, it may be enzymatically degraded in the junctional cleft, or it may be taken up by a prejunctional neuron again before reaching its postjunctional disposition. The latter fate, the combining with prejunctional, or alpha-2, receptors as opposed to the alpha-1 receptors on the smooth muscle cells, regulates the exocytosis of norepinephrine from storage vesicles in as yet an unknown way. Of practical importance is the fact that many drugs interact at the alpha-2 level (including dopamine, clonidine, and yohimbine) and thus inhibit the release of norepinephrine.

HUMAN STUDIES

Clinical experience with antihypertensive drugs suggests an interaction of the sympathetic nervous system and penile erection.

It is recognized that the majority of anti-hypertensive drugs that are used to affect vascular smooth muscle by adrenergic blockade as a means of lowering the systemic blood pressure result in patient complaints of erectile impotence. Although some of the drugs (e.g., α-methyldopa) may have central rather than peripheral effects, others are thought to be effective only at the level of the end organ (e.g., guanethidine). Drugs that effect parasympathetic acetylcholine-mediated activity, particularly those used to control bladder instability, are not commonly associated with impotence. In fact, in a study in which we measured the enzyme responsible for the manufacture of acetylcholine, choline acetyltransferase, the enzyme was not active in the erectile tissue of any of the 16 patients analyzed [9]. The inference is that, as throughout the rest of the body, the vascular smooth muscle of penile erectile tissue is modulated by sympathetic neurons and their associated receptors, and not by acetylcholine-mediated parasympathetic stimulation.

To evaluate the role of norepinephrine in human erectile tissue, we measured the content of norepinephrine in patients who underwent penile surgery [10, 11]. The norepinephrine was determined by a radioenzymatic assay that has a sensitivity as low as 10 pg of norepinephrine per milligram of tissue [5]. Thus, tissue content of norepinephrine is a direct reflection of the sympathetic innervation of that tissue, because all measurable tissue norepinephrine is located only within the neuron.

The majority of patients who were undergoing implantation of a penile prosthetic device did so because of impotence secondary to diabetes, prior radical surgery, Peyronie's disease, or transsexual surgery.

We divided the group of men with diabetes into subsets of those requiring insulin for control of blood sugar and those whose illness was managed by diet alone. The transsexual patients were considered as our controls. However, because they received estrogens before surgery, they cannot be considered truly normal patients. (However, collecting fresh erectile tissue from normal patients is not ethically possible in the United States.)

Our results show the effect of various disease states on the norepinephrine content of corporal tissue (Fig. 3-6). Several inferences can be drawn from the data:

1. Norepinephrine is present in high concentration in the smooth muscle of the penis. The mean value of norepinephrine in patients with Peyronie's disease was significantly lower at 189 ± 58 SE pg/mg and normal in spinal cord injury 696 pg/mg wet weight. The concentration in patients with nondiabetic-induced impotence is approximately 600 to 1000 pg/mg of tissue. These measurements can be compared to a reported value of 300 pg/mg of norepinephrine from a radial artery in humans. Plasma norepinephrine content in resting humans is approximately 250 pg/mg. Thus, penile norepinephrine is present in a concentration greater than would be expected for vascular smooth muscle alone. Furthermore, electron microscopic ultrastructural analysis and gold chloride impregnation studies have demonstrated that terminal axons lie in close proximity to muscle cells throughout the cavernous bodies and are not confined to the walls of the arteries and veins of the penile corpora [10–13].

2. Various diseases, particularly diabetes, significantly reduce the norepinephrine content of human erectile tissue. However, some patients with documented impotence do have high norepinephrine content in their erectile tissue (Fig. 3-7). This may suggest other neurotransmitters or a vascular or endocrine etiology.

Two other factors complicate the analysis of the interaction of norepinephrine content and its role in penile erectile dysfunction. One is that few patients with erectile impotence have total absence of erection. A second factor is the possible effect of aging on catecholamine content.

The data obtained from nocturnal penile tumescence studies, performed by an experi-

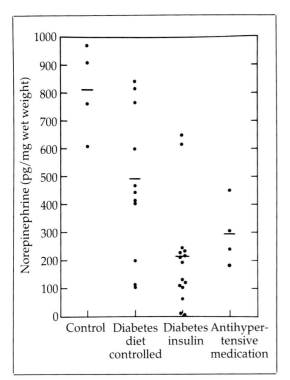

Figure 3-6. The norepinephrine content of penile erectile tissue of impotent men with diabetes of hypertension is shown. The difference between the control and the other groups is significant.

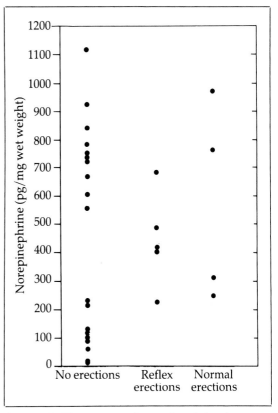

Figure 3-7. The content of norepinephrine from penile tissue is shown, assuming erection as an all-or-none phenomenon.

enced technician, show that men with organic impotence have varying degrees of erection function present. The patients lose penile rigidity, but not all lose tumescence. Thus, it may be improper to compare the neurotransmitter content of the penis of a man who has 30 percent erectile capacity to that of one who has 70 percent capacity. Both are "impotent," but they clearly differ in degree of dysfunction.

With regard to aging, in 1974, Waterson [14] demonstrated decreased catecholamine fluorescence from the gingival tissue of patients 30 to 50 years of age. Berkowitz [2], in a study of rat heart, arteries, and veins, showed a similar decline in norepinephrine content but demonstrated a concomitantly increased activity in the enzyme monoamine oxidase in that tissue. These studies suggest that aging is associated with diminished content of norepinephrine but that the decrease may be secondary to increased degradation.

Another observation from our data is that antihypertensive medication (α-methyldopa and propranolol) did significantly lower the norepinephrine content of the corporal tissue in some impotent men. This finding suggests that decreased intracorporal sympathetic innervation may be a causative factor in diminished potency. However, a drug effect on brain centers may also be of importance.

ANIMAL STUDIES

Because of the observed effect of diabetes mellitus on norepinephrine content of human erectile tissue, we attempted to induce a similar change in a diabetic animal model. Rats were given streptozotocin intravenously as a means of chemically inducing diabetes. Histofluorescent studies of the normal rat penis showed the presence of a dense adrenergic

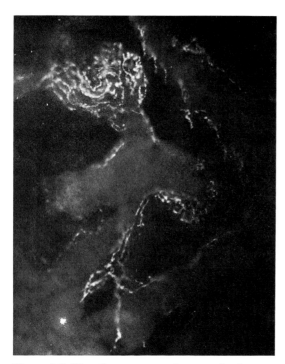

Figure 3-8. Histofluorescence photograph of rat corpora showing vesicles overlying the smooth muscles of the stroma. (Courtesy of Dr. David L. Felten)

innervation of the corporal smooth muscle stoma (Fig. 3-8). However, fluorescence was markedly diminished in animals made diabetic for 29 weeks. Simultaneous erectile function was not measured in that study, but the results suggest that diabetes does, in fact, reduce rat penile catecholamine histofluorescence. In another study, the actual norepinephrine content of streptozotocin-induced diabetic rat penile tissue was measured in rats that had been diabetic for 26 weeks. The mean values of those animals' penile norepinephrine contents were not significantly different from those observed in control animals but were significantly elevated in some animals in which diabetes had been present for 9 months. A significant increase in norepinephrine content was observed in mildly diabetic animals: 1200 ± 184 pg/mg (control: 741 ± 204); severer diabetes (2+ glucosuria) had produced only a mildly elevated norepinephrine content of 793 ± 174 pg/mg. There was no observed functional impairment of

erectile activity in these rats, a finding consistent with the absence of changes in norepinephrine content. Because of the absence of any significant decrease in norepinephrine content, despite markedly diminished fluorescence in rat tissue of diabetic animals, the measurement of norepinephrine content in rat penile corpora must be evaluated further.

We now know that norepinephrine is present in high content in penile erectile tissue of normal men and appears to be altered with disease known to cause impotence. However, the precise interrelationship of disease states with penile norepinephrine content and its effect on penile turgidity is not yet resolved.

REFERENCES

1. Berkowitz, B. A., Tarver, J. H., and Spector, S. Norepinephrine in blood vessels: Concentration, binding, uptake, and depletion. *J. Pharmacol. Exp. Ther.*, 177:119, 1971.
2. Berkowitz, B., and Kohler, C. Vascular Catecholamines and Aging. In J. A. Beran (ed.), *Vascular Neuroeffector Mechanism.* New York: Rover Press, 1980.
3. Dahlstrom, A., Haggendal, T., and Hokfelt, T. The noradrenaline content of the varicosities of sympathetic adrenergic nerve terminals in the rat. *Acta Physiol. Scand.* 67:289, 1966.
4. Eckhard, C. Untersuchgungen Uber Die Erection Des Penis Beim Hunde. *Beit. Anat. Physio.* 3:123, 1863.
5. Henry, D. P., et al. A sensitive radioenzymatic assay for norepinephrine in tissue and plasma. *Life Sci.* 16:375, 1975.
6. Hickler, R. B., Hoskins, R. G., and Hamlin, J. T. The clinical evaluation of faulty orthostatic mechanisms. *Med. Clin. North Am.* 44:1237, 1960.
7. Marshall, J. M. Modulation of smooth muscle activity by catecholamines. *Fed. Proc.* 35:2450, 1977.
8. McConnell, J. A., Benson, G. S., and Wood, J. Autonomic innervation of the mammalian penis: A histochemical and physiological study. *J. Neural Transm.* 45:277, 1979.
9. Melman, A., et al. Alteration of the penile corpora in patients with erectile impotence. *Invest. Urol.* 17:474, 1980.
10. Melman, A., and Henry, D. P. The possible role of the catecholamines of the corpora in penile erection. *J. Urol.* 121:419, 1979.
11. Melman, A., et al. Effect of diabetes upon penile sympathetic nerves in impotent patients. *South. Med. J.* 73:307, 1980.

12. Melman, A., et al. Ultrastructure of human penile erectile tissue in patients with abnormal norepinephrine content. *Invest. Urol.* 19:46, 1981.
13. Vanhoutte, P. M., Verbeuren, T. J., and Webb, R. C. Local modulation of the adrenergic neuroeffector interaction in the blood vessel wall. *Physiol. Rev.* 61:151, 1981.
14. Waterson, J. G., Frewin, D. B., and Saltys, J. S. Age-related differences in catecholamine fluorescence of human vascular tissue. *Blood Vessels* 11:79, 1974.
15. Weiner, N. Multiple factors regulating the release of norepinephrine consequent to some stimulation. *Fed. Proc.* 38:2193, 1979.

Adrenergic Corporal Receptors

ALAN J. WEIN
KEITH VAN ARSDALEN
ROBERT M. LEVIN

Penile erection is generally thought to be a neurovascular phenomenon that occurs within a certain hormonal milieu. Distension of the spaces of the corpora cavernosa with blood during erection has been hypothesized to occur by increased inflow, decreased outflow, or a combination of the two. The opening of arterial shunts at the junction of the arterioles and the cavernosal spaces, the closure of shunt arteries connecting the deep cavernosal arteries with spongiosal vessels, and closure of various venous outflow mechanisms have all been proposed as the final or important vascular event that occurs [2, 4, 9–11, 13].

Classically, the initiation of erection has been thought to be under the control of the parasympathetic nervous system [2, 4, 9–11, 13]. Several lines of evidence, however, suggest that adrenergic mechanisms may play a significant role [1, 3, 5, 7, 8]. To provide further data on a possible adrenergic role in the erectile process, we quantitated alpha- and beta-adrenergic–receptor densities in human corpus cavernosum tissue.

Samples of normal human corpus cavernosum tissue from the midpenis were obtained during surgery from 3 patients who reported previously normal erectile activity. The tissue samples were rapidly frozen in, and stored under, liquid nitrogen until assayed. Assays were performed using recently described methodology that employs ^{3}H-dihydroalprenolol as the beta-adrenergic ligand, ^{3}H-dihydroergocryptine as a nonselective alpha ligand, and ^{3}H-clonidine as a specific alpha-2 (presynaptic) ligand [6]. The specific binding of the ligands to cavernosal tissue was saturable, of high affinity, and had pharmacologic characteristics consistent with the identification of specific alpha- and beta-adrenergic receptors. The density of alpha receptors was nearly 10 times that of the beta receptor density (Fig. 3-9). Approximately 10 percent of the total alpha receptor popu-

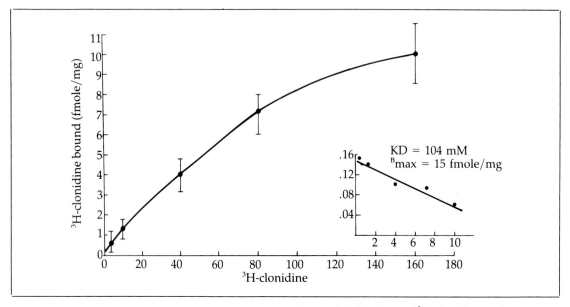

lation was of the alpha-2, or presynaptic, type (Fig. 3-10).

As isolated data, quantitative receptor assays are much more meaningful in organs whose structure and function are better understood [6, 12]. In a structure such as the penis, the obviously missing significant facts are the precise locations of these receptors: Are they in small or large arteries, small or large veins, shunt vessels between the cavernosal arterial and venous systems, shunt vessels between the cavernosal arteries and spongiosal veins, polsters, or the walls of the cavernosal spaces themselves? Virtually any theory of penile erection can be compatible with the participation of an adrenergic mechanism, depending on the selective localization of the various subtypes of receptors demonstrated.

The evidence suggesting that adrenergic mechanisms play a role in penile erection is largely indirect. Histochemical studies [1, 2] have shown numerous catecholamine fluorescent fibers in the human corpora cavernosa, but few in the corpus spongiosum. The adrenergic cavernosal fibers take a circuitous course through the trabeculae and often approach the walls of the cavernous spaces. Catecholamine-containing fibers are seen also in the walls of many penile blood vessels. High concentrations of tissue nor-

Figure 3-9. Binding of ^{3}H-clonidine to human corporal tissue.

Figure 3-10. Binding of ^{3}H-dihydroergocryptine and ^{3}H-dihydroalprenolol to human corporal tissue.

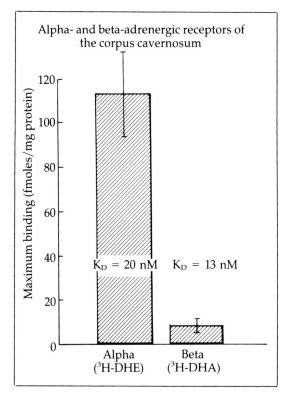

epinephrine have been found in erectile tissue of normal men, and significant reductions of adrenergic neurotransmitter concentration seen in such tissue from patients with several diseases associated with impotence [7, 8]. Muscle-bath experiments with penile erectile tissue from a variety of animals and from humans have shown an alpha-adrenergic excitatory response [1, 2, 5]. Our data support best a hypothesis that suggests that alpha-1-postsynaptic) receptor–mediated smooth muscle contraction participates in the erectile process. Several sites exist at which this might occur in the vascular phenomenon involved. Although "polsters" as such probably do not exist [2], constriction of vessels — whatever their anatomic designation and termination — that normally act to bypass or drain the cavernosal spaces is one possibility. The receptors may be at least in part associated with the walls of the corporal spaces. If so, stimulation and resultant contraction would augment the rigidity of an already engorged penis. Alternatively, the adrenergic effect may be a tonic contractile one in the vessels that supply blood to the cavernosal spaces, a recent and novel suggestion by Wagner [11]. Erection would then involve, among other factors, a release of this alpha-adrenergic tone. This theory is compatible with the observations made by Domer and co-workers, who demonstrated that penile engorgement in the cat occurred in response to alpha-adrenergic blockade or beta-adrenergic stimulation, both phenomena being reversible with alpha stimulation or beta blockade respectively [3]. The quantitative demonstration of beta and presynaptic alpha receptors is also obviously compatible with these results.

It is likely that multiple, and perhaps different, mechanisms are involved in the production of penile tumescence and rigidity and their reversal. Continued and more sophisticated anatomic, neuromorphologic, neurophysiologic, and neuropharmacologic studies may well demonstrate the coexistence of cholinergic, adrenergic, and other neurotransmitter or modulator mechanisms in the erectile process.

REFERENCES

1. Benson, G. S., et al. Neuromorphology and neurophysiology of the human penis. *J. Clin. Invest.* 65:506, 1980.
2. Benson, G. S. Mechanisms of penile erection. *Invest. Urol.* 19:65, 1981.
3. Domer, F. R., et al. Involvement of the sympathetic nervous system in the urinary bladder internal sphincter and in penile erection in the anesthetized cat. *Invest. Urol.* 15:404, 1978.
4. Henderson, V. E., and Roepke, M. H. On the mechanism of erection. *Am. J. Physiol.* 106:441, 1933.
5. Klinge, E., and Sjostrand, N. O. Comparative study of some isolated mammalian smooth muscle effectors of penile erection. *Acta Physiol. Scand.* 100:354, 1977.
6. Levin, R. M., and Wein, A. J. Quantitative analysis of alpha and beta adrenergic receptor densities in the lower urinary tract of the dog and the rabbit. *Invest. Urol.* 17:75, 1979.
7. Melman, A., and Henry, D. The possible role of the catecholamines of the corpora in penile erection. *J. Urol.* 121:419, 1979.
8. Melman, A., et al. Alteration of the penile corpora in patients with erectile impotence. *Invest. Urol.* 17:474, 1980.
9. Newman, H. F., Northrup, J. D., and Devlin, J. Mechanism of human penile erection. *Invest. Urol.* 1:350, 1964.
10. Siroky, M. B., and Krane, R. J. Mechanism of penile erection: A neuropharmacologic study, *Surg. Forum* 30:545, 1979.
11. Wagner, G. Erection. Anatomy, Physiology, Pharmacology. In G. Wagner and R. Green (eds.), *Impotence*. New York: Plenum, 1981. Pp. 7–36.
12. Wein, A. J., and Levin, R. M. Adrenergic receptor density in the human urinary bladder as compared to that of the dog and the rabbit. *Surg. Forum* 30:576, 1979.
13. Weiss, H. D. Physiology of human penile erection. *Ann. Intern. Med.* 76:798, 1972.

Ejaculation and Emission: Normal Physiology, Dysfunction, and Therapy

KAILASH R. KEDIA

A fundamental response included in the copulatory behavior of all male mammals is the ejaculatory response, which results in delivery of spermatozoa into the vagina. Thus, it constitutes an essential link in the behavior chain leading to reproduction and perpetuation of the species. *Ejaculation* may be defined as the expulsion of seminal fluid to the exterior of the organism by the rhythmic contractions of the perineal muscles. The ejaculatory process normally occurs in conjunction with several other reactions that are equally necessary for insemination of the female. These ancillary responses include *penile erection,* a species-specific pattern of postural adjustments and pelvic movements that facilitate the achievement of penis insertion, and the *maintenance of intromission* until ejaculation has been accomplished.

The mechanism of normal ejaculation depends on the integrity of the autonomic nervous system. The inability to ejaculate during the sexual act has received very little attention in the urologic literature. This chapter reviews the pertinent literature as well as some recent clinical observations.

NEUROPHYSIOLOGY: MECHANISM OF ERECTION, EJACULATION, AND ORGASM

Penile erection is controlled by the parasympathetic nerves, or *nervi erigentes.* The parasympathetic activity produces vasodilatation of the penile arteries and occlusion of the penile veins, causing enlargement of the cavernous bodies of the penis and urethra. Ejaculation is a complex process comprised of three discrete phenomena. These events are *seminal emission, anterograde ejaculation,* and *bladder neck closure* (Fig. 4-1). These events are dependent on a neural reflex. In this reflex, afferent sensory stimuli are initially relayed from the genitalia through the dorsal nerve of the penis (a branch of the pudendal nerve). These afferents are carried in the spinothalamic tracts and relay in the thalamus and sensory cortex. The efferent neural fibers travel through the anterolateral column to the thoracolumbar sympathetic outflow, emerging

Carol M. Gibbons, R. N., and Marlene Leib assisted in the preparation of this manuscript.

38

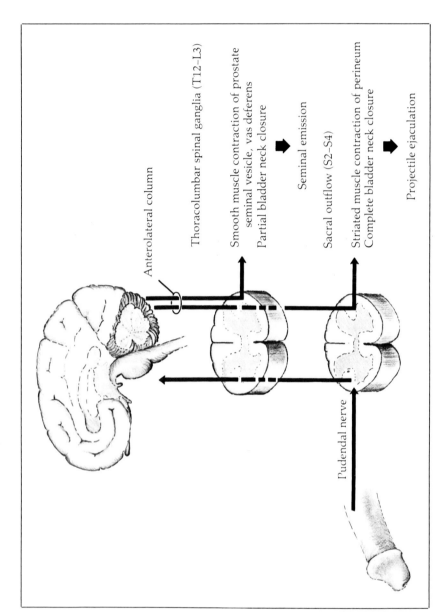

Figure 4-1. Physiology of ejaculation. Afferent stimuli travel to cerebral cortex through the pudendal nerve from the glans penis. Efferent fibers travel through anterolateral column to thoracolumbar sympathetic outflow, emerging through the T12–L3 sympathetic ganglia, which produce smooth muscle contraction of ductus deferens, seminal vesicle, and prostate and partial closure of bladder neck, resulting in seminal emission into posterior urethra. Efferent fibers also continue down to parasympathetic sacral outflow, causing striated muscle contraction of perineum and complete bladder neck closure, and produce projectile ejaculation.

through sympathetic ganglia T12 to L3. The literature indicates that the spinal center of ejaculation exists between the lower thoracic and upper lumbar segments of the spinal cord. This sympathetic neural output produces (1) smooth muscle contraction of the ductus deferens, stimulating peristalsis with propulsion of spermatozoa from the cauda epididymis to the ampulla; and (2) smooth muscle contraction in the ampulla, prostate, and seminal vesicles, with partial closure of the bladder neck, resulting in seminal emission into the posterior urethra. Further efferent neural control is mediated through the parasympathetic sacral outflow (most likely S2–S4) and somatic efferents, which causes clonic contraction of the striated bulbocavernosus and ischiocavernosus muscles and associated movements of the remaining striated muscles of the pelvic floor, lower extremities, and trunk. These responses, together with complete closure of the bladder neck, result in rhythmic, projectile ejaculation through the external urethral orifice [49]. Orgasm is a cortical sensory experience with input from contraction of the smooth muscles of the internal sexual organs as well as the pelvic striated muscles.

The sequence of grossly observable reactions associated with ejaculation in human males differs markedly among individuals and ranges from an almost exclusively genital event, consisting primarily of erection and ejaculation with mild throbbing of the urethra, to a generalized convulsive seizure involving extreme tension and clonic spasms of all extremities and lasting for several minutes [43]. After ejaculation, the male is refractory to further stimulation for a variable period. This period of reduced responsiveness to sexual stimuli is so variable that it ranges from minutes to days in different individuals. This refractory period lengthens with age, with an accompanying reduction in ejaculatory force, frequency, quality, and quantity. This postorgasmic phenomenon occurs only in the male and is probably associated with the emission phase [37].

NEUROANATOMY OF EJACULATION

The nervous control of mammalian autonomic function is highly complex. There are two antagonistic neuronal systems formed by the sympathetic and parasympathetic nerves involved in this control mechanism. The classic experiments of Langley at the end of the nineteenth century gave strong evidence that the peripheral autonomic nervous system is organized as a two-neuron pathway. *Preganglionic fibers* that originate from the central nervous system travel by way of the cranial nerves and central roots of the spinal cord to the peripheral autonomic ganglia. At these sites, they are synaptically connected to nerve cells, constituting the second neuron link. The axons emerging from the ganglia are the *postganglionic fibers.* They in turn innervate the effector organs. It was also shown that the ganglia are located close to the effector organs; this is particularly true of the parasympathetic nerves, so the preganglionic fibers are relatively long, and the postganglionic fibers are short.

In contrast, the sympathetic nervous ganglia are located close to the spinal cord; thus, the postganglionic fibers are relatively long. The concept of chemical transmission of nerve impulses was also studied during the early part of the twentieth century and it was shown that all the parasympathetic and all preganglionic nerves and a small number of postganglionic sympathetic nerves are cholinergic; i.e., the transmitter substance is acetylcholine. The majority of the postganglionic sympathetic nerves, however, are adrenergic, the transmitter substance being noradrenaline.

The peripheral autonomic innervation of the male reproductive tract has considerable functional significance. It was demonstrated as early as 1858 that the stimulation of the inferior mesenteric ganglion, the hypogastric nerve, and the lumbar communicants produced contraction of the rabbit ductus deferens [15]. Similar studies were continued by other investigators, who showed that stimulation of the twelfth thoracic and the first, second, and third lumbar nerves of the rhesus monkey and of the third and fourth lumbar nerves in cats produced contraction of the ductus deferens [54, 72]. The motor response of the ductus deferens and the seminal vesicles in cats and rabbits is transmitted along a pathway running from the lumbar sympathetic outflow through the inferior mesenteric ganglion and the hypogastric nerves [50, 51]. It was also shown that pelvic nerve stimulation did not produce ductus deferens or seminal vesicle contraction. This finding was supported by a demonstration that the emission of seminal fluid is controlled by the hypogastric nerves [71]. The transection of the hypogastric nerves results in sterility in male guinea pigs [66]. By systematic stimulation of the individual roots of the hypogastric nerves, it was established that in men the external genital organs are innervated by sympathetic fibers [52].

Although it was suggested that at least some of the sympathetic preganglionic fibers passed the inferior mesenteric ganglia and ran down in the hypogastric nerve to form synapses with more peripherally located ganglia near the ductus deferens and seminal vesicle, the general opinion long has been that, in most animals, these organs are innervated by postganglionic sympathetic neurons, the cell bodies of which are located in the inferior mesenteric ganglia [51]. This view is based chiefly on the morphology of sympathetic nerves, which have long postganglionic fibers in other parts of the body, and on electrophysiologic findings that indicate that about 90 percent of the fibers in the hypogastric nerve are nonmyelinated C fibers and that there are only a few B fibers [29].

However, the ganglionic blocking agents, e.g., hexamethonium and nicotine, obliterated the motor response of the guinea pig ductus deferens to hypogastric nerve stimulation. Furthermore, while the noradrenaline content of ductus deferens and seminal vesicle could be depleted by reserpine, it could not be reduced by hypogastric denervation [75, 76]. These findings, together with the simultaneous demonstration of an abundant distribution of catecholamine-containing nerve terminals in the ductus deferens of the guinea pig, led to the conclusion that the

original observations of Langley and Anderson were incorrect [22]. The pre- and paravertebral ganglia constitute the classic source of adrenergic nerves to most sympathetically innervated structures, but the internal male genital organs receive a special type of fibers that, in accordance with the anatomic location of the ganglion cells, belong to the system of short adrenergic neurons (Figs. 4-2 and 4-3).

The term *short adrenergic neurons* was introduced by Sjostrand to describe the final postsynaptic sympathetic innervation of the internal male genitalia. This term was used to differentiate the final pathway from conventional "long" adrenergic neurons with their cell bodies in the pre- or paravertebral ganglia. This concept of the adrenergic innervation of the internal genitalia is also strongly supported by recent morphologic, electrophysiologic, histochemical, and pharmacologic investigations. The experimental work on hypogastric and transluminal stimulation of the ductus deferens has shown pharmacologic evidence of a sympathetic relay located close to the effector organs [4, 7]. Similar findings were also reported by Ohlin and Stromblad [64]. Fluorescence histochemistry according to the Falck-Hillarp method has also revealed that the smooth muscles of the ductus deferens, seminal vesicle, and prostate of several species, including humans, receive an extensive adrenergic innervation, and large formations of adrenergic ganglion cells have been demonstrated within or close to these organs [23]. Neither hypogastric nor lumbosacral denervation causes any histochemically visible reduction in the number of fluorescent axons. The number of adrenergic vasomotor nerves is markedly reduced after lumbosacral denervation, but the adrenergic nerve in the smooth muscle coat of the organs disappears only if the peripheral adrenergic ganglion formation is excised [65].

The *short adrenergic neurons* are bundles of preterminal axons that run in the connective tissue space of the smooth muscle coat within the genital organs to ramify into characteristically beaded terminals located along the individual muscle cells. In other organs innervated by sympathetic nerves, general nerve terminals usually run together in each strand

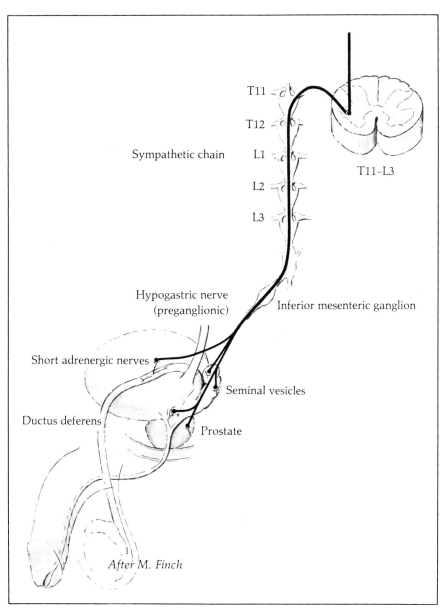

Figure 4-2. Sympathetic innervation of internal male genitalia. Nerve fibers emerge from the dorsolumbar spinal segment and pass through the sympathetic chain and inferior mesenteric ganglion and form the hypogastric nerve. There is no relay of preganglionic fibers in the inferior mesenteric ganglion. Preganglionic fibers relay into ganglia located on the ductus deferens, seminal vesicles, prostate, and the base of the bladder and innervate by so-called short adrenergic neurons.

of the autonomic ground plexus, whereas in the ductus deferens and seminal vesicle most of the strands contain only few varicose terminals. There is a very dense adrenergic in-

nervation of the internal male genitalia, and it has been postulated that most of the smooth muscle cells, somewhere on their surface, have contact with, or lie in close proximity to, varicosities belonging to one or more terminals.

The short adrenergic neurons innervating the internal male genital organs differ in several physiologic and pharmacologic properties from the conventional long adrenergic neurons. They have more sensitivity in vitro to guanethidine [17] and react differently to immunosympathectomy [32]. Their endoge-

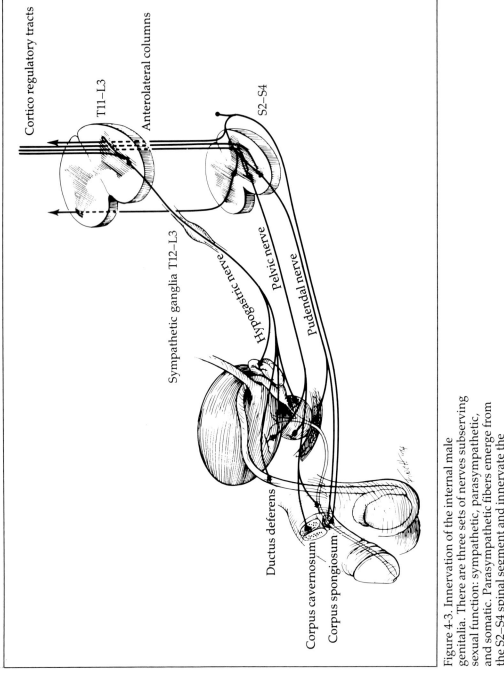

Figure 4-3. Innervation of the internal male genitalia. There are three sets of nerves subserving sexual function: sympathetic, parasympathetic, and somatic. Parasympathetic fibers emerge from the S2–S4 spinal segment and innervate the prostate, base of bladder, prostatic urethra, and corpora cavernosa. Somatic innervation is through the pudendal nerve, which innervates perineal muscles, penile urethra, and corpus spongiosum.

nous noradrenaline content is not increased after decentralization nor is it reduced by nerve stimulation [8, 9]. This suggests that short adrenergic neurons are a unique entity of the sympathetic nervous system innervating the pelvic organs.

Relatively few studies have been done on the human ductus deferens and seminal vesicles. Recently, organ-bath studies using human ductus deferens have shown dose-dependent excitatory responses only to norepinephrine and epinephrine, suggesting that motor innervation is adrenergic and operates through alpha-adrenergic receptors [60]. A fairly high level of norepinephrine in human ductus deferens was also demonstrated, suggesting again that in men the internal genital organs receive adrenergic innervation similar to that observed in many lower species [74].

SUPRASPINAL CONNECTIONS
AND CENTERS
In humans, higher centers alone may suffice for both erection and ejaculation, without genital stimulation. In some animals, there exists an ejaculatory center in the cerebrum, stimulation of which will of itself produce ejaculation. The victim of judicial hanging often ejaculates. The classic withdrawal symptoms associated with morphine addiction in humans include the appearance of spontaneous erections and emissions. In human males, petit mal attacks are sometimes revealed by the occurrence of seminal discharge. Neurophysiologic experiments involving central control mechanism of ejaculation in the squirrel monkey have been undertaken by MacLean and co-workers [55]. From the upper medulla through the pons and midbrain, they found that electrical stimulation of points within the spinothalamic tract resulted in intensive scratching followed by ejaculation. Above the midbrain, positive loci were found in structures lying within the intralaminar region of the thalamus, an area recently shown to receive terminals from the spinothalamic tract. It was shown, in fact, that seminal discharge could occur without even genital manipulation and in the absence

of an erection. Other positive loci were found in the floor of the fourth ventricle, just lateral to the sixth nerve nucleus, and in the floor of the aqueduct. It is assumed that impulses are carried from the thalamus to the limbic system and hypothalamus, to produce pleasurable sensations, and to the sensory cortex, to account for the fact that genital sensations can be consciously perceived, and ejaculation brought under conscious and voluntary control.

NEUROENDOCRINE CONTROL
The exact role of prostaglandins or other biogenic amines in the ejaculatory process has not as yet been established. Some 13 prostaglandins have been detected in human semen. Since these prostaglandins are highly active smooth muscle stimulants, their in vivo role may be to control the frequency of contractions of the prostate and seminal vesicle, because the emptying of the prostate and seminal vesicle leads to a decreased ability of these glands to contract until sufficient freshly formed secretion has reaccumulated [56]. The output of seminal fluid depends on secretory activity in the accessory sex glands, which, in turn, depends on hormone from the testis. Prior to puberty, the gonads secrete a relatively small amount of androgen, and the accessory glands are inactive. For these reasons, seminal emission is lacking in male infants and in prepubertal boys. Nevertheless, genital stimulation has been observed to produce the full sexual response including the normal accompaniments of orgasm without emission in males of every age from 5 months to adolescence [43].

SUMMARY OF MECHANISM
OF EJACULATION
It is generally accepted that the mechanism of ejaculation, which includes three distinct phenomena—seminal emission, ejaculation, and bladder neck closure—depends on normal anatomic and nervous functions. It has been shown that the spinal center of ejaculation exists between the lower thoracic and superior lumbar segments of the spinal cord. The

spinal center is excited by the afferent impulses ascending through the pudendal nerve. Finally, ejaculation occurs when there is summation of afferent stimuli in the ejaculatory center of the cord, to reach threshold level. The efferent stimuli through the sympathetic nerves then cause contraction of the smooth muscle of the epididymis, the ductus deferens, the ampulla of the vas, the seminal vesicles, and the prostate. This produces semen in the posterior urethra (seminal emission). There is also partial closure of the bladder neck. Subsequently, stimulation from the sacral cord (parasympathetic and somatic nerves) through the pudendal nerve induces contraction of the periurethral and perineal musculature, resulting in rhythmic ejections of the seminal fluid from the external urethral orifice (ejaculation).

CLINICAL OBSERVATIONS

Ejaculatory dysfunction in the male may present itself in various forms and grades of severity. The most frequent types of ejaculatory dysfunction are

   I. Aspermia—absence of anterograde ejaculation during coitus — may be due to
      A. Absence of seminal emission
      B. Retrograde ejaculation
      C. Primary anejaculation
  II. Premature ejaculation
 III. Spontaneous ejaculation

SURGICAL SYMPATHECTOMY AND IATROGENIC ASPERMIA

The mechanism of normal ejaculation depends on the intact autonomic nervous system, and bilateral surgical sympathectomy can interfere with ejaculation. In the past, several authors have asserted that sympathectomy disturbs ejaculation by causing bladder neck dysfunction, which allows retrograde emission of semen into the urinary bladder [27, 68, 80]. However, my own experience with patients after surgical sympathectomy has shown that some observations did not fit the conventional concepts described in the literature. Evaluation of patients who

underwent T12 to L3 bilateral sympathectomy performed as a part of retroperitoneal lymphadenectomy for testicular tumors showed that all of them were potent, all experienced normal orgasm, but none had normal ejaculation. The result of this study suggested that these patients do not have retrograde ejaculation [38]. The surgical operation, high retroperitoneal lymphadenectomy, removes all the lymphatic channels and nodes around the renal pedicle and aortocaval areas. This procedure necessarily includes bilateral dorsolumbar sympathectomy, since this type of surgical dissection usually removes both nerves and lymphatics, because they are so intimately intertwined.

Our studies have established that there is no retrograde ejaculation into the bladder, as the postmasturbatory urine sample is consistently negative for sperm and fructose. The ejaculatory failure is probably due to the absence of ductus deferens peristalsis and seminal vesicle contraction. Although all these patients were experiencing normal orgasm, they had no ejaculation and described the sensation of having "dry sex." This is because the bulbocavernosus and ischiocavernosus muscles still contract, as they are innervated by the pudendal nerve. The orgasm thus remains unimpaired.

Reports on the results of sympathectomy vary with regard to sexual function. The lumbar sympathetic ganglia, the rami communicantes, and the abdominal aortic and hypogastric sympathetic plexuses are susceptible to injury during aortoiliac dissection. Lumbar sympathectomy is also performed for peripheral vascular disease. Depending on the extent of the operation and the number of sympathetic ganglia removed, these procedures can result in ejaculatory disturbance. There are also anatomic variations in the innervation of internal male genitalia in terms of distribution of sympathetic fibers. In certain men, the outflow from the first lumbar ganglion, and possibly the lowest of the thoracic ganglia, is of major importance in the innervation of the seminal vesicles and ductus deferens, whereas, in others, the fibers running through the lumbar ganglion are of equal importance. There is no set rule for this distribution, a fact that corresponds with the well-known irregularities in the arrangement of the lumbar ganglia and the tendency to pre- and postfixation of the spinal sympathetic outflow [82]. There was no disturbance of ejaculation with transthoracic sympathectomy when T2 to T11 ganglia were removed, but 27 percent of patients showed permanent loss of ejaculation after dorsolumbar sympathectomy when T12 to L1 sympathetic ganglia were removed on both sides. No loss of ejaculation was seen when the first lumbar ganglion was left on one side. When the upper two lumbar ganglia are resected, 37 percent of patients have permanent loss of ejaculation. After bilateral lumbar sympathectomy, 54 percent of subjects have no ejaculation if the upper three ganglia are resected on one side, and two or more on the other.

Rose [68] investigated the incidence of sterility after lumbar sympathectomy. In 30 cases of bilateral lumbar sympathectomies, in all of which it was certain that the first three lumbar ganglia had been removed bilaterally, 27 patients had no alteration in sexual function. Of eight patients with extensive sympathectomy, seven had no ejaculation. Of the seven with failure to ejaculate, three had retrograde ejaculation into the bladder.

Dorsal or lumbar sympathectomy has also been implicated as a cause of impaired erection, particularly after bilateral resection of the L1 and L2 ganglia [82]. It is difficult to explain this, because the power of erection is under parasympathetic control.

Several reports in the literature show that aortoiliac reconstruction and abdominal aneurysmectomy are prone to cause deterioration of erection as well as impaired ejaculation. May and associates [58] emphasized the importance of maintaining hypogastric arterial blood flow to avert postoperative impotence. Others have advocated a technique that spares the sympathetic nerves during aortic exposure; they claim that this is important in preserving erectile function [18, 81]. In the series reported by May and co-workers, 34 percent of patients with normal preoperative erections developed impaired erectile function after reconstruction for aor-

toiliac occlusive disease. In those with some degree of preexisting erectile impairment, potency was improved postoperatively in 32 percent. Of those with normal preoperative erections, 21 percent developed impaired erectile function after aneurysmectomy. They also reported that 63 percent of the patients undergoing aneurysmectomy and 49 percent of those undergoing reconstruction for aortoiliac occlusive disease developed some ejaculatory changes [31, 81].

I believe that persistence of erectile dysfunction or a deterioration in erectile function may be attributable to the insufficient attention given to the occlusion and stenosis of the internal iliac arteries or parasympathetic denervation. Similarly, retrograde ejaculation is probably due to injury to the parasympathetic nerve fibers that results in relaxation of the internal sphincter and leads to retrograde ejaculation of seminal fluid into the bladder.

MANAGEMENT

Most patients with testicular tumors are young at the time of diagnosis and may not have had a family. The impact of therapy on fertility therefore assumes greater importance. The infertility (due to loss of ejaculation) that follows retroperitoneal lymphadenectomy is a serious problem. In most patients it is a permanent condition. Nerve regeneration may result in an occasional return of function [42, 53]. Preservation of preoperative semen specimens might be considered, but the storage techniques now available are not adequate to guarantee long-term survival of sperm.

Some investigators have reported good results with the use of sympathomimetic drugs. I have tried various sympathomimetic drugs (Sudafed, Actifed, Synephrine, Neo-synephrine) in an attempt to restore normal anterograde ejaculation. Therapy was unsuccessful in all but one patient who had few drops of anterograde ejaculation with only few non-motile spermatozoa [39]. This study clearly demonstrated that sympathomimetic drugs have no effect. Attempts are currently underway to develop an electroejaculator to stimulate ampulla and seminal vesicles locally to cause ejaculation. At present, there is no prevention and no cure for this complication, and it is part of the price that the patient must pay for attempted cure.

CHEMICAL SYMPATHECTOMY

Various pharmacologic agents have been shown to affect the ejaculatory process, but the exact mechanism has never been precisely explained [40]. In the past, several authors have asserted that sympathectomy disturbs ejaculation by causing bladder-neck dysfunction, allowing retrograde emission of semen into the bladder. This thought led many to believe that use of drugs with sympatholytic action might also result in retrograde ejaculation. There are several reports in the literature describing the effect of guanethidine on ejaculation, but the mechanism has never been studied extensively [70]. Bauer and associates [3] suggested that impairment of sexual function in male subjects after guanethidine therapy was similar to that observed after extensive lumbar sympathectomy, although the site and mechanism of action were not described. A possible explanation might be that mitochondria of neurons damaged by guanethidine undergo gross ultrastructural modification. It has been shown that 100 mg/kg doses of guanethidine given 16 to 24 hours before sacrifice of rats results in complete depletion of catecholamines in the adrenergic neurons of the ductus deferens and seminal vesicles [20]. Histologic, fluorescence histochemical, and electron microscope studies have also shown that guanethidine causes degeneration of sympathetic adrenergic neurons with a specific selective action of the short adrenergic nerves of the male reproductive tract [20, 33].

A recent clinical study found infertility in patients on sympatholytic drugs to be caused by ejaculatory failure due to absent contraction of the seminal vesicle, ampulla, and ductus deferens, rather than due to (the previously accepted reason of) retrograde ejaculation [38].

PHENOXYBENZAMINE

Phenoxybenzamine has been used widely for controlling high blood pressure and various peripheral vascular diseases. Recently, excellent results have been obtained by using phenoxybenzamine to treat patients who are unable to empty the bladder due to detrusor dyssynergia [45, 47, 48, 59, 61]. The drug's side effects — particularly on sexual function — are rarely mentioned in the literature. Green and Berman [28] reported ejaculatory failure in four patients treated with phenoxybenzamine; this was attributed to retrograde ejaculation of semen into the urinary bladder. Moser and co-workers [62] reported a "decrease in the amount of seminal fluid" in 26 of 28 patients with occlusive vascular disease who received phenoxybenzamine; libido, erection, and ejaculation were not altered. A recent study refutes the previous reports of retrograde ejaculation [41]. Ejaculatory failure has been shown to be due to an absence of contractions of the seminal vesicle, ampulla, and ductus deferens that results in loss of seminal emission.

PSYCHOACTIVE DRUGS

Recently, several reports have described the effect of psychoactive drugs on ejaculation. Absence of ejaculation has been reported after administration of thioridazine hydrochloride (Mellaril) by Singh [73], Freyhan [24], and Heller [34]. A similar effect has been seen with chlordiazepoxide (Librium) [36].

Other psychoactive drugs affecting the ejaculatory process include: chlorprothixene (Taractan), reserpine, phenelzine (monoamine oxidase inhibitor), and amitriptyline. In a recent report, ε-aminocaproic acid was also shown to produce failure of ejaculation [20]. Drugs with nonspecific actions such as sedatives (alcohol, barbiturates) and narcotics (heroin, morphine, methadone, meperidine, dihydromorphinone, and codeine) may cause ejaculatory dysfunction as well as reduce libido and slow the entire sexual response.

Clearly, many phamacologic agents can

and do affect male sexual function. Drugs with alpha-adrenergic blocking activity probably should be avoided in young patients. We do need more research into the mechanisms and incidence of drug-induced problems of male sexual function before we can make rational choices among drugs.

RADICAL PELVIC SURGERY AND EJACULATION

Sexual dysfunction is known to follow abdominoperineal proctosigmoidectomy. It is generally known that erection is most jeopardized by this operation. The injury to the pelvic autonomic nerve plexuses in the course of radical dissection is probably the main cause of these complications [6, 11, 26]. In the anterior rectal resection operation for cancer, at least 6 cm of distal rectum remains behind, untraumatized, in the deep pelvis and available for the anastomosis. During the limited rectal dissection that takes place in the upper part of the pelvis, no large important nerve fibers of the pelvic plexus are destroyed. However, after the abdominoperineal procedure for cancer with complete extirpation of the rectum, the parasympathetic fibers are totally destroyed. Besides parasympathetic, sympathetic fibers are also likely to be damaged during an excision of the rectum. Presacral nerve containing sympathetic fibers can easily be torn during the separation of the rectum from the front of the sacrum and common iliac vessels. The sympathetic nerves also could be injured in the pelvic plexuses on either side of the pelvis. It is understandable that destruction of these nerve tracts may give rise to disturbances of micturition, potency, and ejaculation. Goligher [26] studied a series of 95 patients who had been sexually active at the time of operation. He found that 72 percent were still capable of erection after the operation, and in 64 percent erection was adequate for intercourse. Although all patients having intercourse reported experiencing more or less normal orgasm, only 61 percent of them actually produced ejacu-

lation. Schellen [78] described a patient with proved retrograde ejaculation after excision of the colon whose erection and orgasm remained unchanged.

There is no prevention or cure for these neurogenic complications after excision of the rectum. They are part of the price that the patient must pay for attempted cure.

RETROGRADE EJACULATION

Retrograde ejaculation is the propulsion of seminal fluid from the posterior urethra back into the bladder. This implies that the seminal fluid reaches the posterior urethra secondarily to contractions of the ductus deferens, ampulla, seminal vesicle, and prostate (seminal emission), but the bladder neck fails to close during ejaculation. This leads to regurgitation of seminal fluid into the bladder in response to contractions of bulbocavernosus and ischiocavernosus muscles. When present in a younger man, retrograde ejaculation may pose problems of fertility.

ETIOLOGY

Retrograde ejaculation may result from congenital or acquired abnormalities of the bladder neck and posterior urethra or from interference with the normal neurologic control of ejaculation. Most authors, believing that surgical or chemical sympathectomy disturbs bladder-neck closure, have assumed that aspermia is the result of retrograde ejaculation of semen into the bladder [27, 68, 80]. In fact, the cause of the complete ejaculatory failure was not studied adequately until recently [38], when it was shown that retrograde ejaculation does not occur after sympathectomy.

The most common cause of retrograde ejaculation is transurethral resection of the prostate, but it has also been noted in congenital anomalies of the posterior urethra, transurethral resection of the bladder neck, open Y-V plasty of the bladder neck, and diabetes.

EJACULATORY FUNCTION AFTER PROSTATECTOMY

Transurethral resection of the prostate may disrupt the mechanism of closure of the bladder neck at the time of ejaculation. It entails excision of segments of the bladder neck muscles (internal sphincter) and destruction of some of the nerve terminals, and leaves in its wake an anatomically and physiologically altered bladder neck. Rieser [67] reported that of 36 patients who had postoperative sexual experience after transurethral prostatectomy, 15 noted retrograde ejaculation. During open surgical enucleation of the prostate, however, there is less destruction of the bladder neck; consequently, open enucleation is much less likely to produce this alteration. After radical prostatectomy or radical cystoprostatectomy, there is no ejaculation, because the ejaculatory structures are surgically removed.

BLADDER NECK REVISION

Surgical revision of the bladder neck to correct bladder dysfunction may also lead to retrograde ejaculation. Ochsner and co-workers [63] reported a follow-up study of 21 adults who had some form of bladder neck revision as children; seven patients (33%) had retrograde ejaculation. They also showed that the type of operative intervention, whether open revision or transurethral resection of the bladder neck, did not influence the outcome. Other investigators [30, 46] have reported normal anterograde ejaculation after anterior Y-V plasty of the bladder neck, with or without posterior bladder-neck revision.

THERAPY

At present, there is no acceptable treatment for retrograde ejaculation that follows iatrogenic destruction of the bladder neck. Abrahams and co-workers [1] reported two patients with retrograde ejaculation (secondary to Y-V plasty) who underwent reconstruction of the internal vesical sphincter and achieved normal ejaculation.

EJACULATORY DYSFUNCTION AND DIABETES MELLITUS

Sexual dysfunction is a common complication of diabetes mellitus in both men and women. In the adult diabetic, impotence is a frequent symptom, and it recently has been shown that the incidence of erectile impotence in the diabetic male at all age levels is 2 to 5 times the normal incidence as reported by Kinsey and co-workers [43]. In addition to impotence, other types of sexual dysfunction may complicate diabetes, including ejaculatory dysfunction. There are several reports in the literature describing retrograde ejaculation as a complication of diabetes [19, 27]. Green and co-workers [27] suggested that diabetic neuropathy resulted in disturbance of the sympathetic nerves supplying the bladder. This in turn prevented closure of the vesical neck and allowed retrograde ejaculation of semen into the bladder. They based their concept on the pattern of anhidrosis (impaired ability to perspire). In two of their patients, anhidrosis of the lower extremities was limited to the feet, suggesting neuropathic involvement of the third lumbar sympathetic ganglion or its peripheral fibers. In the other two patients anhidrosis involved the legs below the knees, suggesting neuropathic involvement of the second and third lumbar sympathetic ganglia or their peripheral fibers. Ellenberg and Weber [19] reported five cases of retrograde ejaculation and stated that medical sympathectomy due to diabetic neuropathy is the cause of this dysfunction. They also reported one case in which the patient had anterograde ejaculation and partial retrograde ejaculation. These findings are at variance with that suggested by Klebanow and co-workers [44]. These authors described nine diabetic males who failed to ejaculate in spite of having normal orgasms, and they attributed this ejaculatory failure to an intrinsic defect of the smooth muscle of the vasa deferentia and seminal vesicles.

Involvement of the nervous system in diabetes has long been recognized. There usually is generalized peripheral neuropathy affecting grossly neglected diabetics as well as those who are in good control. There is ample evidence that neuropathy involves somatic nerves (neuropathic ulcers), parasympathetic nerves (impotence, neurovesical dysfunction), and sympathetic nerves (anhidrosis).

There is no doubt that retrograde ejaculation occurs in patients with diabetes due to failure of closure of the bladder neck at the time of ejaculation. On the other hand, in many patients, *aspermia* (failure of anterograde ejaculation) may not be due to retrograde ejaculation. If the neuropathy involves sympathetic nerves, there would be no seminal emission into the posterior urethra, due to motor denervation of the ductus deferens, ampulla, and seminal vesicles. Although failure of seminal emission was attributed to a smooth muscle degeneration in diabetes, it would be more logical, in view of our understanding of the neurophysiology of ejaculation, to suspect failure of seminal emission as the cause of ejaculatory dysfunction in patients reported by Klebanow and co-workers [44]. Similarly, this also explained the diminution in the volume of ejaculate reported by Rubin and co-workers [69]. Wilson and co-workers [83] reported that calcification of the ductus deferens and ampulla occurred 6 times as frequently in diabetics as in normal individuals. Apparently, they did not comment on the ejaculatory process in these patients. Although the occurrence of retrograde ejaculation has been well documented, the quantity and quality of ejaculate recovered from the bladder has never been studied adequately in these patients. Moreover, it has been assumed that it is probably due to a decrease in adrenergic stimulation of the bladder neck and posterior urethra. It is more likely, however, to be due to parasympathetic denervation of the bladder neck because (1) closure of the bladder neck at the time of ejaculation is mediated by parasympathetic nerves (S2–S4); (2) there is generalized involvement of the parasympathetic nerves resulting in impotence and neurogenic vesical dysfunction; and (3) sympathetic denervation leads to motor paralysis of the ductus deferens, ampulla, and seminal vesicles resulting in failure of seminal emission. In light of our present understanding of neurophysiology and the mechanism of ejaculation, it is evident that, depending on the type and extent of neuropathy, one may encounter retrograde ejaculation, failure of seminal emission, diminution of ejaculate, combined anterograde and retrograde ejaculation, and anterograde ejaculation without any projectile force.

THERAPY

To date, the only effective treatment for retrograde ejaculation has been one of the postcoital catheterization techniques described by Rieser [67], Hotchkiss and co-workers [35], and Bourne and co-workers [12]. Although Green and co-workers [27] have shown that sympathomimetic drugs have been of no avail in the treatment of this complication of diabetes, other investigators have reported that retrograde ejaculation may be reversed by the administration of alpha-adrenergic drugs [14, 79].

SPONTANEOUS EJACULATION

Ejaculation most often occurs as a result of genital stimulation derived from coitus or from some type of masturbation, but it can also take place under other circumstances. The most common example of spontaneous ejaculation is the nocturnal emission, or "wet dream." Kinsey and co-workers [43] estimated that 80 percent of males have nocturnal emissions at some time during their lives, and they observed that such emissions become infrequent after marriage and regular sexual activity. This condition is thought to be due to "psychic stimulation during sleep."

TRAUMATIC LESIONS
OF THE SPINAL CORD

Ejaculatory dysfunctions are common among patients with spinal cord lesions. The level of the spinal cord lesion is important in regard to the incidence and type of ejaculatory dysfunctions. There usually is less involvement in patients with partial than with complete spinal cord lesions. Ejaculation is extremely rare in patients with complete upper motor neuron lesions. Generally, these patients do not ejaculate or have orgasm. Among the lower motor neuron patients with complete lesions, approximately 17 percent have ejaculations and orgasm [10]. Ejaculations are more frequent in patients with incomplete lesions: 29 percent with incomplete upper motor neuron lesions, and as high as 60 percent with incomplete lower motor neuron lesions. These patients have the highest rate of ejaculation when the level of the lesion is below the ninth thoracic segment. Ejaculation among the lower motor neuron group and in patients with cauda equina lesion may be "dripping" ejaculation, because there is no contraction of bulbocavernosus and ischiocavernosus muscles. In rare instances, patients with upper motor neuron lesions and reflexogenic erections urinate instead of ejaculating.

PRIMARY ANEJACULATION

Primary anejaculation is a condition characterized by inability to ejaculate into the vagina despite the presence of a grossly normal genitourinary system. This condition is also known as *ejaculatory incompetence, retarded ejaculation, ejaculatory impotence,* and *ejaculatory sterility.* The patient is capable of developing and maintaining a penile erection for a prolonged period of time but cannot culminate this physiologic response by ejaculation. Men affected by this condition are fertile, yet they have never had a conscious ejaculation during intercourse. They do have nocturnal emissions. According to Kinsey and co-workers [43], primary anejaculation occurs in 0.14 percent of the population. The etiology of this condition is not known exactly. Bergler [5] described primary anejaculation as "psychic masochism" and suggested the term *oral aspermia* because his patients experienced abundant salivation instead of ejaculation. The main characteristic common to these pa-

tients is lack of education. Treatment must be aimed at the underlying conflicts and not at the symptom itself.

PREMATURE EJACULATION

Premature ejaculation is defined as ejaculation that occurs before the person wishes it. Some men with this condition will ejaculate either during foreplay or as soon as their genitals are touched, but most ejaculate either during attempted penetration of the penis into the vagina or during the first few pelvic thrusts. The cause of this dysfunction is thought to be psychologic in a majority of the patients. Taboos against premarital sex and the frequent occurrence of the first intercourse under stressful circumstances are cited as possible background factors. Premature ejaculation during premarital intercourse is common among young men. There has been some speculation that premature ejaculation occurs because of the enhanced stimulation that results from the transition from masturbation to the more exciting involvement with a sexual partner. The method of treatment lies in reassurance, explanation, and urging of frequent coitus. The male is to expect that he will ejaculate prematurely for the first few times, but that will gradually clear with continued coitus. A fairly simple training procedure has also been advocated for alleviating this condition. The method, originally described by Semans [71] and then modified by Masters and Johnson [57], is called the *squeeze technique.* Urologic workup should be undertaken only when specifically indicated on the basis of other urologic disease.

REFERENCES

1. Abrahams, J. I., et al. The surgical correction of retrograde ejaculation. *J. Urol.* 114:888, 1975.
2. Ambache, N., and Zar, M. A. Evidence against adrenergic motor transmission in the guinea pig vas deferens. *J. Physiol.* 216:359, 1971.
3. Bauer, G. E., et al. The reversibility of side effects of guanethidine therapy. *Med. J. Aust.* 1:930, 1973.
4. Bentley, G. A., and Sabine, J. R. The effects of ganglion-blocking and postganglionic sym-

patholytic drugs on preparations of the guinea pig vas deferens. *Br. J. Pharmacol.* 21:190, 1963.

5. Bergler, E. Psychogenic Oral Aspermia. In E. Bergler (ed.), *The Basic Neurosis* (4th ed.). New York: Grune & Stratton, 1949.

6. Bernstein, W. C., and Bernstein, E. F. Sexual dysfunction following radical surgery for cancer of the rectum. *Dis. Colon Rectum* 9:328, 1966.

7. Birmingham, A. T., and Wilson, A. B. Preganglionic and postganglionic stimulation of the guinea pig isolated vas deferens preparations. *Br. J. Pharmacol.* 21:569, 1963.

8. Blakeley, A. G., Dearnaley, D. P., and Harrison, V. The effect of nerve stimulation on the noradrenaline content of the guinea pig vas deferens. *J. Physiol.* 198:106, 1968.

9. Blakeley, A. G. H., Dearnaley, D. P., and Harrison, V. The noradrenaline content of the vas deferens of the guinea pig. *Proc. R. Soc. Lond. (Biol.)* 174:491, 1970.

10. Bors, E., and Comarr, A. E. Neurological disturbances of sexual function with special reference to 529 patients with spinal cord injury. *Urol. Survey* 10:191, 1960.

11. Bors, E., and Comarr, A. E. *Neurological Urology.* Basel: S. Karger, 1971.

12. Bourne, R. B., Kietzschuman, W. A., and Esser, J. H. Successful artificial insemination in a diabetic with retrograde ejaculation. *Fertil. Steril.* 22:275, 1971.

13. Boyd, H., Chang, V., and Rand, M. J. The anticholinesterase activity of some antiadrenaline agents. *Br. J. Pharmacol.* 15:525, 1960.

14. Brooks, M. E., Berezin, M., and Braf, Z. Treatment of retrograde ejaculation with imipramine. *Urology* 15:353, 1980.

15. Budge. Uber das Centrum genitospinale des Nerv sympathicus. *Virchow's Arch. (Zellpathol.)* 15:115, 1858.

16. Burn, J. H., and Rand, M. J. Sympathetic postganglionic cholinergic fibres. *Br. J. Pharmacol.* 15:56, 1960.

17. Burnstock, G., et al. A new method of destroying adrenergic nerves in adult animals using guanethidine. *Br. J. Pharmacol.* 43:295, 1971.

18. DePalma, R. G., Levine, S. B., and Feldman, S. Preservation of erectile function after aortoiliac reconstruction. *Arch. Surg.* 113:988, 1978.

19. Ellenberg, M., and Weber, H. Retrograde ejaculation in diabetic neuropathy. *Ann. Intern. Med.* 65:1237, 1966.

20. Evans, B., Iwayama, T., and Burnstock, G. Long-lasting supersensitivity of the rat vas deferens to norepinephrine after chronic guanethidine administration. *J. Pharmacol. Exp. Therap.* 185:60, 1973.

21. Evans, B. E., and Aledort, L. M. Inhibition of ejaculation due to epsilon aminocaproic acid (letter to the ed.). *N. Engl. J. Med.* 298:166, 1978.

22. Falck, B. Observations on the possibilities of the cellular localization of monoamines by a fluorescence method. *Acta Physiol. Scand.* 56:197, 1962.

23. Falck, B., Owman, C., and Sjostrand, N. O. Peripherally located adrenergic neurons innervating vas deferens and the seminal vesicles of the guinea pig. *Experientia* 21:98, 1965.

24. Freyhan, F. A. Loss of ejaculation during Mellaril treatment. *Am. J. Psychiatry* 118:171, 1961.

25. Furness, J. B., and Iwayama, T. The arrangement and identification of axons innervating the vas deferens of the guinea pig. *J. Anat.* 113:179, 1972.

26. Goligher, J. C. Sexual function after excision of the rectum. *Proc. R. Soc. Med.* 44:824, 1951.

27. Green, L. F., Kellalis, P. O., and Weeks, R. E. Retrograde ejaculation of semen due to diabetic neuropathy. *Fertil. Steril.* 14:617, 1963.

28. Green, M., and Berman, S. Failure of ejaculation produced by Dibenzyline. Preliminary report. *Conn. Med. J.* 18:30, 1954.

29. Grundfest, H., and Gasser, H. S. Properties of mammalian nerve fibers of slowest conduction. *Am. J. Physiol.* 123:307, 1938.

30. Gute, D. B., Chute, R., and Baron, J. A., Jr. Bladder neck revision for obstruction in men: A clinical study reporting normal ejaculation postoperatively. *J. Urol.* 99:744, 1968.

31. Hallbook, T., and Holmquist, B. Sexual disturbances following dissection of the aorta and the common iliac arteries. *J. Cardiovasc. Surg.* 11:255, 1970.

32. Hamberger, B., et al. Monoamines in immunosympathectomized rats. *Int. J. Neuropharmacol.* 4:91, 1965.

33. Heath, J. W., et al. Degeneration of adrenergic neurons following guanethidine treatment: An ultrastructural study. *Virchows Arch.* 11:182, 1972.

34. Heller, J. Another case of inhibition of ejaculation as side effect of Mellaril. *Am. J. Psychiatry* 118:173, 1961.

35. Hotchkiss, R. S., Pinto, A. B., and Klugman, S. Artificial insemination with semen recovered from the bladder. *Fertil. Steril.* 6:37, 1955.

36. Hughes, J. M. Failure to ejaculate with chlordiazepoxide. *Am. J. Psychiatry* 121:610, 1964.

37. Kaplan, H. *The New Sex Therapy.* New York: Brunner/Mazel, 1974.

38. Kedia, K. R., Markland, C., and Fraley, E. E. Sexual function following high retroperitoneal lymphadenectomy. *J. Urol.* 114:237, 1975.

39. Kedia, K. R. Fertility considerations in patients with testicular tumors. American Urological Association (abstract), 1981.

40. Kedia, K. R., and Markland, C. The effect of

pharmacological agents on ejaculation. *J. Urol.* 114:569, 1975.

41. Kedia, K. R., and Persky, L. Effect of phenoxybenzamine (Dibenzyline) on sexual function in man. *Urology* 18:620, 1981.

42. Kedia, K. R., Markland, C., and Fraley, E. E. Sexual function after high retroperitoneal lymphadenectomy. *Urol. Clin. North Am.* 4:523, 1977.

43. Kinsey, A. C., Pomeroy, W. B., and Martin, C. E. *Sexual Behavior in the Human Male.* Philadelphia: Saunders, 1948.

44. Klebanow, D., and MacLeod, J. Semen quality and certain disturbances of reproduction in diabetic men. *Fertil. Steril.* 11:255, 1960.

45. Kleeman, F. J. Use of phenoxybenzamine poorly defined. *Urology* 9:708, 1977.

46. Koraitum, M., and Al-Ghorale, M. Normal ejaculation after Y-V urethrocystoplasty. *Br. J. Urol.* 42:564, 1970.

47. Krane, R. J., and Olsson, C. A. Phenoxybenzamine in neurogenic bladder dysfunction. I. A theory of micturition. *Fertil. Steril.* 110:650, 1973.

48. Krane, R. J., and Olsson, C. A. Phenoxybenzamine in neurogenic bladder dysfunction. II. Clinical considerations. *Fertil. Steril.* 110:653, 1973.

49. Kuntz, A. *The Autonomic Nervous System* (4th ed.). Philadelphia: Lea & Febiger, 1965.

50. Langley, J. N. On the regeneration of preganglionic and postganglionic visceral nerve fibers. *J. Physiol.* 22:215, 1897.

51. Langley, J. N., and Anderson, H. K. The innervation of the pelvis and adjoining viscera. IV, V, and VI. *J. Physiol.* 20:372, 1896.

52. Learmonth, J. R. A contribution to the neurophysiology of the urinary bladder in man. *Brain* 54:147, 1931.

53. Leiter, E., and Brendler, H. Loss of ejaculation following bilateral retroperitoneal lymphadenectomy. *J. Urol.* 98:375, 1967.

54. Loeb, L. Beitrage zur Bewegung der Samenleiter. Ph. D. dissertation, 1866.

55. MacLean, P. D., Dua, S., and Denniston, R. H. Cerebral localization for scratching and seminal discharge. *Arch. Neurol.* 9:485, 1963.

56. Mann, T. *Biochemistry of Semen and of the Male Reproductive Tract.* London: Methuen, 1964.

57. Masters, W. H., and Johnson, V. E. *Human Sexual Inadequacy.* Boston: Little, Brown, 1970.

58. May, A. G., DeWeese, J. A., and Rob, C. E. Changes in sexual function following operation on the abdominal aorta. *Surgery* 65:41, 1969.

59. McGuire, E. J., Wagner, F. M., and Weiss, R. M. Treatment of autonomic dysreflexia with phenoxybenzamine. *Surgery* 115:53, 1976.

60. McLeon, D. G., Reynolds, D. G., and Demaree, G. E. Some pharmacologic characteristics of the human vas deferens. *Invest. Urol.* 10:338, 1973.

61. Mobley, D. F. Phenoxybenzamine in the management of neurogenic vesical dysfunction. *J. Urol.* 116:737, 1976.

62. Moser, M., et al. Chemical blockade of the sympathetic nervous system in essential hypertension. *Proc. Natl. Meet. Am. Fed. Clin. Res.* May, 1952.

63. Ochsner, M. G., Burns, E., and Heinz, H. H., II. Incidence of retrograde ejaculation following bladder neck revision as a child. *J. Urol.* 104:596, 1970.

64. Ohlin, P., and Stromblad, B. C. R. Observations of the isolated vas deferens. *Br. J. Pharmacol.* 20:299, 1963.

65. Owman, C., and Sjostrand, N. O. Short adrenergic neurons and catecholamine-containing cells in vas deferens and accessory male genital glands of different mammals. *Z. Zellforsch. Mikrosk. Anat.* 66:300,1965.

66. Remy, C. H. Nerfs ejaculateurs. *J. Anat. Physiol.* 22:205, 1886.

67. Rieser, C. The etiology of retrograde ejaculation and a method for insemination. *Fertil. Steril.* 12:488, 1961.

68. Rose, S. E. An investigation into sterility after lumbar ganglionectomy. *Br. Med. J.* 1:247, 1953.

69. Rubin, A. J., and Babbott, D. Impotence and diabetes mellitus. *J.A.M.A.* 168:498, 1958.

70. Sah, H. J., Sah, P. P., and Peoples, S. A. The new antihypertensive agent, guanethidine—a review: II. Clinic uses, dosage, and routes of administration, side effects, important notes, summary, bibliography. *Arzneimittelforsch.* 16:199, 1966.

71. Semans, J. H., and Langworthy, O. R. Observation of the neurophysiology of sexual function in the male cat. *J. Urol.* 40:836, 1938.

72. Sherrington, C. S. Notes on the arrangement of some motor fibres in the lumbosacral plexus. *J. Physiol.* 13:1621, 1892.

73. Singh, H. A case of inhibition of ejaculation as a side effect of Mellaril. *Am. J. Psychiatry* 117:1041, 1961.

74. Sjostrand, N. O. The adrenergic innervation of the vas deferens and the accessory male genital glands. *Acta Physiol. Scand.* 65:257, 1965.

75. Sjostrand, N. O. Effect of reserpine and hypogastric denervation on the noradrenaline content of the vas deferens and the seminal vesicle of guinea pig. *Acta Physiol. Scand.* 56:376, 1962.

76. Sjostrand, N. O. Inhibition by ganglionic blocking agents of the motor response of the isolated guinea pig vas deferens to hypogastric nerve stimulation. *Acta Physiol. Scand.* 54:306, 1962.

77. Semans, J. H. Premature ejaculation: A new approach. *South. Med. J.* 49:353, 1956.

78. Schellen, M. C. M. A case of retrograde ejaculation caused by a colon operation. *Fertil. Steril.* 11:187, 1960.

79. Stewart, B. H., and Bergant, J. A. Correction of retrograde ejaculation by sympathomimetic medication: Preliminary report. *Fertil. Steril.* 25:1073, 1974.

80. Walters, D., and Kaufman, M. S. Sterility due to retrograde ejaculation of semen. *Am. J. Obstet. Gynecol.* 78:274, 1959.

81. Weinstein, M. H., and Machleder, H. I. Sexual function after aortoiliac surgery. *Ann. Surg.* 181:787, 1975.

82. Whitelaw, G. P., and Smithwick, R. H. Some secondary effects of sympathectomy with particular reference to disturbance of sexual function. *N. Engl. J. Med.* 245:121, 1951.

83. Wilson, J. L., and Markus, J. H. Calcification of the vas deferens: Its relation to diabetes mellitus and arteriosclerosis. *N. Engl. J. Med.* 245:321, 1951.

5

Neurologic and Neurosurgical Disorders Associated with Impotence

MICHAEL J. TORRENS

Considering the relevance of neurologic observations to the pathophysiology of impotence, scant attention has been paid to the subject, and texts concentrating on neuropathic impotence are rare [31]. It should be remembered that neurologic disease severe enough to be associated with sexual dysfunction is usually physically disabling. This in itself may contribute to psychogenic impotence. Figures relating to the incidence of the problem therefore must be interpreted with care, particularly since authors seldom question the patients in any detail about the exact nature of their dysfunction.

SPINAL INJURIES

More is known about impotence caused by spinal injury than about other neurologic disorders, so it is appropriate to discuss this first. The topographically defined lesions and static clinical state allow a more exact understanding of pathophysiology.

The overall incidence of impotence quoted by Guttmann [22] is 6 to 48 percent; of ejaculation failure, 80 to 97 percent; of failure of intromission, 66 to 76 percent; and of absent orgasm, 86 to 94 percent. Reproduction is possible in only 5 percent of patients. The variability can be explained on the basis of the site and extent of the lesion [60], so the various types will be considered separately.

Higher Cord Injuries

Up to 20 percent of patients with complete upper motor neuron lesions are impotent [5]. Those that are potent have only reflex erections and, frequently, no ejaculation. The level of the lesion influences the type of reflex erection. If the lower level of the lesion extends below T12, the majority of the patients (33 of 41, 80%) will erect only the corpora cavernosa, whereas if the lower level of the lesion is above T12, the majority (36 of 54, 66%) will erect both the corpora cavernosa and the corpus spongiosum [7]. The higher the lesion the greater the chance of reflex erection, and the incidence approaches 100 percent in cervical cord transection.

Table 5-1. Percentages of erection, ejaculation, and significance for coitus

Type of lesion	Number of patients	With no erections (%)	Reflex erections (%)	Psychogenic erections only (%)	Attempt at coitus (%)	Successful at coitus (%)	Able to ejaculate (%)	Able to sire children (%)
Upper motor neuron lesion								
Complete	362	7	93	0	67	49	3	1
Incomplete	163	2	98	0	74	63	28	6
Lower motor neuron lesion								
Complete	142	74	0	26	35	23	16	6
Incomplete	12	18	0	83	83	75	60	10

Source: A. E. Comarr, *The Total Care of Spinal Cord Injuries.* Boston: Little, Brown, 1977.

Intrathecal injection of prostigmine (0.25–0.3 mg) has been used to induce erection and ejaculation, e.g., prior to artificial insemination [22]. Lesions above T11 are more likely to produce testicular atrophy [22], presumably because of changes in vasomotor activity, for the pattern of semen analysis is similar to that of varicocele.

Conus and Cauda Equina Injuries
In contrast to those with higher lesions, about 70 percent of patients with complete lower motor neuron lesions are impotent [5]. This figure is higher than that of Guttmann [22] because it excludes incomplete lesions. When erections do occur, they are psychogenic in type and are not felt by the patient. Clonic ejaculation is almost universally absent, but emission of semen into the urethra, followed by dripping ejaculation, may occur in about 60 percent of cases [7].

The upper level of the lesion affects the incidence of psychogenic erection. It hardly ever occurs with lesions extending above T10, and seldom with lesions above T12 [7]. All of 19 patients with an upper level of lesion below T10 who were potent had testicular sensation of sorts present; impotent patients had not [7]. This is suggested as a method of clinical assessment.

Intermediate Injuries
Logically, patients with complete lesions in which the upper level is below T10 and the lower level is above S2 might be expected

to have a good prognosis for erection of a mixed psychogenic and reflex type. Chapelle and co-workers [7] describe 24 patients in this category, of whom at least 10 had mixed erections.

Incomplete Lesions
The prognosis for erection in incomplete transection of the cord depends very much on the site of the lesion in the cord. The prognosis will be worst with an anterior segmental lesion affecting the cord on both sides. The status of erections and their significance in coitus and reproduction have been studied carefully by Comarr [8] in a series of 679 patients. His results are summarized in Table 5-1. In incomplete lesions, the presence of genital sensation is crucial for the retention of useful potency.

SPINAL CORD DISORDERS
Almost any condition affecting the spinal cord can cause impotence; its effect depends on the rapidity and severity of the history and on the part of the cord affected. Transverse myelitis and anterior spinal artery thrombosis therefore may have a profound effect, whereas subacute combined degeneration is not reported as causing impotence. Tabes dorsalis is particularly likely to induce impotence, and sexual dysfunction has also been recorded in syringomyelia, myelodysplasia, spinal abscess, and arachnoiditis. Bilateral spinothalamic cordotomy

may be responsible if it is too extensive, as may spinal tumors, especially if they are malignant or affect the conus and cauda equina. Dorsal disk prolapse may be a cause because of the morbidity associated with its removal; cervical spondylosis and disk prolapse are seldom causes of impotence. Lumbar disk prolapse will be dealt with separately. Motor neuron disease may not be as significant a cause as one would expect, because of the relative preservation of the intermediolateral cell columns in the lumbosacral region.

Multiple Sclerosis
Multiple sclerosis is a common condition that often causes impotence; the incidence reported varies from 26 [26] to 43 percent [55]. Despite the dissemination of demyelination in this condition, there is evidence that impotence is most often due to spinal cord involvement.

Sexual dysfunction in multiple sclerosis is associated with a longer history of illness and an earlier age of onset. Although impotence is less common as a presenting symptom (3%) than are bladder problems (6%), it becomes relatively more common later in the disease, even in a relatively mildly affected group [26], with an incidence of 26 percent compared with bladder symptoms in 10 percent. It is more positively related to bladder and bowel involvement than to general disability, and this seems to be associated with anterior spinal cord disturbance. Impotent men were found not to sweat in the lower extremities [55]; this leads to the conclusion that descending reticulospinal fibers destined for lateral horn cells had been interrupted by plaques. A further secondary effect has been noted [55] (that of elevated urinary gonadotropins in impotent patients) that has been linked with a presumed deficiency of androgens. This may be related to the testicular atrophy occurring in cord injuries, and consequent to the way the changed sympathetic activity affects testicular vascularity.

Intermediolateral Cell Column Degeneration
A rare syndrome, this degeneration is one of the few conditions specifically causing impotence together with orthostatic hypotension and loss of sweating. It is therefore particularly interesting. Two cases with autopsies have been described by Johnson and coworkers [29]. It is likely to be the significant degeneration causing impotence in the Shy-Drager syndrome [49], and it has neuropathologic associations with olivopontocerebellar atrophy and with idiopathic Parkinson's disease.

PERIPHERAL NERVE DYSFUNCTION
The peripheral nervous system is more accessible than the central nervous system to objective investigation. The recent interest in sacral evoked responses eventually will provide much better documentation of the range of dysfunction, especially of the somatic element.

Sympathectomy
Ganglion-blocking agents used for hypertension had a profound effect on potency, but this is less true of the more recently introduced selective sympathetic blockers. Surgical sympathectomy also has an effect on potency. In 161 cases, Whitelaw and Smethwick [59] noted impaired erection in 27.5 percent and failure of ejaculation in 19.8 percent. The latter symptom may be related to retrograde ejaculation. Retief [44] described erection without ejaculation in 7 of 11 sympathectomies; however, sperm could be isolated from the urine. The incidence of impotence can be reduced greatly by preserving D12–L1 ganglia [59], and perhaps avoided entirely by leaving L2 ganglion as well [44]. Other operations in the retroperitoneal area may damage the relevent nerves; examples are retroperitoneal lymphadenectomy and aortic aneurysm surgery.

Iatrogenic Sacral Nerve Damage
Any trauma, iatrogenic or otherwise, can cause impotence if the relevant nerves are involved [41]. I have observed a man with a gunshot wound affecting selectively S3–S5 nerves whose main complaint was impotence, the bladder being well balanced. The dorsal nerve of the penis is also an important factor in potency [43].

Any sexual function remaining after spinal cord injury is usually abolished by bilateral pudendal neurectomy [8], anterior and posterior rhizotomy, and subarachnoid alcohol block. It is often affected by anterior rhizotomy for spasm even when the lower sacral roots are spared. It is also said to be affected adversely by sacral extradural neurectomy, although there are reports of potency being restored, especially by S3 nerve section, both in paraplegics [36] and in multiple sclerotics [54]. This observation suggests that there may be in some cases a tonic inhibition of vasodilation mediated by the sacral roots.

After rectal excision for benign conditions, erection or ejaculation may be impaired in up to 20 percent of cases [50, 57]. In more radical surgery for malignant disease, the incidence rises to 30 to 100 percent [4, 20, 56]. The effect of cystectomy with prostatectomy and vesiculectomy for bladder cancer is described by Bergman and co-workers [3]. Only 3 of 42 cases retained their erections, one of whom also had a total urethrectomy. However, 21 of 28 cases who had been sexually active postoperatively achieved orgasm, including 2 of 3 who had a total urethrectomy.

Lumbar Disk Prolapse
It is well recognized that central disk prolapse with cauda equina compression can result in impotence and bladder paralysis that may well not recover even after expeditious surgery. Documentation of the syndrome is regrettably sparse [1, 33, 48]. Amelar and Dubin [1] consider impotence to be common in the low-back syndrome, and not due only to massive central disks. In this respect, I believe that the inhibitory effects of pain, both physiologic and psychologic, are most relevant. It would be interesting to study the effect of painful hemorrhoids and their treatment on potency. Impotence in lumbar disk prolapse may occur without bladder dysfunction, and vice versa. Occasionally, disk prolapse is manifested only by impotence and can be relieved by surgery [48].

Peripheral Neuropathy
Disturbances of genitourinary function are encountered most often in diabetic and amy-

loid neuropathy [53]. Failure of erection usually precedes failure of ejaculation. Retrograde ejaculation, as after sympathectomy, however, may be the earliest feature in diabetics [13, 21]. Erectile impotence occurs in diabetics 2 to 5 times more often than in a control population [46]. Twenty-five percent are impotent in the 30- to 34-year age group, and over 50 percent in the 50- to 54-year age group. Impotence may be even more common in primary amyloidosis with neuropathic features. Andersson and Hofer [2] found it in 16 of 24 cases. It may be an early clue to the diagnosis. Ellenberg [12] has emphasized the clinical reasons to believe that impotence in diabetics is neuropathic in origin, showing a strong association between impotence and the presence of a neuropathic bladder and/or other clinical features of peripheral neuropathy. This concept has now been confirmed by sacral evoked responses.

Friedreich's Ataxia
Friedreich's ataxia is a hereditary sensory neuropathy with spinocerebellar degeneration. In Friedreich's original description of 1872 [18], some of his patients with difficulty in emptying the bladder and episodes of sweating and palpitation also were unable to produce penile erection.

CEREBRAL DISORDERS
The role of the olfactory system in sexual behavior was recognized at least as far back as 1873, when Kraft-Ebbing drew attention to the association [32]. The phylogenetic importance of olfaction promoted the evolution of the limbic system. Much recent evidence implicates this system in the central control of sexual activity and erection and of ejaculation in particular [27, 28]. It is here that the "organic" and "psychologic" types of impotence may begin to merge, because the system is involved with many aspects of emotion and behavior.

Temporal Lobe Lesions
The experimental work of Kluver and Bucy [30], which identified the modulating effect of the temporal lobes on sexual activity, has now

been supported by much clinical evidence. Increased sexual activity, perhaps analogous to the Kluver-Bucy syndrome, has been recorded after bilateral temporal lobectomy in humans [52] but is not invariable [15]. In temporal lesions, the sexual activity may be changed rather than increased; fetishism and transvestism have been described in cysticercosis [10] and with other causes of temporal lobe epilepsy [14, 25, 40]. "Sexual seizures" have been described in which coitus may be simulated [9], and seminal emission has been recorded during attacks of petit mal epilepsy [58].

Temporal lobe epilepsy may be more commonly associated with impotence. Gastaut and Collomb [19] noted impotence with decreased libido in two-thirds of 36 hospitalized cases, whereas no patients with other types of epilepsy were impotent. Any contribution by anticonvulsant drugs to impotence was excluded by Hierons and Saunders [23], whose 15 patients with normal libido but decreased potency included cases of cerebral trauma, glioma, aneurysm, angioma, unidentified calcification, and idiopathic temporal lobe epilepsy. This form of epilepsy may be treated by unilateral temporal lobectomy, and an increase in sexuality after the operation is associated with a good prognosis for the epilepsy [15].

Pituitary Tumors

Despite the tendency of pituitary tumors to cause hypothalamic compression, the basis of concurrent impotence is usually endocrinologic. In lesions producing "panhypopituitarism," the cause is often assumed to be the low level of pituitary gonadotropins. This conclusion may need to be reviewed in the light of recent measurement of serum prolactin levels [11]. A raised prolactin concentration may be found in over one-third of "functionless" pituitary tumors [17]. Impotence, with decreased libido and oligospermia, has been described recently in cases of both macro- and microadenomas that produce hyperprolactinemia. The impotence may be cured by transphenoidal microsurgical adenomectomy.

Head Injuries

The diffuse and complex damage occasioned by cerebral trauma makes analysis of specific deficits difficult. Complaints of impotence after head injury are not uncommon [16, 37, 45] (sometimes in relation to litigation), but complaints of personality change are more common, and secondary social factors may be relevant. Stier [51] collected 33 cases of posttraumatic sexual depression. The significant feature was the tendency for the libido to be depressed. Slightly better documentation exists in relation to posttraumatic cerebral atrophy in boxers [35], of whom 3 of 10 patients were impotent.

Stereotaxic Surgery

One of the few studies in humans involving stimulation through stereotaxically implanted electrodes is that of Sem Jacobsen [47]. In 82 patients, with 3632 separate electrodes, reliable sexual responses were recorded only twice, in one case proceeding to ejaculation. In both patients the area was 22 mm lateral to the midline and about 1 cm above and in front of the foramen of Munro in the posterior frontal region. One might be concerned, therefore, that basofrontal leukotomy might cause impotence; but it is our local experience that the reverse is the case, and abolition of anxiety by leukotomy leads to a restoration of potency. This has been observed by others [24].

Impotence has been recorded in 2 of 3 cases treated by open bilateral ansotomy [38]. The lesions were relatively extensive through the dorsomedial hypothalamus to the striothalamic outflow. The medial part of this area is associated with the limbic system.

Other Cerebral States

Various other conditions have been linked with the genesis of impotence, from headaches and vertigo [34] to the presenile dementia of Alzheimer's disease [23] and the use of electroconvulsive therapy [39]. Impotence has been observed in Parkinson's disease, but it is difficult to discount the effect of concomitant personality change and the use of anticholinergic drugs. Certainly, the successful treatment of parkinsonism with L-dopa may lead to "indiscreet sexual advances."

REFERENCES

1. Amelar, R. D., and Dubin, L. Impotence in the low-back syndrome. *J.A.M.A.* 216:520, 1971.
2. Andersson, R., and Hofer, P. A. Genitourinary disturbances in familial and sporadic cases of primary amyloidosis with polyneuropathy. *Acta Med. Scand.* 195:49, 1974.
3. Bergman, B., Nilsson, S., and Petersen, I. The effect on erection and orgasm of cystectomy, prostatectomy and vesiculectomy for cancer of the bladder: A clinical and electromyographic study. *Br. J. Urol.* 51:114, 1979.
4. Bernstein, W. C., and Bernstein, E. F. Sexual dysfunction following radical surgery for cancer of the rectum. *Dis. Colon Rectum* 9:328, 1966.
5. Bors, E., and Comarr, A. E. *Neurological Urology.* Basel: S. Karger, 1971. P. 144.
6. Carter, J. N., et al. Prolactin secreting tumors and hypogonadism in 22 men. *N. Engl. J. Med.* 299:847, 1978.
7. Chapelle, P. A., Durand, J., and Lacert, P. Penile erection following complete spinal cord injury in man. *Br. J. Urol.* 52:216, 1980.
8. Comarr, A. E. *The Total Care of Spinal Cord Injuries.* Boston: Little, Brown, 1977.
9. Currier, R. D., et al. Sexual seizures. *Arch. Neurol.* 25:260, 1971.
10. Davies, B. M., and Morgenstern, F. S. A case of cysticercosis, temporal lobe epilepsy and transvestism. *J. Neurol. Neurosurg. Psychiatry* 23:247, 1960.
11. Editorial. Endocrine basis for sexual dysfunction in men. *Br. Med. J.* 2:1516, 1978.
12. Ellenberg, M. Impotence in diabetes: The neurologic factor. *Ann. Intern. Med.* 75:213, 1971.
13. Ellenberg, M., and Weber, H. Retrograde ejaculation in diabetic neuropathy, *Ann. Intern. Med.* 65:1237, 1966.
14. Epstein, A. W. Relation of fetishism to brain, and especially temporal lobe dysfunction. *J. Nerv. Ment. Dis.* 133:247, 1961.
15. Falconer, M. A., et al. Treatment of temporal lobe epilepsy by temporal lobectomy. *Lancet* 1:827, 1955.
16. Fleck, U. Sexual disturbances following cerebral concussion. *Ztschr f.d. ges Neurol. u. Psychiat.* 165:318, 1939.
17. Franks, S., et al. Hyperprolactinaemia and impotence. *Clin. Endocrinol. (Oxf.)* 8:277, 1978.
18. Friedreich, N. *Uber progressice Muskelatrophie Uber wahre and falsch Muskelhypertrophie.* Berlin: A. Hirschwald, 1873. P. 11.
19. Gastaut, H., and Collomb, H. Etude du comportment sexuel chez les epileptiques psychomoteurs. *Ann. Med. Psychol.* 2:657, 1954.
20. Goligher, J. C. Sexual function after excision of the rectum. *Proc. R. Soc. Med.* 44:824, 1951.
21. Greene, L. F., Kelalis, P. P., and Weeks, R. E. Retrograde ejaculation of semen due to diabetic neuropathy. *Fertil. Steril.* 14:617, 1963.
22. Guttman, L. *Spinal Cord Injuries.* Oxford: Blackwell, 1963. P. 449.
23. Heirons, R., and Saunder, M. Impotence in patients with temporal lobe lesions. *Lancet* 2:761, 1966.
24. Hemphill, R. E. Return of virility after prefrontal leukotomy in case of obsessional neurosis with enlargement of gonads. *Lancet* 2:345, 1944.
25. Hunter, R. A., Logue, V., and McMenemy, W. H. Temporal lobe epilepsy supervening on long standing fetishism and transvestism. *Epilepsia* 4:60, 1963.
26. Ivers, R. R., and Goldstein, N. P. Multiple sclerosis: A current appraisal of symptoms and signs. *Mayo Clin. Proc.* 38:457, 1963.
27. Johnson, J. Sexual impotence and the limbic system. *Br. J. Psychiatry* 111:300, 1965.
28. Johnson, J. *Disorders of Sexual Potency in the Male.* New York: Pergamon, 1968.
29. Johnson, R. H., et al. Autonomic failure with orthostatic hypotension due to intermediolateral column degeneration. *Q. J. Med.* 35:276, 1966.
30. Kluver, H., and Bucy, P. C. Psychic blindness and other symptoms following bilateral temporal lobectomy in rhesus monkeys. *J. Physiol.* 119:352, 1937.
31. Kocketkov, V. D. *Neurologicheskie Aspekty Impotentsii.* Moskva Meditsina, 1968.
32. Kraft-Ebbing, R. *Psychopathia Sexualis.* Rebman: London, 1873.
33. LaBau, M. M. Sexual impotence in men having the low back syndrome. *Arch. Phys. Med.* 47:715, 1966.
34. Mason, I. Headaches and vertigo and their correlation to derangement of sexual function. *Ohio State Med. J.* 41:132, 1945.
35. Mawdsley, C., and Ferguson, F. R. Neurological disease in boxers. *Lancet* 2:795, 1963.
36. Meirowsky, A. M., and Scheibert, C. D. Studies on the sacral reflex arc in paraplegia: III. Clinical observations on inhibitory impulses within the sacral reflex arc. *Exp. Med. Surg.* 8:437, 1950.
37. Meyer, J. E. Sexual disorders in patients with brain injuries. *Arch. Psychiat.* 193:449, 1955.
38. Meyers, R. Three cases of myoclonus alleviated by bilateral ansotomy, with a note on postoperative alibido and impotence. *J. Neurosurg.* 19:71, 1962.
39. Michael, S. T. Impotence during electric shock therapy. *Psychiatr. Quart.* 25:24, 1951.
40. Mitchell, W., Falconer, M. A., and Hill, D. J. Epilepsy with fetishism relieved by temporal lobectomy. *Lancet* 2:626, 1954.

41. Miyazaki, K. Impotence caused by nerve injuries. *Clin. Endocrinol. (Tokyo).* 18:713, 1970.
42. Pont, A., et al. Prolactin-secreting tumours in men: Surgical care. *Ann. Intern. Med.* 91:211, 1979.
43. Rabiner, A. M., and Rubinstein, H. G. Dorsal nerve of penis as a factor in potency. *Trans. Am. Neurol. Assoc.* 70:177, 1944.
44. Retief, P. J. M. Physiology of micturition and ejaculation. *S. Afr. Med. J.* 24:509, 1950.
45. Rojas, L. Post traumatic impotence after fracture of base of skull. *Actas Luso. Espan. Neurol. Psiquiatr.* 6:43, 1947.
46. Rubin, A., and Babbott, D. Impotence and diabetes mellitus. *J.A.M.A.* 168:498, 1958.
47. Sem-Jacobsen, C. W. *Depth Electrographic Stimulation of the Human Brain and Behavior.* Springfield, Ill.: Thomas, 1968.
48. Shafer, N. Occult lumbar disk causing impotency. *N.Y. J. Med.* 69:2465, 1969.
49. Shy, G. M., and Drager, G. A. A neurological syndrome associated with orthostatic hypotension. *Arch. Neurol.* 2:511, 1960.
50. Stahlgren, L. H., and Ferguson, L. K. Influence on sexual function of abdominoperineal resection for ulcerative colitis. *N. Engl. J. Med.* 259:873, 1958.
51. Stier, E. Disturbances of sexual function through head trauma. *J. Nerv. Ment. Dis.* 88:714, 1938.
52. Terzian, H., and Ore, G. D. Syndrome of Kluver and Bucy reproduced in man, by bilateral removal of the temporal lobes. *Neurology* 5:373, 1955.
53. Thomas, P. K. *Clinical Features and Differential Diagnosis in Peripheral Neuropathy* (vol. 1). Philadelphia: Saunders, 1975. P. 503.
54. Torrens, M. J. Management of the uninhibited bladder by selective sacral neurectomy. *J. Neurosurg.* 44:176, 1976.
55. Vas, C. J. Sexual impotence and some autonomic disturbances in men with multiple sclerosis. *Acta Neurol. Scand.* 45:166, 1969.
56. Watson, P. C., and Williams, D. I. The urological complications of excision of the rectum. *Br. J. Surg.* 40:19, 1952.
57. Watts, J. M., de Dombal, F. T., and Goligher, J. C. Long term complications and prognosis following major surgery for ulcerative colitis. *Br. J. Surg.* 53:1014, 1966.
58. Wechsler, I. S. *Clinical Neurology.* Philadelphia: Saunders, 1963. P. 579.
59. Whitelaw, G. P., and Smithwick, R. H. Some secondary effects of sympathectomy. *New Engl. J. Med.* 245:121, 1951.
60. Zeitlin, A. B., Cottrell, T. L., and Lloyd, F. A. Sexology of the paraplegic male. *Fertil. Steril.* 8:337, 1957.

6

Endocrine Disorders Associated with Erectile Dysfunction

LEONARD M. POGACH
JUDITH L. VAITUKAITIS

The ability of a man to achieve an erection depends on a complex interrelationship among emotional, neurologic, vascular, and hormonal factors. Although testosterone is known to be essential for normal male sexual development, the precise relationship between androgens and sexual behavior remains to be elucidated. Whether a "critical" level of testosterone is needed to sustain libido and potency or whether declining levels that remain within the "normal" range account for decreased libido or potency is unclear at this time [3]. Moreover, many studies suffer from a lack of definition of the term *impotent,* which Masters and Johnson define as an inability to achieve an erection in over 25 percent of attempts [47]. Against this background, it is not surprising that the true incidence of endocrine dysfunction as a cause of impotence remains unknown, although it has variably been estimated between 5 and 35 percent [66].

Not only primary disorders of the hypothalamic-pituitary-testicular axis may lead to impotence, but disorders of other endocrine glands may contribute as well. Since endocrinologic dysfunction may result in subtle abnormalities, the clinician dealing with impotence must scrutinize appropriate clinical and laboratory data carefully, lest the patient with a treatable endocrinologic disorder be consigned to months or years of fruitless counseling. On initial screening, the clinician should ascertain whether the defect is congenital or acquired. That differentiation can be made with a combined careful history, physical examination, and appropriate laboratory tests, including serum gonadotropin, prolactin, and testosterone levels, as well as genetic screening when indicated. Moreover, if the patient is capable of collecting an ejaculate for semen analysis, and subsequent analysis reveals normal motility, morphology, and sperm count, an endocrinologic defect is unlikely to be present. Normal spermatogenesis requires normal Leydig cell and seminiferous tubular function; those functions in turn require a normal hypothalamic-pituitary-testicular axis.

The normal range of serum gonadotropins among men varies among laboratories with

Supported in part by NIH grants RR-533 and 5T32AM-07201.

the reference preparation used for dose interpolation as well as with the reagents incorporated in the assay. Consequently, one must be provided the normal adult range for each gonadotropin assay in order to ascertain whether a patient has abnormally high or low gonadotropin levels. The normal adult male range for serum prolactin concentrations in the overwhelming majority of assays does not exceed 30 ng/ml. Finally, the normal adult level for serum testosterone usually ranges between 300 and 1100 ng/dl.

CLINICAL AND
LABORATORY EVALUATIONS

In taking the history, it is important to determine whether the patient had normal developmental milestones and progressed through puberty normally in development of secondary sexual characteristics. In addition to questioning the patient about such development, including axillary, pubic, and facial hair growth, change in voice and body habitus, and phallic enlargement, it may be helpful to have the patient obtain records of his growth pattern. By graphically depicting such records, the physician may detect an abnormality in the growth curve, such as an absent growth spurt that may not otherwise be apparent. A family history of infertility, hypogonadism, or other endocrine disorders should be sought.

A complaint of decreased libido or potency after puberty may be the earliest clue to hypoandrogenism, antedating changes in shaving pattern, loss of axillary or pubic hair, or development of gynecomastia or galactorrhea. Hot flashes, similar to those experienced by women during the climacteric, have been reported to occur in some men concomitantly with declining testicular function [20]. A careful history should be obtained regarding (1) exposure to toxins or radiation; (2) prolonged systemic illnesses; (3) acute febrile illnesses; and (4) drugs, including alkylating agents used to treat some forms of neoplasia and the abuse of alcohol, antihypertensive agents, and marijuana.

On physical examination, one should take note of congenital abnormalities associated with endocrine disorders. Those physical findings include cleft palate, hare lip, cataracts, congenital cardiovascular defects, low-set ears, short stature, ocular abnormalities, and mental retardation. Anosmia is often associated with hypothalamic defects and may be detected only by carefully testing each nostril with specific olfactory stimuli [59]. In addition, the clinician should be aware of the increased incidence of developmental abnormalities affecting the genitourinary tract among patients with congenital abnormalities of reproduction.

If testosterone deficiency antedates puberty, the patient will manifest *eunuchoidal proportions,* defined as an arm span 5 cm or more in excess of height, or a sole-to-pubis length exceeding that of the crown to pubis length by more than 2 cm. Regression of secondary sexual characteristics may be present, as well as galactorrhea and gynecomastia. The latter is characterized by an increase in retroareolar glandular tissue rather than adipose tissue. A biopsy may be necessary to make that distinction. Testicular size should be measured with calipers or a Prader orchiometer and testicular consistency noted. Obviously, signs of systemic illnesses as well as other endocrinologic abnormalities should be sought. A normal clinical evaluation does not exclude underlying endocrinologic pathology and thus mandates laboratory evaluation.

Luteinizing hormone (LH) stimulates the Leydig cells to synthesize and secrete testosterone, whereas follicle-stimulating hormone (FSH) acts on the seminiferous tubules and, through mechanisms poorly understood, stimulates spermatogenesis [16]. Normal Leydig cell and seminiferous tubular function are required for spermatogenesis. The specific effects of prolactin on the male reproductive tract have not been defined, but prolactin clearly affects the system. Pituitary FSH secretion may be inhibited by both testosterone and *inhibin,* an incompletely characterized secretory product of the Sertoli cells [14, 21]. Normal testosterone levels are requisite for normal potency. However, normal testosterone levels but abnormally high prolactin levels may be encountered among some affected men (see Table 6-1) [8].

Table 6-1. Diagnostic evaluation of men with impotence

Test	Clinical application	Comments	Interpretation
Basal hormone levels			
Testosterone [2]	General screening	Level is dependent on alterations of SSBG level, which in turn depends on peripheral metabolism, estradiol, T_3, and T_4 concentrations	Normal: 300–1200 ng/dl. Wide intra- and interindividual variations; low levels with both primary and secondary gonadal dysfunction but may be normal with idiopathic hyperprolactinemia
		Diurnal variation 25% or less; if initial value is low, repeat, or obtain pooled samples	
Free testosterone [75]	Situations in which total testosterone may not correlate with clinical setting	Correlates with clinical state better than total testosterone	Normal: 1–3% of total testosterone concentration
FSH, LH [51]	General screening	Circhoral variation may necessitate multiple or pooled plasma determinations	Normal: 5–25 mIU/ml (IRP 2 hMG);* low or inappropriately low levels occur in hypothalamic or pituitary disorders; elevated levels usually signify primary gonadal failure but may be present in patients with FSH secreting adenomas
		Sensitivity of some radioimmunoassays may not permit distinction between low normal and pathologically low levels	
Prolactin [33]	General screening	Elevations observed after breast manipulation, smoking, stress, and ingestion of numerous medications. Levels increase with dozing or sleeping but remain within the normal range	Normal: 4–26 ng/ml; higher levels have better correlation with pituitary tumor; levels greater than 300 ng/ml virtually pathognomonic of pituitary adenoma
Estradiol [25]	Suspected Leydig or Sertoli cell tumors	Levels dependent on SSBG level, peripheral androgen metabolism, and direct secretion of estradiol	Normal: 20–70 pg/ml
Provocative testing			
hCG administration: (4000 U IM × 4 days) [44]	Measure of testicular Leydig cell reserve	hCG stimulates the actions of LH on Leydig cell function because of its structural homology with LH	Normal: 2.5-fold testosterone level increase above basal; subnormal responses suggestive of impaired gonadal function
		Response may be misleading if patient has had long-standing primary defect of hypothalamic-pituitary axis	

Table 6-1 (continued)

Test	Clinical application	Comments	Interpretation
GnRH (100 μg IV bolus) [57]	Distinguishing hypothalamic from pituitary disease (tenuous)	Test not generally specific enough to distinguish hypothalamic from pituitary disease; best correlation of maximal response appears to be with basal gonadotropin level; not generally useful for single-patient evaluation but exceptions exist	Normal: wide range of responses; serial studies may be useful in selected cases
Clomiphene citrate (100 mg qd × 5) [60]	Distinguishing hypothalamic from pituitary disease (tenuous)	Weak estrogenic compound that has predominately antiestrogenic effect at the hypothalamic level in adults	Normal: twofold increase of LH levels above basal
Chlorpromazine stimulation (25 mg IM) [38]	Differentiation of pituitary tumor from idiopathic hyperprolactinemia	Acts to block dopaminergic receptors	Normal: twofold increase of prolactin levels above basal
TRH stimulation (250 μg IV bolus) [42]	Differentiation of pituitary tumor from idiopathic hyperprolactinemia	Stimulates prolactin-secreting cells to release prolactin directly	Normal: twofold increase in prolactin levels above basal
Radiologic			
Routine skull films (AP and lateral) [15]	General screening for pituitary tumor	Best means to evaluate sella turcica volume but insensitive in detecting microadenomas	Normal: volume 350–1150 cu mm
Sella turcica polytomography [13]	Detection of microadenomas	Best means to evaluate patient for presence of microadenoma (≤10 mm) Sensitivity of procedure dependent on spacing of polytomes (1.0 mm preferable)	Normal: absence of double floor, erosions, demineralization, or ballooning
CAT scan [36] Pneumoencephalogram	Determination of sellar extension of tumors and parasellar masses or cysts as well as determination of "empty" sella	CAT scan with use of intrathecal contrast (metrizamide) may be superior to a conventional pneumoencephalogram for determining suprasellar extension and evaluation of parasellar abnormalities	Normal: absence of suprasellar lesion or marked concavity of diaphragm sella; no air or contrast media within sella; normal ventricles
Chromosomal			
Buccal smear [3]	Evaluation of patients with hypergonadotropic hypogonadism	Two X chromosomes needed to form Barr body	Normal: absence (<4%) of Barr bodies (i.e., chromatin negative-staining)

Table 6-1 (continued)

Test	Clinical application	Comments	Interpretation
Blood or gonadal tissue karyotype [62]	Evaluation of patients with hypergonadotropic hypogonadism	Definitive test for chromosomal aberrations; if patient is suspected of tissue mosaicism, one must examine multiple tissues	Normal: XY karyotype
Semen analysis [54]	General screening of men with hypogonadism	Adequate evaluation must include volume of ejaculate, number of spermatozoa, percent motility, and percent abnormal forms; ejaculate should be collected under standardized conditions (i.e., 2 days' abstinence from sexual activity and laboratory analysis carried out within 2 hours after collection); best to repeat study after several months to ensure exclusion of transient abnormality	Normal: volume 2.5–4.5 ml; sperm count: 10 million/ml; motility: greater than 60%; abnormal forms: less than 30%

*IRP 2 hMG = international reference preparation 2 of human menopausal gonadotropin.

If impotence is secondary to endocrine dysfunction, the clinician must ascertain whether the defect is at the gonadal level or lies at the hypothalamic-pituitary level. Finally, if circulating prolactin levels are abnormally high and the patient has not been taking drugs that increase prolactin secretion, an abnormality of the hypothalamic-pituitary axis must be sought after confirming an abnormal circulating prolactin level under basal conditions. For the purposes of this presentation, we shall focus primarily on acquired endocrinologic abnormalities but shall discuss briefly congenital and heredofamilial disorders leading to altered potency. Table 6-1 summarizes a variety of tests used to evaluate a suspected endocrinologic disorder that might account for the patient's signs and symptoms.

Testosterone, as are all steroid hormones, is transported in the serum primarily bound to albumin and sex steroid–binding globulin (SSBG); only 3 percent of total testosterone is in the free form. Since measurement of total testosterone includes the portion that is protein bound, it is also obvious that the level will be affected by such factors as peripheral metabolism and alterations in sex steroid–binding globulins. Moreover, since only free testosterone is accessible for metabolism at the cellular level, that form correlates best with clinical androgenicity [75]. The test is expensive and difficult to perform, and therefore should be reserved for situations in which the total testosterone concentration may be misleading.

Although the gonadotropin-releasing hormone (GnRH) stimulation test has been proposed to distinguish between low normal and pathologically low gonadotropin levels, or between hypothalamic and pituitary disease, it has not proved to be sufficiently specific to do so [50]. Generally, one observes a larger GnRH-induced release of gonadotropin, especially LH, when a hypothalamic defect is present. However, there is wide overlap between patients with primary hypothalamic and pituitary disorders. Consequently, application of that test on an individual basis is not useful in most clinical settings.

DIFFERENTIAL DIAGNOSIS
Hypothalamic-Pituitary Disorders
Since the hypothalamic-pituitary-gonadal axis is an example of a negative-feedback system, decreased serum testosterone levels should result in a compensatory increase in pituitary LH secretion if the hypothalamus and pituitary function normally. When LH levels are normal or decreased, and circulating testosterone levels are abnormally low, the defect is central and may result either from primary disease of the hypothalamus or pituitary or from systemic disorders secondarily affecting the hypothalamic-pituitary axis.

It should be pointed out here that seminiferous tubular function is more sensitive to any kind of insult than is that of the Leydig cell. Consequently, altered spermatogenesis is usually observed before altered Leydig cell function [67]. If the patient comes to a clinician relatively soon after acquiring a defect of the hypothalamic-pituitary-testicular axis, it will be most likely for infertility rather than impotence.

Men with low serum testosterone levels and normal or abnormally low circulating LH levels usually have hypogonadotropic hypogonadism with an abnormality at the hypothalamic-pituitary level. Table 6-2 summarizes the variety of congenital syndromes, physical findings, and laboratory abnormalities associated with those syndromes. Obviously, patients with congenital abnormalities of the hypothalamic-pituitary axis will most likely come to a pediatrician or endocrinologist with a complaint of delayed or late puberty or absence of pubertal development. The first sign of puberty in a boy is gonadal enlargement, and that event usually occurs at an average age of 10.5 years, with a range of 9 to 14 years [23, 71]. Other early changes include reddening of the scrotal skin in association with the development of sparse pubic hair at the base of the penis. Subsequent pubertal progression results in penile growth and the development of an adult male escutcheon. Normal pubertal boys may have gynecomastia, but this should resolve spontaneously within 2 years.

Table 6-2. Congenital hypothalamic and pituitary disorders associated with impotence

Disorder	Clinical findings	Laboratory findings
Hypothalamic		
Kallman's syndrome (GnRH deficiency) [4]	Classic syndrome consists of hyposmia or anosmia, color blindness, nerve deafness, syndactyly and midline craniofacial abnormalities, and renal agenesis; inheritance: autosomal dominance with incomplete penetrance; affected individuals need not have all signs and need not be hypogonadal	Low serum gonadotropin and testosterone levels; normal pituitary response to GnRH with prolonged or repeated stimulation; may observe developmental abnormalities within hypothalamus at autopsy
Prader-Willi syndrome [76]	Majority of patients recognized in infancy; findings may include massive obesity, neonatal muscle hypotonia, hyperphagia, mental retardation, and hypogonadism	Gonadotropin levels usually low but have been reported to be normal or high; low serum testosterone concentrations
Laurence-Moon-Biedl syndrome [58]	Characterized by high incidence of consanguinity, growth retardation, mental retardation, obesity, syndactyly, and hypogonadism	Low serum gonadotropin and testosterone levels
Alstrom's syndrome [68]	Clinical findings include retinal degeneration, obesity, nephropathy, nerve deafness, hypertriglyceridemia, hyperuricemia, acanthosis nigricans and hypogonadism, and autosomal recessive inheritance	Low serum gonadotropin and testosterone levels
Familial cerebellar syndrome [48]	Findings include cerebellar ataxia, nerve deafness, shortened fourth metacarpals, and hypogonadism	Low serum gonadotropin and testosterone levels
Pituitary		
Prepubertal panhypopituitarism (idiopathic)	Infants are usually of normal length and weight; growth failure usually noted by 1 year of age, but variable onset	Low serum gonadotropin and testosterone levels; variable degrees of GH, TSH, or ACTH deficiency; diagnosis of exclusion
LH deficiency (Pasqualini syndrome) [18, 19]	Patients have eunuchoidal phenotype, absent secondary sexual characteristics, and varying degrees of spermatogenesis	Normal serum FSH, low LH, subnormal testosterone levels, oligospermia or azospermia

Men with an acquired defect of the hypothalamic-pituitary axis usually have a pituitary tumor. The growth of the pituitary tumor is usually very slow and results in insidious clinical changes that the patient, spouse, or other family members may not be aware of. These usually include lethargy, changes in the rate of beard growth as well as axillary or pubic hair growth, impotence, and, sometimes, gynecomastia if the tumor secretes prolactin. Table 6-3 summarizes acquired defects that affect hypothalamic-pituitary function and may result in impotence.

There is a subgroup of patients with impotence who may have normal circulating testosterone and gonadotropin levels but have abnormally elevated serum prolactin concentrations. The incidence of hyperprolactinemia as a cause of impotence is unknown. Moreover, the mechanism by which hyperprolactinemia induces impotence is poorly understood [74]. One should screen the patient carefully for his taking medications known to induce increased prolactin secretion. Those drugs include methyldopa (Aldomet), phenothiazines, and reserpine. Affected men may have no evidence of pituitary tumors. It is interesting that when affected patients are treated with bromocryptine (Parlodel), prolactin levels return to normal, and potency is restored [52].

Table 6-3. Acquired hypothalamic-pituitary disorders associated with impotence

Disorder	Clinical presentations	Diagnostic evaluation*
Hypothalamic		
Idiopathic hypo-gonadism	Signs and symptoms dependent on age of onset; associated with other anterior pituitary hormone deficiencies with their attendant signs and symptoms	Diagnosis of exclusion
Malignant and benign tumors	Adenocarcinoma of the lung most common metastatic tumor; craniopharyngioma most benign tumor and may not be calcified; most patients have growth retardation	Differentiation from pituitary adenomas may be difficult; random loss of factors controlling anterior pituitary function; histologic diagnosis
Infiltrative disorders include sarcoidosis, eosinophilic granuloma, tuberculosis	Loss of libido and fatigue are common with any chronic illness; hence, signs and symptoms of hormonal deficiency should be carefully sought in any disease known to affect the hypothalamic pituitary axis	CSF examination for cytology and culture may be necessary; selected cultures and skin testing
Trauma	Signs and symptoms depend on which tropic hormones are affected	Calcification may be present in hypothalamic area
Cysts	May have growth retardation or arrested pubertal development	CAT scan or pneumoencephalogram may be necessary; must differentiate from solid tumor
Pituitary		
Adenomas		
Nonfunctioning chromophobe	Causes symptoms by virtue of size, hence neurologic findings such as headaches and bitemporal hemianopsia are common; loss of anterior pituitary tropic hormone function occurs randomly	Sellar polytomography; prolactin levels abnormally high in 60% of cases; tests of anterior pituitary function
Prolactinomas [73]	Up to 75% of all chromophobe tumors secrete prolactin; patients exhibit infertility or gynecomastia rather than impotence; galactorrhea is rare in humans	Levels over 200 ng/ml suggestive of tumor; provocative testing of hPr secretion; polytomography may be indicated
Gonadotropin-secreting tumors [40]	Gonadotropin-secreting tumors are rare, but may produce FSH and/or LH; patients may display loss of libido, impotence, and/or infertility; evidence of other hormone deficiencies may be present	FSH and/or LH levels elevated with or without loss of other anterior pituitary hormones; gonadotropin levels may not be suppressible
Cushing's disease [22]	Signs and symptoms may include muscle weakness, fatigue, hypokalemia, hypertension, glucose intolerance, and striae; loss of libido almost always occurs	Urinary free cortisol and dexamethasone suppression tests; sella x rays usually normal
Acromegaly [11]	Prominence of soft tissue occurs before bony overgrowth; patients may be hypertensive and have glucose intolerance	Abnormally high basal GH level; sella x ray often abnormal; may observe paradoxic rise of GH levels with glucose administration

Table 6-3 (continued)

Disorder	Clinical presentations	Diagnostic evaluation*
Aneurysm	Difficult to distinguish from nonfunctioning adenoma by routine clinical laboratory and radiographic evaluations	Arteriogram necessary for diagnosis
Infiltrative disorders include hemochromatosis	See above; infiltrative disorder may also directly affect testis	Evaluation of pituitary and testicular reserve indicated; special histologic strain for iron deposition in testicular biopsy
Meningioma	Rare; usually associated with frontal signs and symptoms	Brain scan or CAT scan helpful; may observe sellar erosion and visual field abnormalities

*All affected patients will have abnormally low circulating testosterone and LH levels as well as other selected tropic hormone abnormalities. Systematic studies of the hypothalamic-pituitary axis are necessary.

Primary Gonadal Disorders

The most common endocrinologic cause of impotence is *primary gonadal failure* that results in abnormally low circulating testosterone levels and high serum LH concentrations. Both seminiferous tubular and Leydig cell functions are abnormal. That state is termed *hypergonadotropic hypogonadism*. Rare instances of elevated FSH levels due to functioning pituitary adenomas have been reported [40]. Table 6-4 summarizes a variety of factors that may cause primary gonadal failure and impotence. *Klinefelter's syndrome,* a genetic disorder that classically is manifested with an XXY karyotype and affects up to 1 in 400 men, may be associated with normal or low circulating testosterone levels [32]. Consequently, patients with that syndrome may not complain of altered potency but are sterile nonetheless. Testicular biopsy from affected men reveals classic changes or peritubular fibrosis together with absence of staining for elastin with specific histologic staining. Some men with Klinefelter's syndrome have a defect in testosterone biosynthesis [69]. Karyotypic analyses are essential in the evaluation of patients having small, firm testes.

Aging

Whether decreased gonadal function occurs as part of the aging process remains unresolved, because of difficulties in defining a cohort of "normal aged men" [26]. A number of investigators have reported declining free and total testosterone levels with age and reciprocally increased LH levels concomitant with degenerative changes in seminiferous tubules and increased Leydig cell pigmentation [56, 61]. In addition, older men may have decreased Leydig cell responsiveness to human chorionic gonadotropin (hCG) stimulation [45]. Together, these findings suggest that in some men normal serum testosterone levels are maintained by compensatory increased serum LH levels in the face of declining Leydig cell reserve.

Although the majority of men have no symptoms, some patients with declining testosterone levels complain of decreased libido, whereas a smaller number may have symptoms similar to those associated with menopause [49]. However, most clinicians are skeptical of that association. Whether the latter is functional or organic has not been determined. It remains unclear whether there is an absolute threshold of serum testosterone level below which such symptoms occur.

TREATMENT

Some patients with primary defects of the hypothalamic-pituitary axis may have potency restored either with exogenous testosterone administration or with human chori-

Table 6-4. Congenital and acquired gonadal disorders associated with impotence

Disorder	Clinical findings	Diagnostic evaluation*
Congenital		
Ullrich-Turner syndrome [9]	Patients display phenotypic characteristics of classic Turner's syndrome: short stature, low-set ears, webbed neck, etc; etiology unknown	Elevated gonadotropin and low testosterone levels; karyotype in XY
Testicular agenesis [37]	Patients fail to undergo puberty; they are usually of short stature; no testes are palpated within the scrotal sac	In pubertal individuals an hCG stimulation test may be necessary to differentiate anorchia from cryptorchidism
Genetic		
Klinefelter's syndrome and variants [32]	Classically affected persons with XXY karyotype; eunuchoidal, with small, firm testes; gynecomastia occurs in 20–80%; evidence of hypoandrogenism in 20–60%; persons who are mosaics have fewer somatic abnormalities; usually have arrested pubertal development	Serum FSH and LH levels elevated; testosterone level low to low normal in most cases; karyotyping mandatory for accurate diagnosis
Acquired		
Orchitis (infections; e.g., mumps, gonorrhea)	Infection is usually postpubertal but may not be recalled; patient may have infertility, impotence, or both; testes may be soft and decreased in volume	Often diagnosis of exclusion; most common cause of primary gonadal failure
Drugs (e.g., chemotherapeutic agents, toxins, alcohol, marijuana, spironolactone) [30]	A careful occupational and geographic history should be obtained; gynecomastia may be present as may stigmata of liver disease	It is necessary to determine whether a specific drug alters the hypothalamic-pituitary axis in addition to being a direct testicular toxin; alcohol may directly affect both the testes and the hypothalamic-pituitary axis
Vascular (e.g., arteriosclerosis, sickle cell disease) [28, 35]	Although impotence is more likely to be secondary to impaired blood flow or neurologic dysfunction, damage to Leydig cells may result in hypoandrogenism	Magnitude of gonadotropin level elevation or decrease in testosterone concentration is dependent on damage to germinal and interstitial cells; Doppler, penile blood pressure of value
Senescence [26]	Whether decreased Leydig cell function occurs independently of associated diseases has not yet been determined; controversial whether aging per se or other factors account for observed abnormalities	Testosterone levels may be low normal, while LH levels may be high normal or elevated; decreased response to hCG
Radiation [43]	Germinal epithelium more radiosensitive than Leydig cell function	Serum FSH level usually elevated, with normal LH and testosterone concentrations; with higher exposure, Leydig cell failure more frequently observed

*All affected men have elevated gonadotropin levels and low serum testosterone concentrations.

onic gonadotropin therapy twice a week in doses of 500 to 4000 IU given intramuscularly [41]. Obviously, the therapy is not undertaken until the underlying defect is defined. Men who are impotent because of hyperprolactinemia but show evidence of pituitary tumor or evidence of other hormonal aberrations may be treated with a dopamine agonist, bromocriptine (Parlodel) [52]. On the other hand, men with primary gonadal failure may have potency restored with exogenous testosterone therapy [12]. When administering exogenous testosterone to older men, one must observe them closely for acute prostatic stimulation, which, in turn, may result in acute urinary outlet obstruction. Consequently it is wise to start older men with a trial of a short-acting or aqueous form of testosterone. If the patient displays no side effects with the short-acting form, a depot form of testosterone can be instituted for long-term therapy. Oral analogues of testosterone are not nearly as effective as parenteral forms of testosterone [46]. Moreover, with the oral testosterone analogues one must carefully monitor liver function because of the well-established hepatotoxic effect of the oral forms.

DIABETES

A number of systemic disorders are capable of inducing impotence, either by secondarily altering the hypothalamic-pituitary-gonadal axis or by causing local neurologic abnormalities. Diabetes is one of the most common causes of impotence, and up to 50 percent of patients are affected during the course of their illness [39]. Endocrine function is normal in the majority of patients, although some investigators have reported decreased serum testosterone concentrations in patients treated with oral agents [63]. Although there may be a role for autonomic neuropathy in the etiology of diabetic impotence [17], the majority of patients are impotent due to a nonneurogenic etiology. Whereas some patients have only an insidious loss of potency but an intact libido, other men will have symptoms of autonomic neuropathy, including those of peripheral neuropathy, neurogenic bladder dysfunction, and nocturnal diarrhea [31]. Similarly, the physical examination may be normal or may provide evidence of peripheral neuropathy, orthostatic hypotension, or decreased testicular sensation. Subclinical autonomic neuropathy may be detected either by lack of R–R variation during the Valsalva maneuver on ECG or by cystometric studies [34].

The treatment of impotence that is secondary to diabetes remains frustrating for both patient and physician. If a patient is debilitated from persistent hyperglycemia, improved blood-sugar control may restore potency, but there is no evidence that tight control will reverse the neurologic lesions [53]. Exogenous testosterone therapy is of no value in this setting.

THYROID DYSFUNCTION

Both *hyper-* and *hypothyroidism* may be associated with decreased potency. According to one recent study, hyperthyroidism may be associated with decreased libido in 71 percent of affected men [36]. Although most younger men will display other signs and symptoms of thyrotoxicosis, older men may be misdiagnosed as being depressed, when, in fact, they may have apathetic hyperthyroidism [72]. Gynecomastia may be observed in 10 to 40 percent of men [6]. The etiology of the decreased libido is not clear but may be due either to the hypermetabolic effects of thyroxine or, perhaps, to increased circulating estrogen levels, which reflect increased peripheral conversion of androgen to estrogen [10].

Patients with hypothyroidism commonly have fatigue and lethargy, which may include complaints of sexual dysfunction. Testosterone secretion is decreased in such individuals, and the metabolic transformation of testosterone is shifted toward etiocholanolone rather than androsterone [27]. In addition, prolactin levels may be elevated in some patients with advanced hypothyroidism, due to either an increase of, or an enhanced response to, thyrotropin-releasing hormone (TRH) [53].

Although a total thyroxine level and T3 resin uptake are usually sufficient to diagnose thyroid disorders, it may be necessary to obtain a total triiodothyronine concentration or thyroid-stimulating hormone (TSH) level. A patient should be euthyroid for several months before reevaluation of persistent impotence is undertaken.

NONENDOCRINE DISORDERS

Finally, nonendocrine systemic illness may result in sexual dysfunction because of alterations in the normal hormonal milieu. Alterations of body weight are observed commonly during chronic illness. Protein calorie malnutrition may lead to low total and free testosterone levels without compensatory elevations of LH levels [65]. In addition, Leydig cell responses to hCG are submaximal. Taken together, those observations suggest a combined primary gonadal and central disorder. Both laboratory and clinical improvement often occur after several months of refeeding. At the other end of the spectrum are men who are pathologically obese and have low testosterone and low gonadotropin concentrations as well as elevated serum estradiol levels [1]. Whether altered gonadotropin secretion is solely the result of altered sex steroid metabolism is poorly understood at the present time.

Patients with chronic renal failure often have complaints of decreased libido and potency, and may have decreased testicular size. Although such patients may have co-existing vascular, neurologic, and nutritional deficits that account for their sexual dysfunction, endocrinologic abnormalities are also prominent. Most uremic patients have low testosterone levels and submaximal testicular responses to hCG [29]. Gonadotropin levels may be inappropriately low, but more commonly are elevated as a result of decreased renal clearance. Estradiol levels often are increased, and, coupled with low androgen, may account for the gynecomastia commonly observed [70]. Finally, hyperprolactinemia may be present in as many as 70 percent of uremic patients on hemodialysis [64]. The reason for this is not clear, although it may be the result of altered dopaminergic function rather than of decreased renal clearance. The hyperprolactinemia also may contribute to the gynecomastia frequently observed in this patient population. Although the use of bromocryptine has achieved some success in improving potency of men on hemodialysis in preliminary studies, its long-term efficacy remains to be proved.

REFERENCES

1. Amatruda, J. M., et al. Depressed plasma testosterone and fractional binding of testosterone in obese males. *J. Clin. Endocrinol. Metab.* 47:268, 1978.
2. Auletta, F. J., Caldwell, B. V., and Hamilton, G. L. Androgens: Testosterone and Dihydrotestosterone. In B. M. Jaffe and H. R. Behrman (eds.), *Methods of Hormone Radioimmunoassay.* New York: Academic, 1979. P. 715.
3. Bancroft, J., and Skakkebaek, N. E. Androgens and human sexual behavior. In *Ciba Found. Symp.* 62:209, 1978.
4. Bardin, C. W., et al. Studies of the pituitary–Leydig cell axis in young men with hypogonadotrophic hypogonadism and hyposmia: Comparison with normal men, prepubertal boys, and hypopituitary patients. *J. Clin. Invest.* 48:2046, 1969.
5. Barr, M. L., and Bertram, E. G. A morphological distinction between neurones of the male and female and the behavior of the nucleolar satellite during accelerated nucleoprotein synthesis. *Nature* 163:676, 1949.
6. Becher, K. L., et al. Gynecomastia and hyperthyroidism: An endocrine and histologic investigation. *J. Clin. Endocrinol. Metab.* 28:277, 1970.
7. Boyar, R. M., et al. Clinical and laboratory heterogeneity in idiopathic hypogonadotrophic hypogonadism. *J. Clin. Endocrinol. Metab.* 43:1268, 1975.
8. Carter, J. N., et al. Prolactin-secreting tumors and hypogonadism in 22 men. *N. Engl. J. Med.* 299:847, 1978.
9. Chaves-Carballo, E., and Haylis, A. B. Ullrich-Turner syndrome in the male: Review of the literature and report of a case with lymphocytic thyroiditis. *Mayo Clin. Proc.* 41:84, 1966.
10. Chopra, I. J., and Tulchinsky, D. Status of estrogen-androgen balance in hyperthyroid men with Graves' disease. *J. Clin. Endocrinol. Metab.* 38:297, 1974.
11. Daughaday, W. H., and Cryer, P. E. Growth

hormone hypersecretion and acromegaly. *Hosp. Pract.* 13:75, 1978.

12. Davidson, J. M., Camargo, C., and Smith, E. R. Effects of androgen on sexual behavior in hypogonadal men. *J. Clin. Endocrinol. Metab.* 48:955, 1979.

13. Deck, M. D. F. Radiographic and Radioisotopic Techniques in the Diagnosis of Pituitary Tumors. In P. O. Kohler and G. T. Ross (eds.), *Diagnosis and Treatment of Pituitary Tumors.* Amsterdam: Excerpta Medica, 1974. P. 71.

14. deJong, F. H. Inhibin: Fact or artifact? *Mol. Cell. Endocrinol.* 13:1, 1979.

15. DiChiro, G., and Nelson, K. B. The volume of the sella turcica. *Am. J. Roentgenol.* 87:989, 1962.

16. Dorrington, J. H., and Armstrong, D. T. Effects of FSH on gonadal function. *Recent Prog. Horm. Res.* 35:301, 1979.

17. Ellenberg, M. Impotence in diabetes: The neurologic factor. *Ann. Intern. Med.* 75:213, 1971.

18. Ewer, R. W. Familial monotropic pituitary gonadotropin insufficiency. *J. Clin. Endocrinol. Metab.* 28:783, 1968.

19. Faiman, C., et al. The fertile eunuch syndrome: Demonstration of isolated luteinizing hormone deficiency by radioimmunoassay technique. *Mayo Clin. Proc.* 43:661, 1968.

20. Feldman, J. M., Postlewaite, R. W., and Glenn, J. F. Hot flashes and sweats in men with testicular insufficiency. *Arch. Intern. Med.* 136:606, 1976.

21. Franchimont, P., et al. Existence of a follicle-stimulating hormone inhibiting factor "inhibin" in bull seminal plasma. *Nature* 257:402, 1975.

22. Gabrilove, J. L., Nicolis, G. L., and Sohval, R. The testis in Cushing's syndrome. *J. Urol.* 112:95, 1974.

23. Grumbach, M. M., et al. Hypothalamic-Pituitary Regulation of Puberty in Man: Evidence and Concepts Derived from Clinical Research. In M. M. Grumbach, G. D. Grave, and F. E. Mayor (eds.), *Control of the Onset of Puberty.* New York: Wiley, 1974. P. 115.

24. Hall, K., and McAllister, V. L. Metrizamide cisternography in pituitary and juxtapituitary lesions. *Radiology* 134:101, 1980.

25. Haning, R., et al. Plasma Estradiol, Estriol, and Urinary Estriol Glucuronide. In B. M. Jaffe and H. R. Behrman (eds.), *Methods of Hormone Radioimmunoassay.* New York: Academic, 1979. P. 675.

26. Harman, S. M., and Tsitouras, P. D. Reproductive hormones in aging men: I. Measurement of sex steroids, basal luteinizing hormone, and Leydig cell response to human chorionic gonadotropin. *J. Clin. Endocrinol. Metab.* 51:35, 1978.

27. Hellman, L., and Bradlow, H. L. Recent advances in human steroid metabolism. *Adv. Clin. Chem.* 13:1, 1970.

28. Herman, A., Adar, R., and Rubinstein, Z. Vascular lesions associated with impotence in diabetic and nondiabetic occlusive disease. *Diabetes* 27:975, 1978.

29. Holdsworth, S., Atkins, R. C., and DeKretser, D. M. The pituitary-testicular axis in men with chronic renal failure. *N. Engl. J. Med.* 296:1245, 1977.

30. Horowitz, J. D., and Goble, A. J. Drugs and impaired male sexual function. *Drugs* 18:206, 1979.

31. Hosking, D. J., Bennett, T., and Hampton, J. R. Diabetic autonomic neuropathy. *Diabetes* 27:1043, 1978.

32. Hsueh, W. A., Hsu, T. H., and Federman, D. D. Endocrine features of Klinefelter's syndrome. *Medicine* 57:447, 1978.

33. Jacobs, L. S. Prolactin. In B. M. Jaffe and H. R. Behrman (eds.), *Methods of Hormone Radioimmunoassay.* New York: Academic, 1979. P. 199.

34. Karacan, I. Diagnosis of erectile impotence in diabetic men: An objective and specific method. *Ann. Intern. Med.* 92:334, 1980.

35. Kempczinski, R. F. Role of the vascular diagnostic laboratory in the evaluation of male impotence. *Am. J. Surg.* 138:278, 1979.

36. Kidd, G. S., Glass, A. R., and Vigersky, R. A. The hypothalamic-pituitary-testicular axis in thyrotoxicosis. *J. Clin. Endocrinol. Metab.* 48:798, 1979.

37. Kirschner, M. A., Jacobs, J. B., and Fraley, E. E. Bilateral anorchia with persistent testosterone production. *N. Engl. J. Med.* 282:240, 1970.

38. Kleinberg, D. L., Noel, G. L., and Frantz, A. G. Chlorpromazine stimulation and L-dopa suppression of plasma prolactin in man. *J. Clin. Endocrinol.* 33:873, 1971.

39. Kolodny, R. C., et al. Sexual function in diabetic men. *Diabetes* 23:306, 1974.

40. Kovacs, K., et al. Pituitary adenomas associated with elevated blood follicle stimulating hormone levels: Histologic, immunologic, and electron microscopic study of two cases. *Fertil. Steril.* 29:622, 1978.

41. Labady, F. Treatment of testicular hypofunction with gonadotropic hormones. *Int. Urol. Nephrol.* 10:125, 1978.

42. Lambert, J. W. J., Birkenhager, J. C., and Kwu, H. G. Basal and TRH-stimulated prolactin in patients with pituitary tumors. *Clin. Endocrinol. (Oxf.)* 5:709, 1976.

43. Lashbaugh, C. C., and Casarett, G. W. The effects of gonadal irradiation in clinical radiation therapy: A review. *Cancer* 37:1111, 1976.

44. Lipsett, M. B., et al. Physiologic basis of disorders of androgen metabolism. *Ann. Intern. Med.* 68:1327, 1968.

45. Longcope, C. The effect of human chorionic gonadotropin on plasma steroid levels in young and old men. *Steroids* 21:583, 1973.

46. Marad, F., and Gilman, A. G. Androgens and Anabolic Steroids. In A. G. Gilman, L. S. Goodman, and A. Gilman (eds.), *The Pharmacological Basis of Therapeutics* (6th ed.). New York: Macmillian, 1975, P. 1448.

47. Masters, W. H., and Johnson, V. E. *Human Sexual Inadequacy.* Boston: Little, Brown, 1970.

48. Matthews, W. D., and Rundle, A. T. Familial cerebellar ataxia and hypogonadism. *Brain* 87:463, 1964.

49. McCullagh, E. P. Climacteric: Male and female. *Cleve. Clin. Q.* 13:166, 1946.

50. Mortimer, R. H., et al. Correlation between integrated LH and FSH levels and the response to luteinizing hormone releasing factor (LRF). *J. Clin. Endocrinol. Metab.* 43:1248, 1976.

51. Moudgal, W. R., Muralidhar, K., and Madhwa Raj, H. G. Pituitary gonadotropins. In B. M. Jaffe and H. R. Behrman (eds.), *Methods of Radioimmunoassay.* New York: Academic, 1979. P. 173.

52. Nagalesparen, M., Ang, V., and Jenkins, J. S. Bromocryptine treatment of males with pituitary tumors, hyperprolactinemia, and hypogonadism. *Clin. Endocrinol. (Oxf.)* 9:73, 1978.

53. Onishi, T., et al. Primary hypothyroidism and galactorrhea. *Am. J. Med.* 63:373, 1977.

54. Paulsen, C. A. The Testes. In R. H. Williams (ed.), *Textbook of Endocrinology.* Philadelphia: Saunders, 1974. P. 323.

55. Pirart, J. Diabetes mellitus and its vascular complications: A prospective study of 4400 patients observed between 1947 and 1973. *Diabetes Care* 1:168, 1978.

56. Pirke, K. M., and Doerr, P. Age related changes in free plasma testosterone, dihydrotestosterone, and oestradiol. *Acta Endocrinol.* 80:171, 1975.

57. Rebar, R., et al. Gonadotropin responses to synthetic LRF: Dose-response relationships in men. *J. Clin. Endocrinol. Metab.* 36:10, 1973.

58. Reinfrank, R. F., and Nichols, F. L. Hypogonadotrophic hypogonadism in the Laurence-Moon syndrome. *J. Clin. Endocrinol. Metab.* 24:48, 1964.

59. Rosen, S. W., Gann, D., and Rogol, A. D. Congenital anosmia: Detection threshholds for seven odorant classes in hypogonadal and eugonadal patients. *Ann. Otol. Rhinol. Laryngol.* 88:288, 1979.

60. Santen, R. J., et al. Short and long term effects of clomiphene citrate on the pituitary-testicular axis. *J. Clin. Endocrinol. Metab.* 33:970, 1971.

61. Sasano, N., and Ichijo, S. Vascular patterns of the human testis with special reference to its senile changes. *Tohoku J. Exp. Med.* 99:269, 1969.

62. Seabright, M. A rapid banding technique for human chromosomes. *Lancet* 2:971, 1971.

63. Shahwan, M. M., et al. Differences in pituitary and testicular function between diabetic patients on insulin and oral antidiabetic agents. *Diabetologia* 15:13, 1978.

64. Sievertsen, G. D., et al. Metabolic clearance and secretion rates of human prolactin in normal subjects and in patients with chronic renal failure. *J. Clin. Endrocrinol. Metab.* 50:846, 1980.

65. Smith, S. R. The pituitary-gonadal axis in men with protein calorie malnutrition. *J. Clin. Endocrinol. Metab.* 41:60, 1975.

66. Spark, R. F., White, R. A., and Connolly, M. S. Impotence is not always psychogenic. *J.A.M.A.* 243:750, 1980.

67. Steinberger, E. Management of male reproductive dysfunction. *Clin. Obstet. Gynecol.* 22:187, 1979.

68. Steinberger, E. Disorders of Testicular Function (Male Hypogonadism). In L. DeGroot (ed.), *Endocrinology.* New York: Grune & Stratton, 1979. P. 1549.

69. Stewart-Bentley, M., and Horton, R. Leydig cell function in Klinefelter's syndrome. *Metabolism* 22:875, 1973.

70. Swerdloff, R. S., Kantor, G., and Korenman, S. G. Gynecomastia of hemodialysis: Consideration of pathogenesis. *J. Clin. Invest.* 49:94a, 1970.

71. Tanner, J. M., and Whitehouse, R. H. Clinical longitudinal standards for height, weight, height velocity, weight velocity, and stages of puberty. *Arch. Dis. Child.* 51:170, 1976.

72. Thomas, F. B., Mazzaferri, E. L., and Skillman, T. G. Apathetic thyrotoxicosis: A clinical and laboratory entity. *Ann. Intern. Med.* 72:679, 1970.

73. Thorner, M. O. Prolactin: Clinical Physiology and the Significance and Management of Hyperprolactinemia. In L. Martin and G. Besser (eds.), *Clinical Neuroendocrinology.* New York: Academic, 1977. P. 320.

74. Thorner, M. O., et al. Prolactin and Gonadotropin Interaction in the Male. In P. Troen and H. R. Nankin (eds.), *The Testis in Normal and Infertile Men.* New York: Raven, 1977, P. 351.

75. Vermeulen, A., Stoica, T., and Verdonck, L. The apparent free testosterone concentration: An index of androgenicity. *J. Clin. Endocrinol. Metab.* 33:759, 1971.

76. Zellweger, H., and Schneider, H. J. Syndrome of hypotonia-hypomentia-hypogonadism-obesity (HHHO) or Prader-Willi syndrome. *Am. J. Dis. Child.* 115:588, 1968.

7

Impotence in Diabetes Mellitus

IRWIN GOLDSTEIN
MIKE B. SIROKY
ROBERT J. KRANE

Diabetes mellitus may be considered as a genetically and clinically heterogeneous group of disorders that share glucose intolerance as a common feature [54]. Historically, prior to the use of insulin, diabetic patients often had impaired potency [62, 64, 76]. Unfortunately, despite the discovery of insulin, this complication has persisted [12, 16, 30, 37, 41, 65, 68]—so much so that in diabetic men impotence is more common than either retinopathy or nephropathy [38]. By current estimates [80], roughly half of male diabetics, or approximately 2.0 to 2.5 million diabetic American men, complain of sexual dysfunction.

There is a clear clinical need to understand the relationship between diabetes and sexual dysfunction, but there is an equal need to identify the pathogenesis of the erectile dysfunction [45]. Without such information, it is not possible to prevent this complication.

In the past, sexual disorders in the disease have been evaluated by history taking alone. Recently, however, objective erectile function testing has been applied [33]. Several areas of controversy now exist on the subject of sexual dysfunction in the diabetic:

1. What is the pathophysiology of erectile dysfunction in diabetes?
2. Why is it that most complications in diabetes, i.e., microangiopathy, retinopathy, and neuropathy, are related to both the severity and increased duration of the diabetes, whereas impotence "apparently" is not [12, 30, 65]?
3. Why has the incidence of impotence not decreased despite improvement in the treatment of diabetes?
4. Why does the incidence of impotence increase with increasing age?
5. Is impotence in diabetes a specific complication of the disease or is it related to the general condition of "having a chronic disease" and not "feeling completely well"?

In this chapter, the mechanisms involved in these controversial areas will be addressed on the basis of previous series and our own review of 71 impotent diabetic patients (Table 7-1).

Table 7-1. Survey of 71 impotent diabetic men

Average age (years)	52 (range 25–67)
Average duration of diabetes (years)	11 (range 1–30)
Insulin-independent	48%
Diet treatment	34%
Oral hypoglycemic	14%
Insulin-dependent	52%
Average duration of impotence (years)	4.3 (range 1 month to 25 years)
Smoking	63%
Hypertension	57%
Absent morning erections	45%
Claudication symptoms	39%
Loses erections with coital movement	40%
Libido preserved	67%

PATHOPHYSIOLOGY

Penile erection depends on a complex interaction of psychologic and physiologic factors. An intact autonomic and somatic nervous system, adequate penile arterial flow with adjusted venous outflow, and a functioning hypothalamic-pituitary-gonadal hormonal axis all contribute to the physiologic process of erection [70]. Impairments in one or more of these factors in diabetes may result in organic impotence. Psychologic factors may be primary or secondary to an organic dysfunction [13, 47, 67, 69]. Evaluation of impotent patients with diabetes must take into account all of the above considerations.

ARTERIAL VASCULAR IMPOTENCE

Recent studies on the physiology of erection have demonstrated that full erection requires a marked increase in both resting penile blood flow and intracorporeal pressure. A spectrum of partial erections therefore results when the arterial bed of the penis is unable to deliver the necessary changes in resting penile blood flow sufficient to generate appropriate intracorporeal pressures [56–59].

Vascular disease in diabetic patients has long been recognized as a major contributor to the morbidity and mortality of diabetes [1, 26, 35, 66]. Historically, small vessel changes in diabetics were reported 4 years after the invention of the opthalmoscope (1851) [29]. The diabetic microangiopathy has received wide research attention, and, although the exact mechanisms for microvascular changes remain unresolved, several alterations in the microvascular physiology have been identified. In sequential development, one can observe in the microcirculation increased local blood flow [25], progressive venule dilation (greater than that required to carry the increased blood flow [10]), periodic arteriole vasoconstriction [7], and eventual sclerosis of the walls of arterioles, capillaries, and venules [2, 10, 22]. In time, the alteration and decompensation of local microvascular blood flow become irreversible. Endothelial cell metabolism and function, thickened vessel wall basement membrane, and such additional microvascular factors as oxygen transport, blood flow properties, and hemostasis have all been documented as altered in diabetic microangiopathy [53].

Similarly, large-vessel disease is strongly associated with diabetes mellitus. Intimal, medial, and luminal changes observed in obliterative atherosclerosis have been well described [73, 82].

In impotent male diabetics, vascular lesions have been found by autopsy series [66], aortography [26], and phalloarteriography [58, 60]. In Ruzbarsky and Michal's [66] series of 15 diabetic men, postmortem examination revealed numerous penile arterial vascular abnormalities, including fibrous proliferation of the intima, medial fibrosis, calcification, and narrowing and obliteration of the lumen. Those authors concluded that these vascular alterations in the penile arteries necessarily impeded blood flow to the cavernous bodies at the time of erection and were thus responsible for the erectile impairment. Michal [56] and others [42, 50] also have identified large-vessel vascular lesions by arteriography.

Noninvasive vascular testing in impotent diabetic patients has been performed in numerous series [1, 20, 33, 35]. The incidence of suspected vascular pathology has varied from 33 percent to 87 percent.

In our own series of 71 impotent diabetics, penile blood flow was assessed by Doppler

Table 7-2. Doppler testing in 67 diabetic patients

Total patients	Resting Doppler only (n = 14)	Pelvic steal testing (n = 53)
Abnormal studies	3	42
Abnormal resting Dopplers	3(21%)	12(22%)
Abnormal fall in index with exercise		20(38%)
Abnormal exercise Doppler index		10(19%)

determination in 67 (94%) [24]. Overall, vasculogenic impotence was strongly suspected in 67 percent of the patients (see Table 7-2). It is our feeling that vascular abnormalities play a major role in the pathogenesis of impotence in diabetes mellitus. Presumably, high association of vascular risk factors, a tendency toward atherosclerosis, and diabetic microangiopathy all contribute to high impedance of blood flow in the arterial bed of the penis.

NEUROLOGIC IMPOTENCE
Multiple levels of the nervous system are thought to play a role in male sexual function; at the peripheral level there are the pudendal nerve, the pelvic parasympathetic nerves, and the thoracolumbar sympathetic nerves. Stimulation of the parasympathetic fibers (S2–S4) results in shunting of arterial blood into trabecular spaces within the corpora cavernosa. The final pathway of this corporal vasomotor control may be through postganglionic neurons that release a noncholinergic neurotransmitter [70]. The pudendal nerves (S2–S4) supply sensation from the penile skin and motor innervation to the bulbocavernosus, ischiocavernosus, and external urethral sphincter muscles. The thoracolumbar sympathetic nerves supply the vas deferens, seminal vesicles, posterior urethra, and penile vasculature; their stimulation results in contraction of the posterior urethra and seminal emission. It appears that the thoracolumbar nerves do not play a major role in generating erectile activity [39].

Diabetic autonomic and/or somatic neuropathy afflicts approximately 50 percent (or 4–5 million) of diabetic patients in the United States [80]. The autonomic neuropathy tends to involve multiple visceral structures and to produce not only impotence but also postural hypotension and bowel and bladder symptoms [3,11,14]. The somatic neuropathy is primarily a symmetric sensory polyneuropathy associated with loss of lower extremity deep tendon reflexes [53]. Neurophysiologic studies on autonomic unmyelinated diseased nerve fibers have been few [52]. In contrast, diseased myelinated fibers characteristic of somatic neuropathies have been evaluated in detail [80]. Neurophysiologic studies in these latter nerves have demonstrated decreased nerve conduction velocity and altered temporal patterns of impulse transmission. The net effect of these conduction aberrations is neuronal asynchrony within the central nervous system [80]. It appears that damage to somatic nerve fibers in diabetic neuropathy is a result of segmental demyelination secondary to Schwann cell degeneration [74]. The pathophysiology (that is, whether it is a metabolic or vascular phenomenon) remains controversial [53].

Nerve damage in impotent diabetic males has been documented by autopsy series [16], corpus cavernosal biopsy [54, 55], cystometrography [12, 13], perineal electromyography [75], and sacral latency (bulbocavernosus reflex latency) testing [33, 75]. In Faerman's [16] series of five impotent diabetic men, postmortem analysis of corpus cavernosal tissue revealed morphologic alterations of nerve fibers not present in potent, nondiabetic patients. Melman [54, 55], however, demonstrated intact nerve fibers in corpus cavernosal biopsies of 16 impotent diabetic men, but they had reduced content of neurotransmitters (norepinephrine) as compared to nondiabetic patients.

Ellenberg [12] performed cystometrography on 45 impotent diabetic males and found detrusor areflexia in approximately 75 percent. He concluded that, since the parasympathetic nerves concerned with potency and micturition were identical, a significant neuropathic factor existed in diabetic impotence. While this may in fact be true, it has been shown clearly that detrusor areflexia can occur without any neurologic lesion [40]. Furthermore, parasympathetic denervation could have been more directly demonstrated with bethanechol supersensitivity testing [41], which was not performed.

Vacek [75], Karacan [33], and others have performed sacral latency testing in impotent diabetic patients. Abnormal values usually indicative of pudendal sensory diabetic polyneuropathy were identified in 60 [33] and 85 percent [75] of patients studied.

In our series, neurologic evaluation was assessed by perineal electromyography and sacral latency testing (53 patients, 72%). In our patient population, clinical symptoms of *neurologic* detrusor areflexia such as urinary retention, urinary incontinence, and abdominal straining were not commonly observed. Abnormally prolonged sacral latency studies were identified in 16 of 53 patients (30%). In all these patients, perineal electromyography (EMG) demonstrated characteristics of peripheral denervation, i.e., neuropathic potentials and a decreased interference pattern. Another five patients had an abnormal perineal EMG, but subsequent sacral latency values were within normal limits. It is not known whether these patients had sufficient nerve injury to account for neurologically induced impotence. Neurologic impotence was suspected in our series in 30 percent of the impotent diabetic men. Although this is a significant organic factor in the genesis of erectile dysfunction, it apparently is not as common as abnormal arterial vasculogenic factors. This may, however, be related to the method of neurologic testing, which does not directly evaluate the integrity of the penile parasympathetic nerves.

ENDOCRINE CAUSES

Although erection may be considered as a neurologic reflex resulting in major penile hemodynamic alterations, the role of hormones in this process cannot be ignored. The particular hormonal system thought to play the most significant role in the sexual act is the hypothalamic-pituitary-gonadal axis. Clinically, disturbances within this hormonal system have resulted in abnormal sexual function [17, 18, 46, 72]. Furthermore, in numerous cases, correcting the disturbance has resulted in reversal of the erectile dysfunction [46, 72].

The exact role of testosterone or other gonadal steroids in the generation of normal erectile function, however, has not yet been established.

In impotent diabetics, studies in the 1940s, 1950s, and the early 1960s demonstrated a possible endocrine etiology. Reports based on the urinary excretion of both pituitary gonadotropin and 17-ketosteroids as well as on testis biopsies appeared to indicate hypogonadotropic hypogonadism as a leading cause of diabetic impotence [4, 27, 60, 68]. Since the advent of radioimmunoassay analyses, no endocrine abnormalities have been detected in impotent diabetic patients. No significant difference in LH, FSH, prolactin, testosterone, and estradiol values were found between impotent patients and potent nondiabetic controls [16, 30, 33, 37, 81]. The search for an endocrine abnormality, however, continues. A recent report [21] demonstrates a significantly increased testosterone-binding capacity and a significantly lower plasma testosterone after a 3-day stimulization with human chorionic gonadotropin in impotent diabetic patients compared to nondiabetic potent controls. The significance of this, however, remains unclear.

In our series, endocrine evaluation was performed by measuring levels of serum testosterone (mean value: 409.9 ng/dl ± 199), serum luteinizing hormone (mean value: 9.8 m/u/ml ± 5.9), and serum prolactin (mean value: 8.7 ng/ml ± 4.5). The mean values in all impotent diabetic patients were not significantly different from those in nondiabetic controls.

Seven patients had elevated estradiol and decreased testosterone-estradiol ratios. The significance of these findings remains unclear. In summary, endocrine impotence does not appear to play a major role in the overall pathogenesis of diabetic impotence. It is still recommended, however, that endocrine screening be done in impotent patients, because a recognized hormonal dysfunction may be amenable to medical treatment.

PSYCHOGENIC CAUSES

Any organic dysfunction related to a genital organ is almost inevitably accompanied by a psychologic response to that dysfunction [32, 47, 67, 79]. This is of special significance in diabetic men who are often "waiting their turn" for complications of the diabetes to be unveiled [68]. Thus, in diabetic men in whom organic factors may take years to develop—if they do at all—psychologic factors may play a more prominent role in a primary sense [63, 67, 79].

The psychologic response to a sexual dysfunction is usually influenced by such factors as personality, cultural and social upbringing, sexual experiences, skills, and information, and the patient's reaction to the sexual abnormality [67].

That this psychologic response is able to inhibit erectile capacity and sexual activity is well documented in the literature. Numerous case reports demonstrating obsessive concern over performance, affective depression, fear of rejection, failure, and abandonment, and feelings of anger, hostility, and shame all noted impotence reversal after appropriate psychologic treatment [47, 63, 79]. The exact mechanisms of how psychologic factors promote erectile dysfunction is, however, not yet known [31].

Much is written of the typical history of the man whose impotence is primarily psychologic. His onset of erectile dysfunction is abrupt, commonly situational, and associated with stress, anger, or depression. It also appears not to impair masturbation or morning erections [67]. In our series, this "classic" individual has not been commonplace. Patients with documented *organic disease* also can have a relatively abrupt onset of impotence and can have morning erections [24]. Patients with primary psychologic disease can, on the other hand, have slow-onset progressive impotence, not situational and

impairing masturbation [63, 67].

In performing erectile function testing, one does not intend to establish a diagnosis of either absolutely organic or absolutely psychologic impotence. Instead, attention is focused on the relative contribution of organic factors that are thought to exist in the sexual dysfunction. It is assumed that, in most cases, some psychologic contribution already exists in the dysfunction. Erectile function testing is used to clarify the objective contributions of organic abnormalities.

In our series, 40 percent of the 71 diabetic patients underwent psychologic assessment by direct interview. Sufficient psychologic factors to produce impotence were thought to exist in 55 percent of these cases. Additional organic factors coexisted in 90 percent of these cases (72% vascular, 9% vascular-endocrine, 9% neurologic).

DURATION OF DIABETES

It has long been recorded that the incidence of impotence does not *appear* to increase with increasing duration of diabetes. Rubin [65] reported that the incidence of impotence in diabetes of less than 1 year's, of between 1 to 5 years', and of more than 5 years' duration was 70, 43, and 45 percent, respectively. Ellenberg [12] showed similar results in that the incidence of impotence in diabetes of 0 to 5 years', 5 to 10 years', and 10 to 15 years' duration was 60, 60, and 58 percent, respectively.

Several explanations have been proposed for this observation, e.g., the frequent occurrence of psychologic factors (anxiety, distress, etc.) early after the initial diagnosis of diabetes [67].

In many series, organic factors have played a prominent role in the pathogenesis of diabetic impotence [33–35, 37]. Since diabetic microangiopathies and neuropathies often take 10 to 20 years to manifest [6], why is not the duration of diabetes more significant? A possible explanation is that organic factors can occur in a relatively short time frame. Healthy, genetically nondiabetic kidneys, for example, when transplanted into diabetics

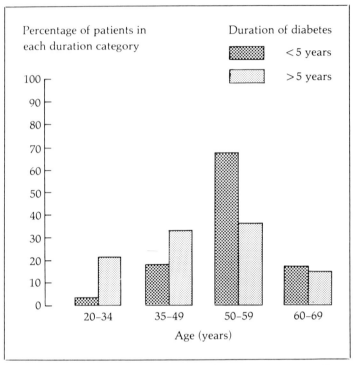

Figure 7-1. Percentage of impotent patients of less than 5 years' and more than 5 years' duration of diabetes in four age cohorts.

with renal failure can show characteristic renovascular lesions in as little as 2 to 3 years [49].

Ruben [65] commented that most of the patients who both were impotent and had diabetes for less than 1 year were over age 50, and he found a 54 percent incidence of impotence in the group between 50 and 54 years of age. He therefore concluded that the high incidence of impotence in diabetics with a short duration of diabetes was possibly due to the inclusion of older patients, who had a high likelihood of being impotent.

McCullough [51] further tested this hypothesis and separated out age-group cohorts when he compared duration of diabetes to the incidence of impotence. In this manner, he did find an increasing prevalence of impotence with increasing duration of diabetes.

In our series, the average duration of diabetes was 11 years (range 1–30 years). Since our patients were all impotent, we could not assess an incidence of impotence with any factors such as increasing duration of diabetes. We did, however, note the observations of Rubin and McCullough. There were several men who had diabetes of less than 5 years' duration who were more than 50 years old. These patients tended to have significant hypertension and smoking histories and a high incidence of vasculogenic impotence. The inclusion of these patients in a large series of diabetics might lead to erroneous conclusions concerning the incidence of impotence and the duration of diabetes (Fig. 7-1).

In summary, when age is accounted for, there does appear to be a greater risk of developing impotence with increasing duration of diabetes [51, 66]. This observation supports the contention that, since organic disease worsens with increasing duration of the disease, organic disease plays an important role in the pathogenesis of diabetic impotence.

INCIDENCE

In the preinsulin era, Von Noorden [76] and Naunyn [62] noted the high frequency with which diabetic males became impotent. After

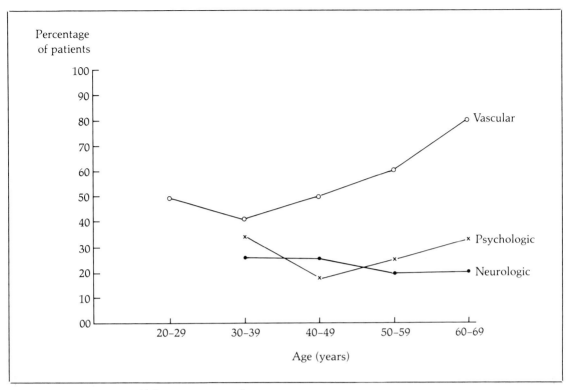

Figure 7-2. Positive erectile function tests in five age groups.

the discovery of insulin by Banting and Best in 1922, it was generally assumed that sexual disorders would become less common. A review of a large number of diabetic patients in 1958 [65] revealed a 55 percent incidence of impotence. Since then, in various series in several countries, the incidence has been reported as 51 percent [63] in 1963, 59 percent [12] in 1971, 43 percent [30] in 1979, and 35 [51] and 23 percent [43] in 1980.

It is possible that with better management of the diabetic patient in terms of more rigid control of the plasma glucose, the incidence of impotence will fall. The controversy over whether strict control of plasma glucose prevents or delays diabetic complications remains unresolved [6]. Retinopathy, neuropathy, and nephropathy often progress despite apparently satisfactory management of plasma glucose [69]. Until the mechanisms of diabetic microangiopathy and neuropathy are more completely understood, the proper application of present-day management or future management to control the long-term complications of diabetes (including impotence) will remain unsolved.

AGING

Kinsey [36], Masters and Johnson [48], and others have demonstrated a higher incidence of impotence with progressive aging in a nondiabetic population. In these epidemiologic studies, the incidence of impotence apparently rose exponentially with age, usually progressing after age 50.

Several surveys of large numbers of diabetic patients have noted a similar phenomenon, except that the increased incidence of impotence with age in diabetics is more accentuated than that for the corresponding normal nondiabetic population [16, 51, 65]. These series have shown that impotence appears to rise exponentially at age 40. In Rubin's series [65], the incidence of impotence at age 45 was 13 percent, whereas in McCullough's series [51], it was 28 percent.

This is compared to Kinsey [36], who found a 3 percent incidence of impotence.

In Ruzbarsky and Michal's [66] autopsy series of 15 diabetic males, they noted pathologic penile arterial changes that worsened with increasing age. They compared the changes in diabetic patients to those in men without diabetes and concluded that the pathologic findings in both groups were qualitatively the same but that the penile vessels in diabetics showed accelerated progression at the same age. They summarized by stating that diabetes mellitus "appeared" to accelerate the aging process in the penile vasculature.

In contrast, Faerman [15] performed an autopsy series, analyzing the autonomic nerve fibers by light microscopy. He found the same morphologic abnormalities in the nerve fibers of patients of ages 19 and 26 as he did in patients of ages 51, 65, and 67. No increased abnormality with aging was identified.

In our series, there was a marked increase in vasculogenic impotence with increasing age (42% under age 50; 67% above age 50) (Fig. 7-2). Risk factors such as hypertension, smoking, claudication, and losing erections with coital movement all were more frequent with increasing age.

Neither psychologic nor neurologic impotence increased with age (23% under 50 years, 27% over 50 years, 27% under 50 years, and 20% over 50 years, respectively) (see Fig. 7-2).

In summary, it appears that diabetic vascular aberrations account for the dramatic increase in incidence of impotence with increasing age.

CONCLUSIONS

Impotence is a relatively common complication of diabetes mellitus. Numerous organic and psychologic factors in diabetes interact to create this erectile dysfunction. To help identify the contribution of each organic component to the genesis of the impotence, objective erectile function testing has been most useful.

In our series, it was discovered that vascular, neurologic, and psychologic abnormalities could be identified in 79, 30, and 55 percent of cases studied.

The major cause of diabetic impotence appeared to be vascular disease. Neurologic impotence as evaluated by perineal electromyography and sacral latency testing appeared to be the second major organic cause. There appeared to be an increased incidence of diabetic impotence with increasing age and was best explained by progressive involvement with vascular disease. Finally, the incidence of impotence in diabetes does appear to increase with increasing duration of the disorder.

REFERENCES

1. Abelson, D. Diagnostic value of the penile pulse and blood pressure: A Doppler study of impotence in diabetics. *J. Urol.* 113:636, 1975.
2. Ashton, N. Vascular changes in diabetics with particular reference to the retinal vessels: Preliminary report. *Br. J. Opthalmol.* 33:407, 1949.
3. Bennett, T., Evans, D. F., and Hosking, D. J. Physiological investigation of male diabetics complaining of impotence. *J. Physiol.* 272:190, 1977.
4. Bergquist, N. The gonadal function in male diabetics. *Acta Endocrinol. [Suppl.] (Copenh.)* 18:3, 1954.
5. Bradley, W. E. Introduction and workshop summary. *Ann. Intern. Med.* 92:293, 1980.
6. Bressler, R. Should you control glucose in the older diabetic? *Geriatrics* 34:41, 1979.
7. Chazan, B. I., et al. Capillaries of the nailfold of the toe in diabetes mellitus. *Microvasc. Res.* 2:504, 1970.
8. Cooper, A. J., et al. Androgen function in "psychogenic" and "constitutional" types of impotence. *Br. Med. J.* 3:17, 1970.
9. Deutsch, H., and Sherman, L. Previously recognized diabetes mellitus in sexually impotent men. *J.A.M.A.* 244:2430, 1980.
10. Ditzel, J. Functional microangiopathy in diabetes mellitus. *Diabetes* 17:388, 1968.
11. Duchen, L. W., et al. Pathology of autonomic neuropathy in diabetes mellitus. *Ann. Intern. Med.* 92:301, 1980.
12. Ellenberg, M. Impotence in diabetes: The neurologic factor. *Ann. Intern. Med.* 75:213, 1971.
13. Ellenberg, M. Sexual function in diabetic patients. *Ann. Intern. Med.* 92:331, 1980.
14. Ewing, D. J., Campbell, I. W., and Clark, B. F. Mortality in diabetic autonomic neuropathy. *Lancet* 1:601, 1976.
15. Faerman, I., et al. Impotence and diabetes: Histological studies of the autonomic nervous

fibers of the corpora cavernosa in impotent diabetic males. *Diabetes* 23:971, 1974.

16. Faerman, I., et al. Impotence and diabetes: Studies of androgenic function in diabetic impotent males. *Diabetes* 21:23, 1972.
17. Franklin, S., Jacobs, S. H., and Martin, N. Hyperprolactinemia and impotence. *Clin. Endocrinol.* 8:277, 1978.
18. Franks, S., Nabarro, J. D. N., and Jacobs, H. S. Prevalence and presentation of hyperprolactinemia in patients with "functionless" pituitary tumors. *Lancet* 1:778, 1977.
19. Furlow, W. L. Diagnosis and treatment of male erectile failure. *Diabetes Care* 2:18, 1979.
20. Gaskell, O. The importance of penile blood pressure in cases of impotence. *Can. Med. Assoc. J.* 105:1047, 1971.
21. Geisthövel, V. N., et al. Androgenstatus bei Männlichen Diabetikern. *Med. Klin.* 70:1417, 1975.
22. Gibson, G. G., and Smith, L. W. Retinal phlebosclerosis. *Arch. Opthalmol.* 26:840, 1941.
23. Glassman, C. N., Rife, C. C., and Wilson, C. B. Prolactin-added dimension in male genitosexual disorders. *Urology* 15:49, 1980.
24. Goldstein, I., et al. Vasculogenic impotence: Role of the pelvic steal test. *J. Urol.* 128:300, 1982.
25. Haggendale, E., Steen, B., and Suanborg, A. Blood flow in subcutaneous fat tissue in patients with diabetes mellitus. *Acta Med. Scand.* 187:49, 1970.
26. Herman, A., Adar, R., and Rubinstein, Z. Vascular lesions associated with impotence in diabetic and nondiabetic arterial occlusive diabetes. *Diabetes* 27:975, 1978.
27. Horstmann, P. The excretion of androgens in human diabetes mellitus. *Acta Endocrinol.* 5:261, 1950.
28. Hosking, D. J., et al. Diabetic impotence: Studies of nocturnal erection during REM sleep. *Br. Med. J.* 2:1394, 1979.
29. Jäger, E. Beiträge zur Pathologie des Auges. Vienna, 1855.
30. Jensen, S. B., et al. Sexual function and pituitary access in insulin-treated diabetic men. *Acta Med. Scand. [Suppl.]* 624:65, 1979.
31. Johnson, J. Sexual impotence and the limbic system. *Br. J. Psychiatry* 111:300, 1965.
32. Kaplan, H. S. *The New Sex Therapy.* New York: Brunner & Masel, 1974.
33. Karacan, I. Diagnosis of erectile impotence in diabetes mellitus: An objective and specific method. *Ann. Intern. Med.* 92:334, 1980.
34. Karacan, I., et al. Nocturnal erections, differential diagnosis of impotence and diabetes. *Biol. Psychiatry* 12:373, 1977.
35. Karacan, I., et al. Impotence and blood pressure in the flaccid penis: Relationship to nocturnal penile tumescence. *Sleep* 1:125, 1978.
36. Kinsey, A. C., Pomeroy, W. B., and Martin, C. E. *Sexual Behavior in the Human Male.* Philadelphia: Saunders, 1948.
37. Kolodny, R. C., et al. Sexual dysfunction in diabetic men. *Diabetes* 23:306, 1974.
38. Koncz, L., and Balodimos, M. C. Impotence in diabetes mellitus. *Med. Times* 98:159, 1970.
39. Krane, R. J., and Siroky, M. B. Neurophysiology of erection: Symposium on male sexual dysfunction. *Urol. Clin. North Am.* 8:91, 1981.
40. Krane, R. J., and Siroky, M. B. Psychogenic Voiding Dysfunction. In R. J. Krane and M. B. Siroky (eds.), *Clinical Neuro-Urology.* Boston: Little, Brown, 1979.
41. Lapides, J., et al. Denervation supersensitivity as a test for neurogenic bladder. *Surg. Gynecol. Obstet.* 114:241, 1962.
42. Leriche, R., and Morel, A. The syndrome of thrombotic obliteration of the aortic bifurcation. *Ann. Surg.* 127:193, 1948.
43. Lester, E., Grant, A. J., and Woodroffe, F. J. Impotence in diabetic and nondiabetic hospital out-patients. *Br. Med. J.* 281:354, 1980.
44. Levine, S. B. Marital sexual dysfunction: Erectile dysfunction. *Ann. Intern. Med.* 85:342, 1976.
45. Levine, S. B. Sexual dysfunction and diabetes, behavior and psychosocial issues in diabetes. *NIH Pub.* 80:183, 1980.
46. Lundberg, P. O., and Wide, L. Sexual function in males with pituitary tumors. *Fertil. Steril.* 29:175, 1978.
47. Martin, L. M. Impotence in diabetes: An overview. *Psychosomatics* 22:318, 1981.
48. Masters, W. H., and Johnson, V. E. *Human Sexual Inadequacy.* Boston: Little, Brown, 1970.
49. Mauer, S. M., Barbosa, J., and Vernier, R. L. Development of diabetic vascular lesions in normal kidneys transplanted into patients with diabetes mellitus. *N. Engl. J. Med.* 295:916, 1976.
50. May, A. G., DeWeese, J. A., and Rob, C. G. Changes in sexual function following operation on the abdominal aorta. *Surgery* 65:41, 1969.
51. McCulloch, D. K., et al. The prevalence of diabetic impotence. *Diabetologia* 18:279, 1980.
52. McDonald, W. I. The effects of experimental demyelination on conduction in peripheral nerve: A histological and electrophysiological study. II. Electrophysiological observations. *Brain* 86:501, 1963.
53. McMillian, D. E. Deterioration of the microcirculation in diabetes. *Diabetes* 24:944, 1975.
54. Melman, A., et al. Alteration of the penile corpora in patients with erectile impotence. *Invest. Urol.* 17:474, 1980.
55. Melman, A., et al. Effect of diabetes upon penile sympathetic nerves in impotent patients. *South. Med. J.* 73:307, 1980.

56. Michal, V., Kramer, R., and Pospichal, J. Femaropudendal bypass, internal iliac thromboendarterectomy and direct arterial anastomosis to the cavernosus body in the treatment of erectile impotence. *Bull. Soc. Int. Chir.* 33:343, 1974.

57. Michal, V., et al. Arterial epigastricocavernosus anastomosis for the treatment of sexual impotence. *World J. Surg.* 1:515, 1977.

58. Michal, V., and Pospichal, J. Phalloarteriography in the diagnosis of erectile impotence. *World J. Surg.* 2:239, 1978.

59. Michal, V., et al. Vascular surgery in the treatment of impotence: Its present possibilities and prospects. *Czech. Med.* 3:213, 1980.

60. Miller, S., and Mason, H. L. The excretion of 17-ketosteroids by diabetics. *J. Clin. Endocrinol.* 5:220, 1945.

61. National Diabetes Data Group. Classification and diagnosis of diabetes mellitus and other categories of glucose intolerance. *Diabetes* 28:1039, 1979.

62. Naunyn, B. *Der Diabetes Mellitus.* Vienna: Alfred Holder, 1906.

63. Renshaw, D. C. Impotence in diabetics. *Dis. Nerv. Syst.* 36:369, 1975.

64. Rollo, J. *An Account of Two Cases of Diabetes Mellitus: With Remarks as They Arose During the Progress of the Case.* London: C. Dilly, 1797.

65. Rubin, A., and Babbott, D. Impotence and diabetes mellitus. *J.A.M.A.* 168:498, 1958.

66. Ruzbarsky, V., and Michal, V. Morphologic changes in the arterial bed of the penis with aging: Relationship to the pathogenesis of impotence. *Invest. Urol.* 15:194, 1977.

67. Schiavi, R. C. Psychological treatment of erectile disorders in diabetic patients. *Ann. Intern. Med.* 92:337, 1980.

68. Schöffling, K., et al. Disorders of sexual function in male diabetics. *Diabetes* 12:519, 1963.

69. Siperstein, M. D., Foster, D. W., and Knowles, H. C., Jr. Control of blood glucose and diabetic vascular disease. *N. Engl. J. Med.* 296:1060, 1977.

70. Siroky, M. B., and Krane, R. J. Physiology of Male Sexual Function. In R. J. Krane and M. B. Siroky (eds.), *Clinical Neuro-Urology.* Boston: Little, Brown, 1979.

71. Sotile, W. M. The penile prosthesis and diabetic impotence: Some caveats. *Diabetes Care* 2:26, 1979.

72. Spark, R. F., White, R. A., and Connolly, P. B. Impotence is not always psychogenic: Newer insights into hypothalamic-pituitary-gonadal dysfunction. *J.A.M.A.* 243:750, 1980.

73. Stojanovic, V. K., et al. Diabetic arteriopathies. *J. Cardiovasc. Surg.* 15:51, 1974.

74. Thomas, P. K., and Lascelles, R. G. Schwann cell abnormalities in diabetes neuropathy. *Lancet* 1:1355, 1965.

75. Vacek, J., and Lachman, M. Bulbocavernosus reflex in diabetes with erectile disorders. Clinical and electromyographic study. *Cas. Lek. Cesk.* 116:1015, 1977.

76. Van Noorden, C. *Die Zuckerkrankheit und ihre Behandlung.* Berlin: August Hirschwald, 1903.

77. Wabrek, A. J. Sexual dysfunction associated with diabetes mellitus. *J. Fam. Pract.* 8:730, 1979.

78. Waller, B. F., et al. Status of the coronary arteries at necropsy in diabetes mellitus with onset after age 30 years. *Am. J. Med.* 69:498, 1980.

79. Waxberg, J. D. Sexual therapy of diabetic impotence. *Conn. Med.* 42:555, 1978.

80. Waxman, S. G. Pathophysiology of nerve conduction: Relation to diabetic neuropathy. *Ann. Intern. Med.* 92:297, 1980.

81. Wright, A. D., London, D. R., and Holden, G. Luteinizing release hormone tests in impotent diabetic males. *Diabetes* 25:975, 1976.

82. Zannini, G. Diabetic arteriopathy. *J. Cardiovasc. Surg.* 15:68, 1974.

Peyronie's Disease

MAX K. WILLSCHER

Peyronie's disease is characterized by the development of a fibrous plaque in the dorsum of the penis. Clinically, this fibrosis results in dorsal or lateral curvature of the penis that makes intercourse painful and, in many cases, prevents intromission. It is difficult to overestimate this disability. The first published report of this condition was by Peyronie, who, in 1873, described the presence of plaques in the dorsum of the penis that caused the upward bend of the organ during erection [66]. François de la Peyronie, count, physician to Louis XIV, thought that this disorder was often associated with gonorrhea or syphilis and that it was useless to treat this condition until the venereal disease was eradicated. Once the venereal disease was eradicated, he recommended that patients bathe in the Bargege Spa in the Pyrenees [3]. Because of the variable natural history of this disease as well as its uncertain etiology, various therapeutic regimens have evolved since the original description.

CLINICAL SYMPTOMS

Most cases of Peyronie's disease involve men in their fourth or fifth decade. However, patients as young as 18 and as old as 80 years have been recorded [16, 20, 22, 32, 43].

Why patients seek the advice of the physician may be reduced to three main complaints: (1) the presence of a plaque or induration within the penis, (2) penile curvature during erection, and (3) painful intercourse.

Series vary as to which symptoms are most common. Dorsal curvature of the penis is most common (80–100% of cases), whereas ventral chordee is rare [22, 39]. Pain is less common in older patients, yet several authors have reported its presence in approximately 70 percent of their cases, whereas Martin reported pain in only 11 percent of patients [17, 28, 32, 49, 72]. In Martin's series, 22 percent also had preoperative impotence [42]. Whether this is due to actual plaque invasion of the corpora cavernosa or to anxiety created by pain on penile curvature is unclear.

Plaque size may vary but it is usually 1 to 2 cm in width and 2 to 4 cm in length [8, 20].

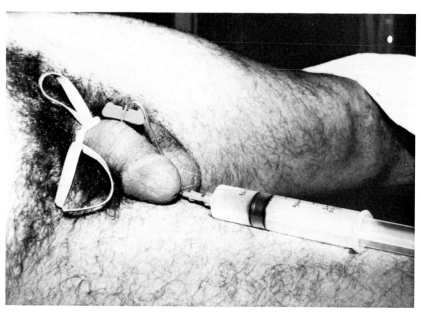

Figure 8-1. After injection of local Xylocaine anesthesia, a 21-gauge scalp needle is inserted into the corpora cavernosa. An elastic tourniquet is in place.

Most commonly, they are located in the proximal shaft, although 15 percent may involve the entire penis [28]. Only 3 percent are distal. Ventral plaques also have been described [28]. Martin found the average (estimated) penile deformity erection to be 60-degree dorsal curvature. If lateral plaques were present, an average lateral curvature of 13 percent occurred.

Peyronie's disease often has been associated with multiple other pathologic disorders including Dupuytren's contracture, fibrous degeneration of the external ear cartilage, osteoarthritis, urethritis, prostatitis, and alcoholism [28, 38, 76].

DIAGNOSIS

On physical examination, the dorsal or lateral plaque is readily palpable. The plaque is usually located between the two corpora cavernosa in the area of the dorsal vein, and it is usually discretely nodular and hard, quite unlike the rest of the normal-feeling fascial envelopes of the corpora cavernosa. The defect may be short, or it may extend dorsally between the two divisions of the corpora. X-ray films can be of help in that 20 percent of the cases have calcification [38].

Cavernosography may be a useful clinical tool in evaluating the extent of plaque. This technique has been advocated by Gittes and McLaughlin [26]. They use a 21-gauge scalp needle, which is directed into the corporal body at the base of the penis [26] (Fig. 8-1). Local lidocaine is used for anesthesia. Normal saline with added heparin is slowly injected by hand with a large syringe, until a full erection is achieved (Fig. 8-2). Usually, about 60 to 100 ml are used. Because of the communication between both corpora cavernosa, usually only one side is injected. This technique clearly defines the extent of the penile curvature (Fig. 8-3). Hamilton has found that by simultaneous injection of meglumine diatrizoate (Renografin), x rays may define the extent of the plaque [31]. The best radiographs are usually obtained after injection of about 20 ml of dye. If more than this is injected, distention is produced, and defects may be missed. The usual findings are nonopaque defects corresponding in position to the plaques. Occasionally, one finds unsuspected areas of involvement, and a common

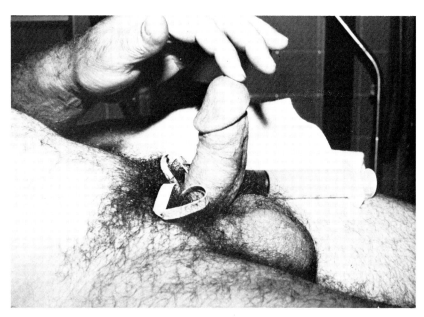

Figure 8-2. Heparinized saline is injected, and an erection simulated. This patient has only a mild deformity.

Figure 8-3. A technique similar to that in Figure 8-2 carried out at surgery. Note severe curvature.

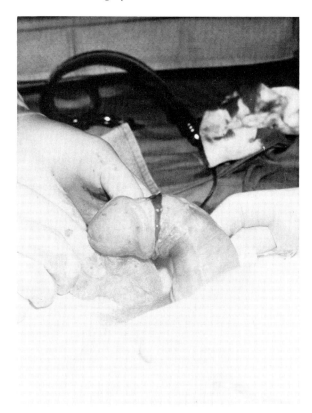

finding is widening of the septum between the corpora. In a normal study, two smooth and equal sides of the corpora cavernosa can be seen with a narrow septum between them.

PATHOLOGY

Most early reports state that the fibrosis in Peyronie's disease occurs between Buck's fascia and the tunica albuginea. Smith in 1966 [66], studied the slides of 26 patients with Peyronie's disease at the Armed Forces Institute of Pathology. In comparison to 30 patients with normal penile anatomy studied at autopsy, he found that the earliest pathologic finding was a vasculitis in the loose areolar tissue beneath the tunica albuginea surrounding the erectile tissue of the corpora. At surgery, if the tunica albuginea is carefully elevated in the area where no plaque is found, an easy cleavage plane can be achieved outside the erectile tissue of the corpora. The areolar layer that surrounds the erectile tissue is made up of hyaluronic acid, the significance of which is unknown. Early lesions show a lymphocytic and plasmocytic infiltrate in this area. The inflammatory infiltrate is mainly perivascular. As the lesion progresses, endoproliferation and perivascular fibrosis can be seen. Advanced increased fibrous formation in the area of the areolar layer with invasion of the erectile tissue follows. Hyaline degeneration is present in many cases [38], whereas less common are deposits of calcium, bone, cartilage, and even bone marrow formation [66]. Recently Ariyan has demonstrated by electron microscopy the presence of myofibroblast in the fibrous plaque of Peyronie's disease removed at surgery [1]. As anticipated, the adjacent normal tunica albuginea showed only the presence of normal fibroblast with smooth nuclear membranes with an absence of myofilaments. *Myofibroblasts* contract like smooth muscle cells and have been identified in a variety of chronic and open wounds. The myofibroblast has been reported as a cause of wound contraction. These same authors demonstrated myofibroblasts in Dupuytren's contractures and suggest that the myofibroblast may account in part for the high association of these two disorders.

ETIOLOGY

The etiology of Peyronie's disease remains unclear. It is thought to be related to or caused by a variety of urologic systemic disorders. Bilig's recent review presents little evidence to support the often-cited associations with venereal disease, atherosclerosis, diabetes mellitus, gout, osteoarthritis, or degree of sexual activity [5]. Peyronie's disease, however, has been associated with a more generalized fibrotic tendency. For example, patients with this disorder have an increased incidence of Dupuytren's contractures and often display fibrous degeneration of the external ear cartilage [15, 28, 76]. Peyronie's disease may also be a feature of carcinoid syndrome together with profound fibrotic changes seen in the retroperitoneum [6]. In a report of six patients with carcinoid syndrome by Zarafonetis and Horrax [79] two were noted to have Peyronie's disease. In both individuals, 5-hydroxyindoleacetic acid (5HIAA) was elevated. Each man had a long history of pain and curvature of the penis on erection. At autopsy, one also had fibrosis of the cardiac valves. Since carcinoid syndrome also is associated with fibrosis in other areas, such as the endocardium and peritoneum, these authors postulated that Peyronie's disease may be secondary to excess of 5HIAA in some cases [82].

Most recently, the histocompatibility antigen (HLA-B27) has been associated with diseases that exhibit characteristic localized fibrotic manifestations. It is one of a group of immunologically similar B-locus antigens that include B7, BW22, B27, and BW42. Collectively, they are called the *B7 cross-reacting* group because of the tendency of component antigens to cross-react in a standard lymphocytotoxicity tissue-typing assay. In some cases, B7 and BW22 antigens may predispose to clinical syndromes thought previously to be related only to B27 [2, 34] (Table 8-2).

Genetically determined host factors may play a role in determining clinical syndromes characterized by excess fibrosis reaction. The histocompatibility antigen HLA-B27 has been linked to a variety of such disorders. Ankylosing spondylitis is a disease strongly associated with this antigen and has a distinctive type of upper-lobe pulmonary fibrosis [35]. There also is an increased incidence of pulmonary fibrosis in HLA-B27–positive patients with asbestosis [47]. Rotator cuff fibrosis (frozen shoulder syndrome) likewise has been associated with the presence of the HLA-B27 antigen [11].

The B7 cross-reacting antigen group also may play a role in the development of retroperitoneal fibrosis in black males. In three separately reported cases, two black males with idiopathic retroperitoneal fibrosis were HLA-B27–positive, whereas one carried the B7 antigen [14, 53, 74] (Table 8-1).

In anticipation of finding a link between HLA-B27 or its cross-reacting antigens with Peyronie's disease, eight patients with Peyronie's disease were studied [75] using a standard microlymphocytotoxicity assay. As noted in Figure 8-2, seven patients, or 88 percent, possessed an antigen of the B7 cross-reacting group. In contrast, the incidence of the B7 cross-reacting group as a single entity in the general population is not greater than 36 percent, a worst-case figure obtained by summing component B-locus frequencies (B7, 18%; BW22, 5%; B27, 10%; and B42, 1%) (Fig. 8-4). This is a significant association (p = 0.05). When individual antigens in this group of patients are considered, four had B7 (50%), two had B27 (25%), and one had B22 (13%). Their frequencies are not significantly different from those of the general populations with the small sample used. Likewise, there was no significant association found for any of the other 22 antigens tested. Three patients with Peyronie's disease with a definite history of trauma sustained during intercourse also were studied. None possessed an antigen of the B7 cross-reacting group as compared to seven of eight (88%) of those with idiopathic fibrosis (p = 0.024).

The relation of Peyronie's disease to immunologically similar antigens rather than to a single antigen has significance beyond mere association. One can surmise that a specific molecular configuration shared by all antigens of the B7 cross-reacting antigen group expressed on the surface of host cells in some way predisposes to the development of this illness.

There are three generally held concepts as to why the above should occur. One possibility is the *molecular mimicry* hypothesis, which supposes that the cell surface of an invading organism is immunologically similar to the HLA antigens of the host. The supposition is that the host cannot distinguish the invading organism from itself, and this re-

Table 8-1. Tissue types of three black males with retroperitoneal fibrosis

	HLA antigens			
Olsson [14]				B27
Norton [53]	A		B7	
Willscher [74]	A3	A9	B8	B27

Table 8-2. HLA typing of eight patients with idiopathic Peyronie's disease

Patient	HLA antigens			
E. V.	A1	A3	B7	B8
G. N.	A1	A2	B7	B8
F. S.	A3	AW30, W31, W32	B7	B8
S. J.	A3	A10, W26	B7	B12
H. W.	A3		B27	BW35
H. C.	A2	A9, W23, W24	B27	BW15
J. P.	A1	A9	BW22	BW5
J. S.	A2	A10		B12
	A2	A9, 10, W26		B12

Figure 8-4. Incidence of HLA-B7 cross-reacting antigens in normal population.

Antigen	%
HLA-B7	18
HLA-BW22	7
HLA-B27	10
HLA-BW42	0-1 (Blacks only)
	36%

sults in a compromised immune response, and clinical disease. For instance, studies indicate that a cross reaction exists between HLA-B27 and species of *Klebsiella-Enterobacter*. Ankylosing spondylitis is strongly associated with the HLA-B27 antigen as well as positive stool cultures for *Klebsiella* species [18]. Such studies suggest that certain antigens may genetically predispose individuals to certain diseases.

The second possibility is that the HLA antigens may act as receptor sites for certain viruses or pathogens that cause disease. And lastly, certain nonimmunologic, nonviral ligands such as drugs and hormones may enhance or alter receptor sites of the host cells and cause a disease state. For instance, it has been shown that a positive response of schizophrenics to chlorpromazine is highly dependent on the presence of HLA-A1. This drug can be shown to bind selectively to HLA-A1–positive lymphocytes in vitro [65]. Thus, it appears that Peyronie's disease may be a syndrome of aberrant fibrosis associated with the HLA-B27 cross-reacting group.

Two other etiologic possibilities are noteworthy. Recently, 150 patients have been described by four separate authors linking Peyronie's disease to beta blockers, particularly propranolol [54] (Table 8-3). In Pryor's series of 146 patients, 19 had Peyronie's disease. Seven were taking practolol and 13 were taking propranolol [58]. They point out that practolol has been associated with fibrotic lesions of the peritoneum, eye, and, in four cases, Peyronie's disease. It may be surmised that these beta-blocking agents act as a ligand in patients who are genetically predisposed [54, 58, 70, 78]. Specifically, those who are positive for one of the antigens of the B27 cross-reacting group may be at greater risk.

As an etiologic factor in the development of Peyronie's disease a good case also can be made for minor trauma. Small-vessel rupture leading to hematomas eventually may be replaced by fibrosis. Smith substantiated this argument by studying normal penile anatomy in 100 consecutive autopsies [67]. Histologic sections of these individuals revealed mild inflammatory changes in the loose areolar connective tissue of 23 patients compatible with early Peyronie's disease. Perivascular inflammation with lymphoid cells and in several actual fibrosis-forming nodules in areas were demonstrated. Finding these changes in a large group of normal individuals would suggest that a common etiologic factor such as trauma may play a significant role in the development of this disease.

In summary, although the exact etiology of Peyronie's disease remains obscure, perivascular inflammation is its earliest manifestation. This well may be an immunologically mediated phenomenon progressing to fibrosis in patients who are predisposed to the development of the disease. Recently, beta-blocking agents such as propranolol have been associated with the development of Peyronie's disease. Minor trauma also has been implicated as being of possible importance in the pathogenesis of the disease.

Table 8-3. Association of Peyronie's disease and beta blockers

Author	Number of patients	Number of patients receiving beta blockers
Osborne [54]	2	2
Pryor [58]	146	19
Wallis [70]	1	1
Yudkin [78]	1	1
Totals	150	23

NATURAL HISTORY

It is clear that the natural history of Peyronie's disease is variable [50]. Whereas several authors state that the disease progresses with time, others have stated the opposite. Furlow followed 26 patients who received no therapy [25]. He found that there was improvement of the curvature of the penis in 52 percent. He also noted that if a lump was present on the penis, improvement was noted in 58 percent of patients receiving no therapy. The average time from diagnosis to follow-up was 9.2 years. Bystrom found that of seven patients who received no treatment, six had significant improvement [13]. Three had moderate curvature, two had small plaques, but none of them had pain. These patients were followed from 1 to 7 years. Ashworth, however, points out that the course of the disease, including pain and curvature, may decrease as a consequence of a progressive loss of potency [3]. In eight untreated patients followed for 5 years, two became impotent and six almost so [42]. As the potency decreased, so did their symptoms. It would seem logical that, as the disease progresses and as intercourse becomes more painful and difficult, desire for sexual intercourse by both partners would decrease, and consequently so would the complaints registered by patients. Soiland points out that only 1 of 19 patients who were not treated for Peyronie's disease had any significant improvement [68].

Mira in his recent review tries to demonstrate that the natural history of the disease is mostly one of spontaneous improvement [50]. However, he himself points out that multiple nonspecific modalities have been used to judge the end results of this disease. Nor is the extent of corporal involvement with the fibrotic process clearly defined. Objective analysis is often difficult because many reports are unspecific in defining improvement parameters.

It is self-evident that some patients with minimal manifestation of this disease will show some improvement, whether real or subjective. Others with a marked deformity causing severe curvature of the penis and pain on erection will continue to have progressive symptomatology resulting in loss of sexual function. My own experience suggests that there is a continuum of pathologic findings in Peyronie's disease. Many patients have minimal problems that will improve with time, whereas others display a significant pathologic process that will worsen.

DIFFERENTIAL DIAGNOSIS

Although the history and physical findings are usually characteristic in patients with Peyronie's disease, one should exclude the possibility of malignant infiltration of the penis secondary to metastatic disease as has

Table 8-4. Medical treatment of Peyronie's disease

Author	Year	Treatment
Scardino [60]	1949	Vitamin E
Bodner [7]	1954	Cortisone-hyaluronidase
Zarafonetis [79]	1959	Potoba (para-aminobenzoate)
Griff [29]	1967	Radiation
Persky [56]	1967	DMSO (dimethyl sulfoxide)
Frank [20]	1971	Ultrasound
Martin [42]	1972	Radiation
Furlow [25]	1975	Radiation
Winter [77]	1975	Dexamethasone by Dermo-Jet
Morales [51]	1975	Parathormone
Morgan [52]	1978	Procarbazine

been reported with prostate carcinoma. Such infiltration, however, is usually diffuse and involves both corpora equally. The corpora are usually hard and do not have the characteristic dorsal fibrosis. Severe fibrosis secondary to urethritis also may mimic Peyronie's disease. This usually is seen with some ventral curvature, and induration felt along the length of the urethra. Penile infiltration also has been reported with lymphogranuloma venereum [15]. Lymphogranuloma venereum results in "plastic" induration of the penis and usually occurs only in countries where this disease is prevalent [43].

TREATMENT
Medical Treatment
Because the etiology of Peyronie's disease has not been defined clearly, the treatment has been equally divergent. As Table 8-4 indicates, many different forms of treatment have been advocated. However, it is difficult to recommend a particular treatment since all methods seem to be successful to some extent [50]. Since each of these treatments is accompanied by some slight risk, considering the probable benign course of Peyronie's disease, therapy with low risk of complications should be tried first. None of the treatments listed in Table 8-4 above seems to have an advantage

over the others. Two, however, need special mention because they are used most commonly. Scardino suggested in 1949 that vitamin E is helpful in the treatment of Peyronie's disease in that it maintains the normal connective tissue metabolism by acting as a "normalizer" for hydration by preventing an accumulation of tissue fluid in local areas that may have either high acid or high alkaline surroundings causing, first, swelling of the tissue contents and, later, fragmentation of adjoining muscle fibers [60]. He further states that connective tissue is a "repair" tissue and that a deficiency of vitamin E would interfere with subsequent normal repair, leaving scar tissue in a state of contraction. Thus, vitamin E has been recommended by Wild and co-workers [71] as an initial treatment of Peyronie's disease. Ordinarily, 100 mg of vitamin E 3 times a day is recommended. Wild and co-workers used vitamin E as primary therapy in all their patients and warned them not to expect results for at least 3 to 6 months. In their series, 20 percent were cured, and improvement was noted in 33 percent [71].

Para-aminobenzoate was used initially for manifestations of scleroderma, pulmonary fibrosis, and Dupuytren's contracture. Zarafonetis and Horrax treated 21 patients with Peyronie's disease with Potaba [79]. Of 16 organs with curvature, 3 became straight and 11 improved. The dosage is 12 gm per day in 4 divided doses.

Dimethyl sulfoxide (DMSO) recently has been released for the treatment of interstitial cystitis, and interest may awaken for its use in the treatment of Peyronie's disease. Persky and Stewart reported on the use of this drug in 13 patients with Peyronie's disease [56]. The drug is applied locally, to the skin. Fifty percent had significant improvement.

SURGICAL TREATMENT

There are three major surgical approaches to the treatment of Peyronie's disease. The first involves *excision* of the fibrotic plaque and replacement with some noncontractile tissue that allows for normal healing. The second is placement of a rigid or inflatable *penile implant*, with or without incision of the Peyronie's plaques. The third is *removal* of a diamond-shaped piece of *fascia corpus* from the opposite normal *corporum* (Nesbit procedure) to allow straightening of the penis.

Since 1950, over 255 patients with Peyronie's disease have had their plaques excised and replaced with a variety of grafts (Table 8-5). Initially, Losley and Boyce described replacement of the excised area with fat. They reported excellent results in 20 patients, good results in 10 and only three had a poor outcome. More recently, Wild and co-workers have used a deepithelialized dermal graft with good results in 70 percent of their patients operated on and poor results in the remaining 30 percent [71] (Fig. 8-5). Kalami [36] has used dura as a replacement for the fibrotic plaque, whereas others such as Brushimi have used fascia [9]. This collective series indicated that 132 patients had excellent to good results (61%), whereas 52 (39%) had poor results (Table 8-5). These figures compare favorably to those reported by Wild and co-workers [71] in their large series of 50 patients.

It should be noted although authors such as Wild and co-workers [71], Martin [42], and Hicks and co-workers [33] uniformly report good results, others, such as Hall [30], Melman [46], and Bruskevitz [10] report dismal results with this procedure. Special surgical techniques as well as enthusiasm for the procedure therefore must play some role in its outcome. Furthermore, the procedure is not without complication. Green and Martin described partial anesthesia of the glans occurring in 15 percent of his patients, penile shortening in 30 percent, and impotence in 5 percent [28]. Eleven of those operated on continued to have pain on erection. Of these complications, the most severe is anesthesia of the glans penis due to injury of the dorsal nerves. This injury is usually permanent and can be best avoided by careful attention to surgical detail. Impotence can be rectified by the insertion of a penile prosthesis.

The second major surgical approach in Peyronie's disease is implantation of a *penile prosthesis*. In a review of the major series re-

Table 8-5. Various grafting procedures for correction of Peyronie's disease

Author	Year	Number of patients with Peyronie's	Number of patients with a graft	Type of graft	Excellent	Good	Poor
Lowsley and Boyce [38]	1950	50	33	Fat	20	10	3
Bruschimi [9]	1972	4	4	Fascia	4		
Bystrom [12]	1973	15	15	13 Dermal		10	3
				2 Fascia			2
Taranger [69]	1975	7	2	Dermal		2	
Hall and Turner [30]	1977	5	5	Dermal		5	
Melman [46]	1978	7	7	Dermal			7
Hicks [33]	1978	15	15	Dermal		12	3
Wild [71]	1979	50	50	Dermal		35	15
Martin [28]	1979	27	27	Dermal		18	7
Medgyesi [44]	1979	4	4	Corpus cavernosum		3	
Bruskevitz and Raz [10]	1980	24	5	Dermal			5
Kelami [36]	1980	22	7	Dura	7		
Palomar [55]	1980	25	10	Dermal	2	1	7
Totals		255	184		29	103	52

Figure 8-5. The fibrotic plaque has been removed, and a deepithelialized graft inserted. Note dorsal retraction of neurovascular bundle.

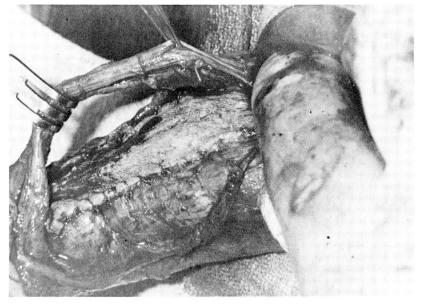

Table 8-6. Selected literature review of penile implants, 1973–1980

Author	Year	Prosthesis	Number of patients implanted	Number of patients with Peyronie's disease	Number of patients with Peyronie's disease who had implants	Results		
						Excellent	Good	Poor
Scott [61]	1973	Inflatable	5	0	0			
Melman [45]	1976	Small-Carrion	13	0	0			
Merrill [48]	1976	Small-Carrion	15	0	0			
Finney [19]	1977	Hinged	27	1	1		1	
Malloy [40]	1977	Inflatable	39	0	0			
Gottesman [27]	1977	Small-Carrion	61	7	7	Not reported		
Small [63]	1978	Small-Carrion	260	11	11	10	1	
Furlow [24]	1978	Inflatable	249	6	6	Not reported		
Paulson [37]	1979	Small-Carrion	76	6	6	Not reported		
Scott [62]	1979	Inflatable	245	18	18	Not reported		
Kelami [36]	1980	Small-Carrion	22	22	15		15	
Palomar [55]	1980	Small-Carrion	25	25	6		5	
Malloy [41]	1980	Small-Carrion	45	0	0			
Malloy [41]	1980	Inflatable	105	0	0			
Barry [4]	1980	Hinged	25	3	3	Not reported		
Bruskevitz [10]	1980	Small-Carrion	24	24	19		17	2
Total			1236	123	93	10	39	2

ported since 1973, over 1236 patients have had penile prostheses implanted. Of these patients, 123 had Peyronie's disease, of whom 93 received a penile implant. The majority of these had a rigid prosthesis implanted, while 24 received an inflatable prosthesis. Results were uniformly excellent (Table 8-6). The major advantage of implantation of a penile prosthesis, as recommended by Raz, is that only one operative procedure is required and that anesthesia of the glans penis as well as postoperative impotence are avoided [10]. The obvious disadvantage of this procedure is that the patient no longer has a normally functioning sexual organ.

Disagreement exists as to whether the fibrotic plaques need to be incised at the time of implantation of the penile prosthesis. Raz generally has recommended the incision of the penile plaques, whereas Kelami [36] and Small [63] have found that this is usually not necessary. A slight bend in the penis after implantation of the device usually straightens with time. Sometimes this bend can be modified by placing a different-size prosthesis in each corpus. The hinged prosthesis developed by Finney [19] can be trimmed at each end to allow for a different prosthetic length

to be placed in each corpus, thereby straightening the penis. If curvature of the penis after implantation is severe, Small has recommended a 1- to 2-in. vertical incision on the dorsum of the penis carried down the corpora bilaterally. The neurovascular bundle should be identified on each side and spared. A transverse incision is then made across the plaque in the corpus on one side, and then the other if necessary. These incisions may be multiple and may cut through to the implanted penile prosthesis. The only complication noted from multiple incisions is penile edema, which usually resolves in time. Furlow [24] has noted that, when one is implanting an inflatable prosthesis into a patient with Peyronie's disease, it is necessary not only to incise the plaque to achieve straightening but it is in fact necessary to make many linear incisions distal to the plaque to provide satisfactory erections without significant curvature. Mild degrees of Peyronie's disease, however, may permit satisfactory erections after implant without significant curvature. Since the degree of inflation can be regulated with an inflatable penile prosthesis, significant rigidity often can be obtained without significant curvature. Furlow also describes no sensory loss or impairment of circulation if the dorsal neurovascular bundle is dissected carefully prior to incision of the plaques.

The third alternative to surgical repair of patients with Peyronie's disease was described by Pryor and Fitzpatrick in 1978 [57]. They reported 23 patients whose penises were straightened by employing the *Nesbit procedure*. The skin and Colles' fascia are peeled back to the base of the penis, and the corpora inflated in the manner described by Gittes and McLaughlin [26]. A marking suture is inserted in the tunica albuginea at the point of maximum curvature. If the deformity is toward the abdomen, pointing dorsally, it is necessary to dissect the corpus spongiosum away from the corpora cavernosa, and the urethra is elevated with tapes. Diamond-shaped pieces of fascia are then excised at the opposite point of maximum curvature. These ellipses are then closed in a vertical fashion with No. 1 nonabsorbable monofilament sutures. The penis is reinflated, and a further ellipse is removed if the deformity has not been corrected. The skin of the shaft of the penis is reapproximated to the subcoronal edge once the penis has been straightened. In a series of 23 patients, 20 had excellent results, providing satisfactory coitus. All were potent.

CONCLUSIONS

Peyronie's disease is a problem that is not infrequently seen in the urologist's office. Its resultant plaque causes dorsal or lateral curvature of the penis, making coitus difficult, if not impossible. Its pathogenesis, although not totally clear, appears to be a manifestation of a generalized fibrotic tendency in patients who are genetically predisposed for the development of this disease. The B7 cross-reacting antigen group has been closely associated with development of Peyronie's disease. Patients who are positive for one of these antigens through an altered immunologic response may develop dorsal penile fibrosis. Additionally, trauma sustained during intercourse may cause Peyronie's disease.

The disease to some extent appears self-limited and improves with time. However, other patients may develop progressive penile curvature resulting in pain and, in some cases, total impotence. Because of the varying natural history of this disease, medical treatment of Peyronie's disease has been difficult to assess. Vitamin E and para-aminobenzoate (Potaba) seem to have some clinical rationale as treatment.

Surgical correction usually is limited to patients in whom the disease has progressed to the point where coitus is nearly impossible. Excision of the plaque, followed by grafting procedures, appears to be the procedure of choice in young patients in whom the fibrotic plaque is short and well defined. The Nesbit procedure also may be a reasonable alternative in this group. Patients who are over 60 years of age or have an extensive fibrotic change in the dorsum or lateral aspect of the penis are probably best treated with a penile implant, and a straightening procedure if necessary.

REFERENCES

1. Ariyan, S., Emriguez, R., and Krizek, T. J. Wound contraction and fibrocontractive disorders. *Arch. Surg.* 113:1034, 1978.
2. Arnett, F. C., Jr., Hochberg, M. C., and Bias, W. B. Cross reactive HLA antigens in B27-negative Reiter's syndrome and sacroileitis. *Johns Hopkins Med. J.* 141:193, 1977.
3. Ashworth, A. Peyronie's disease. *Proc. R. Soc. Med.* 53:642, 1960.
4. Barry, J. M. Clinical experience with hinged silicone penile implants for impotence. *J. Urol.* 123:178, 1980.
5. Bilig, R., et al. Peyronie's disease. *Urology* 6:409, 1975.
6. Bivens, C. J., Marecek, R. L., and Feldman, J. M. Peyronie's disease: A presenting complaint of the carcinoid syndrome. *N. Engl. J. Med.* 289:844, 1973.
7. Bodner, H., Howard, A. H., and Kaplan, J. H. Peyronie's disease: Cortisone — hyaluronidase — hydrocortisone therapy. *J. Urol.* 72:400, 1954.
8. Buford, E. H., Glen, J. E., and Burford, C. E. Therapy of Peyronie's disease. *Urol. Cutan. Rev.* 55:337, 1951.
9. Brushimi, H., and Mitre, A. I. Peyronie's disease: Surgical treatment with muscular aponeurosis. *J. Urol.* 13:505, 1979.

10. Bruskevitz, R., and Raz, S. Surgical considerations of Peyronie's disease. *Urology* 15:134, 1980.

11. Bulger, D. Y., Hazelman, B. L., and Voak, D. HLA-B27 and frozen shoulder. *Lancet* 1:1042, 1976.

12. Bystrom, J., et al. Induratio penis plactica (Peyronie's disease). *Scand. J. Plast. Reconstr. Surg.* 7:137, 1973.

13. Bystrom, J., and Rusio, C. Induratio penis plastico (Peyronie's disease). *Scand. J. Urol. Nephrol.* 10:12, 1976.

14. Case records of Massachusetts General Hospital. *N. Engl. J. Med.* 294:712, 1976.

15. Chesney, J. Plastic induration of the penis in Peyronie's disease. *Br. J. Urol.* 35:61, 1963.

16. Desanctis, P. N., and Furey, C. A. Steroid injection for Peyronie's disease. *J. Urol.* 97:114, 1967.

17. Dugan, H. E. Effect of x-ray therapy on patients with Peyronie's disease. *South. Med. J.* 65:1192, 1972.

18. Ebringer, R., et al. Ankylosing Spondylitis and Presense of HLA B27 Cross-Reacting *Klebsiella* A-Pneumonial Species. In *Proceedings of 14th International Congress of Rheumatology.* 1977. P. 179.

19. Finney, R. P. New hinged silicone penile prosthesis. *J. Urol.* 116:585, 1977.

20. Frank, I. N., and Scott, W. W. The ultrasonic treatment of Peyronie's disease. *J. Urol.* 106:883, 1971.

21. Frank, I. N., and Winfield, W. S. The ultrasonic treatment of Peyronie's disease. *J. Urol.* 106:883, 1971.

22. Furey, C. A. Peyronie's disease: Treatment by the local injection of meticortelone and hydrocortisone. *J. Urol.* 77:251, 1957.

23. Furlow, W. L. Inflatable penile prosthesis: Mayo Clinic experience with 175 patients. *Urology* 13:166, 1970.

24. Furlow, W. L. Peyronie's disease and penile implantation. Letters to editor. *J. Urol.* 120:647, 1978.

25. Furlow, W. L., Swenson, H. E., Jr., and Lee, R. E. Peyronie's disease: A study of its natural history and treatment with ortho voltage radiotherapy. *J. Urol.* 114:69, 1975.

26. Gittes, R. F., and McLaughlin, A. P., III. Injection technique to induce penile erection. *Urology* 4:473, 1974.

27. Gottesman, J. E., et al. The Small-Carrion prosthesis for male impotency. *J. Urol.* 117:289, 1977.

28. Green, R., and Martin, D. C. Treatment of Peyronie's disease by dermal grafting. *Plast. Reconstr. Surg.* 64:208, 1979.

29. Griff, L. C. The role of radiation therapy and a general review. *AJR* 100:916, 1967.

30. Hall, W. T., and Turner, R. W. Experience with Devine-Horton dermal patch graft for Peyronie's disease. *Urology* 9:407, 1977.

31. Hamilton, R. W., and Swann, J. C. Corpus cavernosography in Peyronie's disease. *Br. J. Urol.* 39:409, 1967.

32. Helvie, W. W., and Ochsner, S. F. Radiation therapy in Peyronie's disease. *South. Med. J.* 65:1192, 1912.

33. Hicks, C. C., et al. Experience with the Horton-Devine dermal graft in the treatment of Peyronie's disease. *J. Urol.* 119:504, 1978.

34. Hochberg, M. C., Bias, W. B., and Arnett, F. C. HLA-A28 and HLA-B7, cross-reacting antigens in HLA-B27 associated arthritis. *Clin. Res.* 25:520A, 1977.

35. Jessamine, A. G. Upper lobe fibrosis in ankylosing spondylitis. *Can. Med. Assoc. J.* 98:25, 1968.

36. Kelami, A. Peyronie's disease and surgical treatment. *Urology* 15:559, 1980.

37. Kramer, S. A., et al. Complications of Small-Carrion penile prosthesis. *Urology* 13:49, 1979.

38. Lowsley, O. S., and Boyce, W. H. Further experiences with an operation for cure of Peyronie's disease. *J. Urol.* 63:888, 1950.

39. Lowsley, O. S., and Gentile, A. An operation for the cure of certain cases of plastic induration (Peyronie's disease). *J. Urol.* 57:552, 1947.

40. Malloy, T. R., and Von Enschenbach, A. C. Surgical treatment of erectile impotence with inflatable penile prosthesis. *J. Urol.* 118:49, 1977.

41. Malloy, T. R., Wein, A. J., and Carpiniello, V. L. Comparison of the inflatable penile and the Small-Carrion prosthesis in the surgical treatment of erectile impotence. *J. Urol.* 123:678, 1980.

42. Martin, C. L. Long-term study of patients with Peyronie's disease treated with irradiation. *AJR* 114:492, 1972.

43. McRoberts, J. W. Peyronie's disease. *Surg. Gynecol. Obstet.* 129:1291, 1969.

44. Medgyesi, S. Surgical treatment of induratio plastica (Peyronie's disease) with a corpus cavernosum graft. *Br. J. Plast. Surg.* 32:129, 1979.

45. Melman, A. Experience with implantation of the Small-Carrion penile implant for organic impotence. *J. Urol.* 116:49, 1976.

46. Melman, A., and Holland, T. F. Evaluation of the dermal graft inlay technique for the surgical treatment of Peyronie's disease. *J. Urol.* 120:421, 1978.

47. Merchant, J. A., et al. The HLA system in asbestos workers. *Br. Med. J.* 1:189, 1975.

48. Merrill, D. C., and Swanson, D. A. Experience with the Small-Carrion penile prosthesis. *J. Urol.* 115:277, 1976.

49. Mira, J. G. The value of radiotherapy for Peyronie's disease: Presentation of 56 new case studies and review of the literature. *Int. J. Radiat. Oncol. Biol. Phys.* 6:161, 1980.

50. Mira, J. G. Is it worthwhile to treat Peyronie's disease? *Urology* 16:1, 1980.

51. Morales, A., and Bruce, A. W. The treatment of Peyronie's disease with parathyroid hormone. *J. Urol.* 114:901, 1975.

52. Morgan, R. J., and Pryor, J. P. Procarbazine (Natulane) in the treatment of Peyronie's disease. *Br. J. Urol.* 50:111, 1978.

53. Norton, J., III. Idiopathic retroperitoneal fibrosis: Letter to the editor. *J. Urol.* 121:689, 1979.

54. Osborne, D. R. Propanolol and Peyronie's disease. *Lancet* 1:1111, 1977.

55. Palomar, J. M., Halikiopoulos, H., and Thomas, R. Evaluation of the surgical management of Peyronie's disease. *J. Urol.* 123:680, 1980.

56. Persky, L., and Stewart, B. H. The use of dimethylsulfoxide in the treatment of genitourinary disorders. *Ann. N. Y. Acad. Sci.* 141:551, 1967.

57. Pryor, J. P., and Fitzpatrick, J. M. A new approach to the correction of the penile deformity in Peyronie's disease. *J. Urol.* 122:622, 1979.

58. Pryor, J. P., and Khan, O. Beta blockers and Peyronie's disease [letter]. *Lancet* 1:331, 1979.

59. Raz, S. Peyronie's disease and penile implantation. [Letters to editor.] *J. Urol.* 119:709, 1978.

60. Scardino, P. L., Scott, W. W., and Ant, M. The use of tocopherols in the treatment of Peyronie's disease. *Ann. N. Y. Acad. Sci.* 52:310, 1949.

61. Scott, R. B., Bradley, W. E., and Timm, G. W. Management of erectile impotence: Use of implantable inflatable prosthesis. *Urology* 2:80, 1973.

62. Scott, F. B., et al. Erectile impotence treated with an implantable, inflatable prosthesis. *J.A.M.A.* 241:2609, 1979.

63. Small, M. P. Peyronie's disease and penile implantation. Letters to editor. *J. Urol.* 119:579, 1978.

64. Small, M. P. The Small-Carrion prosthesis. *Urol. Clin. North Am.* 5:549, 1978.

65. Smeraldi, E., and Scorza-Smeraldi, R. Interference between HLA antibodies and chlorpromazine. *Nature* 260:532, 1976.

66. Smith, B. J. Peyronie's disease. *Am. J. Clin. Pathol.* 45:670, 1966.

67. Smith, B. H. Subclinical Peyronie's disease. *Am. J. Clin. Pathol.* 52:385, 1969.

68. Soiland, A. Peyronie's disease or plastic induration of the penis. *Radiology* 42:183, 1944.

69. Taranger, L. A., Robson, C. J., and Barkim, M. The surgical approach to Peyronie's disease. *J. Urol.* 114:404, 1975.

70. Wallis, A. A., Bell, R., and Sutherland, P. W. Propranolol and Peyronie's disease. *Lancet* 1:980, 1977.

71. Wild, R. M., DeVine, C. J., and Horton, C. E. Dermal graft repair of Peyronie's disease: Survey of 50 patients. *J. Urol.* 121:47, 1979.

72. Williams, J. L., and Thomas, G. G. The natural history of Peyronie's disease. *Proc. R. Soc. Med.* 61:876, 1968.

73. Williams, R. E., et al. Experience with the Small-Carrion penile prosthesis in the treatment of organic impotence. *J. Urol.* 115:280, 1976.

74. Willscher, M. K., Novicki, D. E., and Cwaska, W. F. Association of HLA-B27 antigen with retroperitoneal fibrosis. *J. Urol.* 120:631, 1978.

75. Willscher, M. K., Cwaska, W. F., and Novicki, D. E. The association of histocompatibility antigens of the B7 cross-reacting group with Peyronie's disease. *J. Urol.* 122:34, 1979.

76. Winter, C. C. *Practical Urology.* St. Louis: Mosby, 1969. P. 229.

77. Winter, C. C., and Khanna, R. Peyronie's disease results with Dermo-Jet injection of dexamethasone. *J. Urol.* 114:898, 1975.

78. Yudkin, J. S. Peyronie's disease in association with metoprol. *Lancet* 11:1355, 1977.

79. Zarafonetis, C. J., and Horrax, T. Treatment of Peyronie's disease with potassium para-aminobenzoate (POTABA). *J. Urol.* 81:770, 1959.

Priapism

RALPH deVERE WHITE
HARRIS M. NAGLER

The term *priapism* is derived from the name of the Roman god Priapus, a god of excessiveness, male sexuality, fertility, hunting, fishing, and agriculture.

Priapism is a prolonged, generally extremely painful, erection that is not associated with stimulation or sexual desire, although it may be precipitated by sexual activity.

PATHOPHYSIOLOGY

Since the physiology of erection has been dealt with thoroughly in Chapters 1, 2, and 3, it will not be discussed in detail here.

In the flaccid state, as described by Conti, arterial blood bypasses the erectile tissue of the penis. With stimulation, arterial blood is shunted into potential spaces of the corpora cavernosa. Initially, blood entering the penis is greater than that exiting, but soon a steady state is established, with maintenance of an erection [26]. Newman and co-workers feel that venous obstruction is not necessary for erection and have demonstrated experimentally that venous occlusion, rather than leading to erection, causes edema and cyanosis [44]. The process of erection may be aided by a decrease in blood to erectile penile tissues. Detumescence may be passive due to opening of shunts or may be an active process in which vasoconstriction of vessels supplying the penis is accomplished by activation of the sympathetic nervous system.

In priapism, penile engorgement is prolonged. The mechanism of this prolongation may vary. There may be a mechanical or a physiologic obstruction that has not yet been defined. Nevertheless, the final pathway remains the same. There is increasing carbon dioxide tension, acidosis, and blood viscosity. The normal corporal septa become edematous, and further occlusion occurs. This becomes a self-perpetuating phenomenon. Fibrosis supervenes and impotence may result.

ETIOLOGY

The etiology of priapism is varied, and although certain specific causes may be identified readily and influence the patient's initial management, one must be aware that such cases are in the minority.

Idiopathic Causes

As in many other conditions, the primary cause in priapism is idiopathic; it accounts for 58 percent of the 28 patients in Winter's series [69] and 43 percent of the 23 patients in Darwish's report [13].

Sickle Cell Anemia

Sickle cell hemoglobinopathy is the second most prevalent etiology of priapism. Nelson and Winter report 23 percent of their patients had sickle cell disease; of the children with priapism, 63.3 percent had sickle cell disease [43]. In the series of Larocque and Cosgrove [34], 29 percent of the black patients with priapism had sickle cell disease.

It would appear from Seeler's work that, in children, the chance of impotence after sickle cell–induced priapism is considerably less than that in other etiologies of priapism [54]. Although sickle cell disease is a common cause of priapism, only 3.6 percent of the affected patients ever develop priapism [24]. It should be borne in mind that recurrent episodes are a hallmark of sickle cell–induced priapism [43].

The pathophysiology of priapism in sickle cell disease is easily understood. Localized sickling occurs as a result of the decreased blood flow rate that is present in the stable erection [4, 65]. This localized sludging leads to increased hypoxia and acidosis, which cascades to further sickling and sludging and results in further decrease in venous outflow. This vicious cycle is further aggravated by perivascular edema. With progression, there is thrombosis of vascular spaces and eventual fibrosis that will lead to irreversible impotence [69]. It is not clear why this process does not occur in children as often as in their adult counterparts.

Inflammatory Causes

Many kinds of inflammatory lesion have been implicated in priapism. In 1954, Dahlin reported a case of priapism secondary to tularemia [12]. Mumps has been implicated in the etiology of at least two cases, one with and one without clinical orchitis. The postulated mechanisms in these disorders is a perivascular lymphocytic response with resultant impediment to venous outflow [18, 29]. Rabies and Rocky Mountain spotted fever also have been implicated [69]. An alleged episode of allergic priapism in response to tetanus antitoxin was reported in 1952 by Lipton and Toomey [37]. The causality of the tetanus antitoxin was accepted by a compensation court. Pelvic thrombophlebitis secondary to local suppuration has been indicted as a mechanism of priapism [6]. To put inflammatory causes of priapism in perspective, in Winter's series, they accounted for only 1 percent of the cases [69].

Infiltrative Diseases

Infiltrative disease is a relatively recently appreciated category in the varied etiology of priapism. In 1973, Wilson and co-workers reported two cases of priapism considered to be secondary to Fabry's disease [68]. Fabry's disease, an X-linked deficiency of the enzyme ceramide trihexosidase, results in lipid deposition in blood vessels, ganglia, and perineural cells of the autonomic nervous system, connective tissues, and kidneys. Priapism in this setting is attributed to blood vessel narrowing and motor unresponsiveness due to lipid deposition. Other characteristic aspects of Fabry's disease are renal failure and a singular skin rash consisting of flat, punctate, purple red papules symmetrically distributed between umbilicus and knees.

Amyloidosis, another infiltrative disease of questionable etiology, recently has been incriminated as the cause of priapism [32].

Neoplasm

Neoplasm resulting in priapism can be divided into two major categories: solid tumors and leukemias.

SOLID TUMORS. Extensive local tumor or metastatic disease may lead to priapism by causing outflow obstruction and corporal body replacement. So-called malignant priapism secondary to metastatic disease is an extremely rare occurrence [14]. Only 160 cases of metastatic disease of the penis were reported by 1977 [56]. In Smith and Bonacarti's series, all reported cases of renal metastases to the penis were associated with priapism [56]. This, however, is not a feature of all metastatic carcinoma to the penis, as evidenced by Abeshouse and Abeshouse's report in which priapism occurred in 38.1 percent of 140 cases of metastatic carcinoma to the penis; the primary tumors were renal, testicular, pulmonary, and osseous [1]. The majority of their cases of malignant priapism were caused by local tumor growth. Of the 52 cases they reviewed, 17 were of bladder origin, 14 prostate, and 5 rectal.

LEUKEMIA. Although priapism has been stated to occur in up to 10 percent of all leukemic patients, leukemia accounts for only 5 percent of all cases of priapism, and 15 percent of those occurring in children [1, 69].

Chronic granulocytic leukemia is the major culprit, although chronic lymphocytic, acute lymphoblastic, and acute myeloblastic leukemias also have been implicated [53]. Leukemia causes priapism by direct infiltration of the corpora blocking outflow, although central and peripheral neurologic effects also have been implicated by Vadakan and Ortega [63] and Williams and co-workers [67].

Trauma

Trauma seldom causes priapism. Darwish and associates include no case of trauma-induced priapism in their 20 cases [13]. Winter attributes 5 percent of all priapism to trauma, and that estimation excludes sexual excessiveness [69]. Persky and Kursh reviewed seven cases of posttraumatic priapism in 1977; however, the specific mechanisms of the trauma were not described [48]. Nevertheless, it is easy to visualize how direct trauma to the phallus or perineum may cause thrombosis of the corpora and subsequent priapism. Wear and associates reported a case of straddle injury causing a vascular corporal shunt, the secondary increase in arterial blood flow resulting in priapism. They utilized autologous clot to embolize the left internal pudendal artery with resolution of the priapism [64].

If prolonged excessive sexual behavior were included in this category, the numbers would certainly increase. Central nervous system trauma will be dealt with under Neurologic Causes section.

Hematologic Causes

This section will exclude sickle cell disease and the leukemias, since these were dealt with in the preceding sections.

Two hematologic procedures recently have been associated with priapism: leukapheresis and dialysis [11]. Heparin, which is used in both these procedures, has been shown to induce antiplatelet antibodies and complement-mediated leukostasis [3, 38]. These aggregates could cause obstruction to drainage of the corpora and could cause priapism.

Another extremely rare entity causing priapism is primary thrombocythemia or hemorrhagic thrombocythemia [35]. It is associated with abnormal bleeding (which is due to a functional abnormality of the platelets) and, paradoxically, with pathologic thrombosis. The mechanism of priapism is presumed to be the same as that described previously.

Multiple myeloma has been reported as the cause of priapism in a single case [51]. Its pathophysiology is thought to be an increased plasma viscosity, which experimentally has been demonstrated to lead to red cell agglutination. The other symptoms usually linked with plasma hyperviscosity have been associated with this phenomenon.

Neurologic Causes

According to Winter, neurologic causes account for only 1 percent of all cases of priapism [69]. These cases do not include drugs with central nervous system effects. In Ookoshi's series of 156 patients [47], 2.1 percent were secondary to cerebrospinal lesions.

Priapism has been reported to have occurred consequent to a ruptured intracranial aneurysm [60]. Cauda equina compression from a herniated disk has been linked causally to a case of priapism, and priapism secondary to spinal canal stenosis has responded to laminectomy [33, 49]. Becker and Mitchell list multiple sclerosis, tabes dorsalis, and trauma (mechanical or inflammatory) to both the spinal cord and brain as potential etiologies [6]. Even the trauma of hanging has been reported to cause priapism; it occurs at the moment of hanging and persists 1½ hours after death [2]. Thus, it appears that many irritative central nervous system processes can lead to priapism. All these neurologic lesions may cause prolonged pathologic stimulation of either cerebral or spinal erectile centers, leading to priapism through what would otherwise be normal pathways.

Local irritative phenomena, i.e., phimosis and condyloma accuminatum, have been implicated by Hinman as causing reflex neurogenic priapism [25]. Other reflex neurogenic causes in the literature include urethritis and vesical or urethral calculi [2]. Epilepsy has been associated with priapism, which responded to antiepileptic medications [9]. The association of various neurologic conditions with priapism is often no better than tenuous. Nevertheless, certain neurologic conditions can be the cause of priapism and one's index of suspicion should be high.

Medicinal and Chemical Causes

The list of medications implicated in priapism grows steadily. Emodi (1906) noted episodes of priapism in a printer with lead poisoning [9]. Reports of priapism induced by aphrodisiacs containing canthariden, yohimbin, turpentine, androgen, phosphorus, zinc, and strychnine appear in the literature [9]. More recently, psychotropic drugs, including phenothiazines, methaqualone, marijuana, and alcohol have been blamed [15, 40, 69]. Antihypertensive medications, including hydralazine, prazosin, and guanethidine may lead to priapism [3, 7, 69]. Heparin as a cause of priapism was disucssed under Hematologic Causes, above.

MEDICAL TREATMENT

The treatment of priapism should be based on the presence or absence of a definable under-

lying etiology, i.e., primary as distinguished from secondary priapism. With certain clearly defined causes, specific treatments may be administered. Generally, treatments that are etiologically specific are medical; the nonspecific are medical or surgical. If the specific medical therapies are unsuccessful, surgical treatment must be instituted before irreversible fibrosis and impotence supervene. In addition, certain specific medical treatments aimed at the underlying pathophysiology may be started in concert with nonspecific surgical treatment.

There are several nonspecific medical treatments of priapism that will be dealt with first:

1. Sedation is a cornerstone of the treatment of priapism. The pain of priapism may be excruciating.
2. Hydration, although used in all forms of priapism, is most important in sickle cell disease because dehydration may lead to further sickling.
3. Thermal treatments with either ice or warm-water enemas have no place. Cold causes vasoconstriction and decreased blood flow from the penis. Warmth only leads to increased blood flow to an already overperfused organ. These methods are unsuccessful.
4. Continuous compression as a part of a treatment regimen is to be condemned, as is evidenced by the reports of Weiss and Ferguson [66]. They report three cases of penile necrosis secondary to compression. Instead, intermittent compression or gentle binding should be used, generally, in association with needle aspiration.
5. Fibrinolytic agents (streptokinase) have theoretic advantages in early priapism. Dissolution of clots, and prevention of further propagation can reverse the process. Eriksson and co-workers [17] report successful use of streptokinase in two of three patients, resolving priapism and maintaining potency. The most serious drawback with this treatment is the need to defer surgical intervention for at least 3 to 4 days if there is no response, and thus, greatly increase the chance of impotence. Treatment

is reported to be successful in approximately 50 percent of cases if it is begun within 24 hours of the onset of priapism.

6. General anesthesia, ketamine anesthesia, and epidural anesthesia have not withstood the test of time and have been abandoned as primary treatment modalities [26, 46].

7. Controlled hypotension induced by trimethaphan camsylate (Arfonad) and by sodium nitroprusside has been used successfully by Ulm [62] and Sozer [57] respectively. These were employed in conjunction with other, nonspecific treatments, making assessment of their effectiveness difficult [57]. Hypotensive anesthesia without adjunctive measures causes detumescence when the systemic pressure is maintained below 70 mm Hg. This is not without considerable risk and difficulty, because of the prolonged periods of hypotension that are necessary [41].

8. Hormonal manipulation with either estrogenic compounds or adrenal hormones has long been regarded as ineffectual [23].

9. Other agents, such as succinylcholine or antispasmodic and ganglionic blocking agents, also yield no predictable response.

ETIOLOGY-SPECIFIC MEDICAL MANAGEMENT

The causes of priapism that lend themselves to specific treatments are sickle cell disease, malignant priapism, and some traumatic cases.

Sickle Cell Disease

In these cases, primary therapy consists of hydration, alkalinization, and analgesia. If these measures fail to bring about resolution, hypertransfusion is utilized. Hypertransfusion was first suggested in 1962 by Hasen [24]. Seeler demonstrated a reduction in spleen size after acute sequestration crisis with transfusion [55]. The results of treatment for sickle cell disease were reviewed recently by Baron and Leiter [4]. The treatment with hypertransfusion yielded 100 percent potency (8 of 8) in those patients in whom there was adequate follow-up. Cavernosum saphenous vein shunts also yielded 100 percent potency in a group with adequate follow-up. The potency rate for cavernosum spongiosum shunts was 60 percent. Aspiration as the sole treatment had a 40 percent potency rate. The potency rate for all therapies in those with adequate follow-up was 77 percent.

Baron and Leiter [4] suggest initial treatment with hydration, alkalinization, and analgesia while obtaining hemoglobin electrophoresis. Then, if there is no detumescence, the patient should be hypertransfused to a hematocrit of 2 times normal. If the priapism persists after an observation period of 24 hours, a shunting procedure should be performed. By using the following formula, the amount necessary to hypertransfuse can be calculated readily, assuming the hematocrit [55] of packed red cells is 75 to 80% and the blood volume is 75 to 80 cc/kg.

$$\text{Hematocrit} = \frac{\text{hematocrit of packed cells} \times \text{volume transfused}}{\text{patient's blood volume}}$$

Exchange transfusion has been used for the treatment of symptomatic crisis of sickle cell disease [8]. Since this is not technically feasible or sufficiently rapid in an adult, red blood cell exchange pheresis was used by Rifkind and associates with success [50]. If these maneuvers are unsuccessful, surgical intervention should be carried out.

Malignant Priapism

Malignant priapism is a secondary cause that at times can be treated quite specifically. Leukemic infiltrates may be treated with alkylating agents and radiotherapy [20]. Radical surgery (penectomy) may be necessary for debridement of extensive necrotic tissue [42].

Trauma

Traumatic priapism occasionally may be amenable to specific intervention, as is reported by Wear and associates [64]. In their case, autologous clot was successfully used to embolize a traumatic shunt, with cessation of priapism.

Hematologic Causes

Multiple myeloma causing priapism has been treated successfully with plasmapheresis. This reduced the plasma hyperviscosity that was the presumed mechanism of the priapism [51].

Inflammatory Causes

Priapism secondary to pelvic inflammation may require specific treatment in addition to surgical intervention.

SURGICAL TREATMENT

The surgical treatment of priapism also can be considered as either specific or nonspecific intervention.

The specific surgical treatments are few. Malignant priapism, alluded to in the previous section, can at times, be handled by penectomy. Certain central nervous system lesions causing priapism require surgical intervention that is directed both at the underlying process and at the priapism [49, 60].

The vast majority of the cases of priapism require nonspecific surgical intervention, which has become the mainstay of the therapy of priapism. As was indicated in the preceding sections, the etiology of priapism is often idiopathic, and the nonspecific medical therapies are usually unsuccessful. Even the specific treatments may be unsuccessful, and a surgical procedure ultimately may be necessary.

Throughout history, there have been many surgical approaches to the treatment of priapism:

1. *Ligation of the dorsal artery of the penis* was reported by Lewis in 1897. Obviously, the need for blood supply to the corporal bodies makes this an unreasonable approach [2]. The erectile tissues are supplied mainly by the terminal branches of the internal pudendal arteries directly entering the corpora cavernosa [36].

2. *Divisions of ischiocavernosus* muscles is not a rational approach to the treatment of priapism. At one time, it was thought that these muscles enabled erection by causing mechanical venous outflow obstruction. This has not proved to be a valid concept. The ischiocavernosus muscles are not required for erection [45].

3. *Incision and drainage of the corpora cavernosa* has been reported as long ago as 1824 by Calloway [2]. Hinman, in 1914, reported 31 of 33 cases of priapism treated successfully in this manner [25].

4. *Aspiration of corporal bodies* was first described in 1928 by McKay and Colston. Essentially a modification of the incision and drainage of the corpora cavernosa, it was followed by application of a compression dressing [39]. Modifications of this technique continued to be used widely in conjunction with other surgical techniques. Harrow, with good results, combined aspiration with T-binding of the phallus in flexed state [23].

5. In 1961, Bolliger noted that since the corpora spongiosa remains flaccid in the erection of priapism, it may be used to provide satisfactory egress for the turgid blood trapped in the corpora cavernosa [59]. In 1963, Quackels performed the first *cavernospongiosum shunt*. The shunt was performed at the base of the penis. This procedure was subsequently modified with a perineal approach by Sacher and associates in 1972, which permitted greater safety because of abundant spongiosa tissue protecting the urethra and the ease of anatomic dissection [52].

6. *The saphenocavernosum shunt* was performed by Grayhack and associates in 1963. They felt that unless some detumescence has been gained by irrigation, this procedure should not be employed [21]. The saphenous vein was isolated and divided distally to the junction with the femoral vein, leaving an 8- to 10-cm segment that is tunneled to the area of the corpora cavernosa. A widely patent elliptic anastomosis is carried out after irrigation of the corporal bodies with a dilute heparin and saline solution. Saphenous vein shunts have several major disadvantages. Cases of pulmonary emboli secondary to thrombosis of the shunt

appear in the literature [13, 28]. Moreover, in this era of bypass vascular surgery, the saphenous vein is a valuable natural resource, not to be used unnecessarily. In 1975, Gruber, in a single case, used the inferior epigastric artery to increase blood flow through the corpora cavernosa to maintain patency of the saphenous shunt [22]. No further reference to this was encountered in the literature. It is well known that the saphenous shunt does not maintain its patency, and, if it does, it paradoxically may cause impotence, due to excessive shunting of blood away from the corporal bodies.

7. J. Barry described a procedure creating a *shunt* from the *corpora cavernosa* to the *dorsal vein* of the penis. In the two cases reported, this led to successful detumescence. The deep or superficial dorsal vein was unilaterally anastomosed in a spatulated macroscopic fashion to the corpora cavernosa [5].

8. An *external shunt* procedure was proposed by Ten Cate and co-workers [61] in 1975. This was an outgrowth of a case reported by Boerema in 1964 of continuous corporal drainage successfully treating priapism. In the external shunt procedure, the corpora are irrigated; polyethylene tubes then are placed proximally within each corporal body. Large infusion needles are positioned in the distal end of both corpora, and a continuous irrigation system is instituted. When bright red blood is exiting, the distal end of the polyethylene drainage tubes are inserted into the veins of the lower arms. This system is maintained for 4 days of detumescence. This was successful in three patients reported, although one developed a penile abscess.

9. *Unilateral internal pudendal artery ligation* has been reported to cure priapism [69]. Three case reports of internal pudendal artery ligation appear in the literature. Two of these patients were impotent [64]. It is well known that after bilateral renal transplantation when both internal iliac arteries are interrupted, there is a significant incidence of impotence on a vasculogenic basis [19].

10. The concept of shunting to the corpora spongiosum has been used in other procedures as well. Winter, using the concept of shunting outflow through the corpora spongiosum, in 1976 reported using a *Travenol Tru-Cut Biopsy Needle* to create a *fistula* between the glans penis (corpora spongiosum) and corpora cavernosa bilaterally [71]. Relatively easily and quickly performed, it has become the surgical treatment of choice. It is usually carried out under local anesthesia. It spares the saphenous vein and is based on sound physiologic principle. The procedure is performed through the dorsal aspect of the glans after detumescence of the erection has been achieved by irrigation. The Tru-Cut Biopsy Needle passed through the anesthetized tract removes a core of tissue between the glans and the most distal portions of both corpora cavernosa, creating a patent fistula. This operation, as described by Winter, is really a modification of that proposed by Ebbehoj in 1975. Ebbehoj's operation created a fistula by puncturing the glans with a narrow knife blade instead of the biopsy needle [16].

RESULTS OF SURGICAL TREATMENT

The results of treatment for priapism are difficult to assess. As has been mentioned, the major sequela of priapism is impotence. Hinman stated in 1914 that if no treatment is utilized, the patient will almost inevitably be impotent [25]. In spite of this, many reports do not include this information. For instance, Baron and Leiter, in reviewing the literature on priapism and sickle cell disease, found 57 percent of 79 patients had no follow-up data [4]. The results of specific medical treatment have been covered in previous sections of this chapter.

A review by Darwish and co-workers [13] in 1974 retrospectively examined 21 episodes of priapism. This group includes eight patients with sickle cell disease or trait who

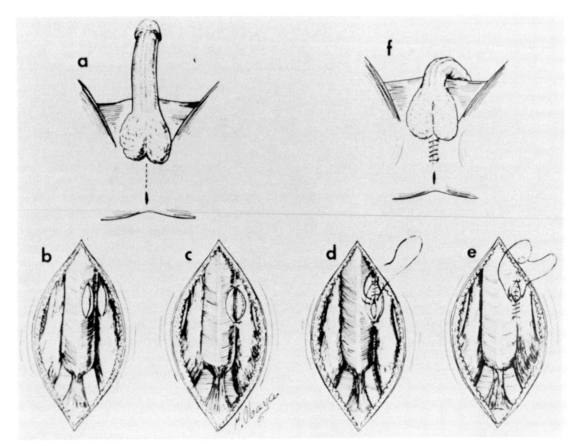

Figure 9-1. Creation of arteriovenous fistula (cavernospongiosal shunt). A. Perineal incision. B. Longitudinal incisions in corpus spongiosum and corpus cavernosum. C. Apical sutures placed for alignment. D., E. Closure with running 5-0 prolene. F. Skin closure. (Reprinted from Wasmer, J. M., et al. Evaluation and treatment of priapism. *J. Urol.* 125:204, 1981. With permission of Williams & Wilkins.)

were initially treated conservatively with nonspecific medical regimens. Only two achieved detumescence with conservative measures, and one of these patients was potent. The remaining 13 patients then underwent needle aspiration and irrigations. Ten (50%) of these responded with flaccidity; however, the potency rate was only 22 percent. Of the eight nonresponding patients, four underwent "successful" corporosaphenous shunts; only one was potent (25%). Four underwent corporospongiosum shunts; three (75%) were potent postoperatively.

Moloney and associates report 5 patients managed conservatively (including irrigations) with a potency rate of 60 percent [41].

Eleven patients underwent a saphenocavernosus shunt. All patients undergoing surgery within 36 hours had a "good result." If an attempt at aspiration had been made, "good results" could be obtained after as much as 48 hours of priapism. The definition

of "good results" was not offered. Eighteen months after corporosaphenous shunts, two impotent patients were demonstrated radiologically to have patent shunts. Ligation of these shunts restored potency. This implies that in potent patients, there is spontaneous thrombosis of the saphenous shunts [41].

In 1972, Klein, Hall, and Smith found 29 reported patients who underwent corporosaphenous shunts. Fourteen of these were potent postoperatively (48%) [30].

Srougi and co-workers performed cavernospongiosum shunts in 10 patients (3 bilateral). There was a 60 percent detumescence

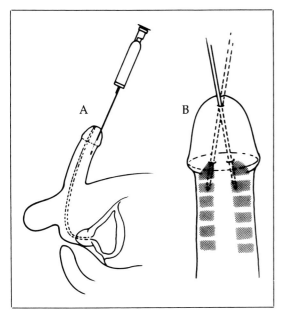

Figure 9-2. A. Sagittal view of biopsy needle entering corpus cavernosum through glans, thus creating fistula. B. Dorsal view showing biopsy needle entering each corpus cavernosum. (Reprinted from Winter, C. C. Priapism cured by creation of fistulas between glans penis and corpora cavernosa. *J. Urol.* 119:227, 1978. With permission of Williams & Wilkins.)

rate and a 50 percent potency rate. Those having early surgical intervention had a greater degree of detumescence and preservation of potency. All patients with priapism of longer duration than 48 hours were impotent postoperatively [58].

LaRocque and Cosgrove (1974), in reviewing their 40 patients, found a 55 percent potency rate among nine patients with medical treatment and adequate follow-up. There did not seem to be any relationship among etiology, duration, and results in this group. Of 11 patients with priapism of greater than 24 hours' duration treated with aspiration, only two of eight (25%) with adequate follow-up were potent. Five of nine patients (55%) undergoing cavernosaphenous or cavernospongiosum shunts were potent. Results did not differ with the type of shunt employed. It is very interesting that all successful shunts were performed in patients who had priapism for longer than 48 hours [34].

The formation of a fistula between the glans penis and corpora cavernosa, as described in the preceding section, has met with early success. Winter reported in 1979 a 60 percent potency rate in five patients, and he alludes to nine other patients successfully treated but not reported [70].

There does not appear to be any difference between cavernosaphenous and cavernosum spongiosum shunts (Figs. 9-1 and 9-2) [43]. Certainly, the latter is a simpler procedure. The cavernosum spongiosum shunt procedure can be complicated by urethrocavernosus fistula, a relatively minor complication as compared to the potential pulmonary emboli associated with cavernosaphenous shunts [13, 31, 70]. Moreover, the preservation of the saphenous veins in this era of elaborate vascular reconstruction is a serious consideration. Both these procedures should be *preceded* by the Winter procedure (transglandular spongiosum cavernosum fistula formation) because of its simplicity and comparable results in early reports.

CONCLUSIONS
The etiologies of priapism are multitudinous. The treatments are many. None has proven to be ideal in terms of preserving potency, and some are associated with severe complications. In a few processes, specific medical treatment can reverse the underlying pathophysiology leading to detumescence. However, in the majority of patients, a short period of conservative management should be quickly followed by surgical interventions as described by Winter. The creation of the transglandular fistula leaves the patient with the greatest chance of preserving potency with the smallest risk; therefore, it is the procedure of choice.

REFERENCES
1. Abeshouse, B. S., and Abeshouse, G. A. Metastatic tumors of the penis: A review of the literature and a report of 2 cases. *J. Urol.* 86:99, 1961.
2. Abeshouse, B. S., and Tankin, L. True priapism: Report of 4 cases and review of literature. *Urol. Cutan. Rev.* 54:449, 1950.

3. Babcock, R. B., Dumper, C. W., and Scharfman, W. B. Heparin-induced immune thrombocytopenia. *N. Engl. J. Med.* 295:237, 1976.

4. Baron, M., and Leiter, E. The management of priapism in sickle cell anemia. *J. Urol.* 119:610, 1978.

5. Barry, J. M. Priapism: Treatment with corpus cavernosum to dorsal vein shunts. *J. Urol.* 116:754, 1976.

6. Becker, L. E., and Mitchell, A. D. Priapism. *Surg. Clin. North Am.* 45:152, 1965.

7. Bhalla, A. K., et al. Prazosin and priapism. *Br. Med. J.* 2:1039, 1979.

8. Brody, J. I., et al. Symptomatic crisis of sickle cell anemia treated with limited exchange transfusion. *Ann. Intern. Med.* 72:327, 1970.

9. Calloman, F. T. Phenomenon of priapism: Diagnostic significance. Initial review. *Urol. Cutan. Rev.* 54:144, 1950.

10. Conti, G. L'erection du penis human et ses bases morphologico-vasculaires. *Acta. Anat.* (Basel) 14:217, 1952.

11. Dahkle, M. B., et al. Priapism during leukapheresis. *Transfusion* 19:482, 1979.

12. Dahlen, C. P., Kaplan, L., and Goodwin, W. E. Priapism occurring as a complication of tularemia. *Surg. Clin. North Am.* 72:1192, 1954.

13. Darwish, M., Atassi, B., and Clark, S. S. Priapism: Evaluation of treatment regimen. *J. Urol.* 112:92, 1974.

14. Deacock, A. H. Malignant priapism due to secondary carcinoma in the corpora cavernosa. *Northwest. Med.* 37:143, 1930.

15. Dorman, B. W., and Schmidt, J. D. Association of priapism in phenothiazine therapy. *J. Urol.* 116:51, 1976.

16. Ebbehoj, J. A new operation for priapism. *Scand. J. Plast. Reconstr. Surg.* 18:241, 1975.

17. Eriksson, A., et al. Priapism: Surgical or medical treatment? *Scand. J. Urol. Nephrol.* 13:1, 1975.

18. Foreman, J. M. Priapism as a complication of mumps. *Med. J. Aust.* 47:378, 1960.

19. Gittes, R., and Waters, B. Sexual impotence: The overlooked complication of a second renal transplant. *J. Urol.* 121:719, 1979.

20. Grayhack, J. T. Early Shunting Procedures in the Treatment of Priapism. In R. Scott, Jr. (ed.), *Current Controversies in Urologic Management.* Philadelphia: Saunders, 1972. P. 377.

21. Grayhack, J. T., et al. Venous bypass to control priapism. *Invest. Urol.* 1:509, 1964.

22. Gruber, H. The treatment of priapism: Use of inferior epigastric artery. A case report. *J. Urol.* 108:882, 1972.

23. Harrow, B. Simple technique for treating priapism. *J. Urol.* 101:71, 1969.

24. Hasen, H. B., and Rainis, L. Priapism associated with sickle cell disease. *J. Urol.* 88:71, 1962.

25. Hinman, F. Priapism: Report of cases and a clinical study of the literature with reference to its pathogenesis and surgical treatment. *Ann. Surg.* 60:639, 1914.

26. Hotchkiss, R. S., and Fernandez-Leal, J. The nervous system as related to fertility and sterility. *J. Urol.* 78:173, 1957.

27. Jaffe, N., and Kim, B. S. Priapism in acute granulocytic leukemia. *Am. J. Dis. Child.* 118:619, 1969.

28. Kandel, G., Bender, L., and Grove, J. Pulmonary embolism: A complication of corpus-saphenous shunt for priapism. *J. Urol.* 99:196, 1968.

29. Katz, E. R., Politano, V., and Scandittio, M. Priapism: An unusual complication of parotitis without orchitis. *J. Urol.* 115:613, 1976.

30. Klein, L. A., Hall, R. L., and Smith, R. B. Surgical treatment of priapism with a note on heparin-induced priapism. *J. Urol.* 108:104, 1972.

31. Klugo, R. C., and Olsson, C. A. Urethrocavernous fistula: Complication of cavernospongiosal shunt. *J. Urol.* 108:750, 1972.

32. Laden, D. I., et al. Amyloidosis presenting as priapism. *Urology* 15:167, 1980.

33. Laha, R. K., Dujovny, M., and Huang, P. Intermittent erection in spinal canal stenosis. *J. Urol.* 121:123, 1979.

34. LaRocque, M., and Cosgrove, M. Priapism: A review of 46 cases. *J. Urol.* 112:770, 1974.

35. Leifer, W., and Leifer, G. Priapism caused by primary thrombocythemia. *J. Urol.* 121:254, 1979.

36. Lich, R. J., Howerton, L. W., and Amin, M. Anatomy and Surgical Approach to the Urogenital Tract in the Male. In J. H. Harrison, et al. (eds.), *Campbell's Urology* (vol. 1). Philadelphia: Saunders, 1978. P. 2526.

37. Lipton, B., and Toomey, J. J. Priapism: An unusual complication of tetanus antitoxin injection. *J. Urol.* 60:371, 1952.

38. MacGregor, R. R. Granulocyte adherence changes induced by hemodialysis, epinephrine, and glucocorticoids. *Ann. Intern. Med.* 86:35, 1977.

39. McKay, R., and Colston, J. Priapism: A new method of treatment. *J. Urol.* 19:121, 1928.

40. Merkin, T. E. Priapism as a sequela of chlorpromazine therapy. *J.A.C.E.P.* 6:367, 1977.

41. Moloney, P. J., Elliott, G. B., and Johnson, H. W. Experiences with priapism. *J. Urol.* 114:72, 1975.

42. Narayana, A. S., Kelly, D. G., and Duff, F. A. Malignant priapism. *Br. J. Urol.* 49:326, 1977.

43. Nelson, J., and Winter, C. Priapism: Evolution of management in 48 patients in a 22 year series. *J. Urol.* 117:455, 1977.

44. Newman, H. F., Northrup, J. D., and Devlin, J. Mechanism of human penile erection. *In-*

vest. Urol. 1:350, 1964.

45. Newman, H. F., Northrup, J. D., and Devlin, J. Mechanism of human penile erection. *Invest. Urol.* 1:350, 1964.

46. Nieder, R. Ketamine treatment of priapism. *J. A. M. A.* 221:195, 1972.

47. Ookoshi, M. (ed.). *Priapism.* Tokyo: Nankodo, 1950. Pp. 1-75.

48. Persky, L., and Kursh, E. Posttraumatic priapism. *J. Urol.* 118:397, 1977.

49. Ravindran, M. Cauda equina compression presenting as spontaneous priapism. *J. Neurol. Neurosurg. Psychiatry* 42:280, 1979.

50. Rifkind, S., et al. The exchange pheresis for priapism in sickle cell disease. *J. A. M. A.* 242: 2317, 1979.

51. Rosenbaum, E. H., Thompson, H. E., and Glassberg, A. B. Priapism in multiple myeloma: Successful treatment with plasmapheresis. *Urology* 12:201, 1978.

52. Sacher, E., et al. Cavernospongiosum shunt in the treatment of priapism. *J. Urol.* 108: 97, 1972.

53. Schreibmen, S. M., et al. Management of priapism in patients with chronic granulocytic leukemia. *J. Urol.* 111:786, 1974.

54. Seeler, R. A. Intensive transfusion therapy for priapism in boy with sickle cell anemia. *J. Urol.* 110:360, 1973.

55. Seeler, R. A., and Sbwiaki, M. Z. Acute splenic sequestration crisis (ASSC) in young children with sickle cell anemia. *Clin. Pediatr.* (Phila.) 11:704, 1972.

56. Smith, M. J. V., and Bonacarti, A. F. Malignant priapism due to clear cell carcinoma: A case report and review of the literature. *J. Urol.* 92:297, 1964.

57. Sözer, I. T. The treatment of priapism by a new antihypertensive drug: Sodium nitroprusside and penile aspiration. *J. Urol.* 99:311, 1968.

58. Srougi, M., et al. Cavernospongiosum shunt in management of priapism: Is it a reliable method? *Int. Urol. Nephrol.* 10:229, 1978.

59. Stein, J., and Martin, D. Priapism. *Urology* 111:8, 1974.

60. Takaku, A., Fukawa, O., and Suzuki, J. A case of priapism with ruptured intracranial aneurysm. *J. Neurol.* 221:279, 1979.

61. Ten Cate, H. W., Gallas, P., and Thé, P. The external shunt in the treatment of idiopathic priapism. *J. Urol.* 114:726, 1975.

62. Ulm, A. H. The treatment of primary priapism with Arfonad. *J. Urol.* 81:291, 1959.

63. Vadakan, V. V., and Ortega, J. Priapism in acute lymphoblastic leukemia. *Cancer* 30:373, 1972.

64. Wear, J. B., Jr., Crummy, A. B., and Munson, B. O. A new approach to the treatment of priapism. *J. Urol.* 117:252, 1977.

65. Weiss, H. The physiology of human penile erection. *Ann. Intern. Med.* 76:793, 1972.

66. Weiss, J. M., and Ferguson, D. Priapism: The danger of treatment with compression. *J. Urol.* 112:616, 1974.

67. Williams, H. M., Diamond, H. D., and Craver, L. F. The pathogenesis and management of neurological complications in patients with malignant lymphomas and leukemia. *Cancer* 11:76, 1953.

68. Wilson, S. K., Klonsky, B. L., and Rhamy, R. K. A new etiology of priapism: Fabry's disease. *J. Urol.* 109:646, 1973.

69. Winter, C. Priapism. *Urol. Surv.* 28:163, 1978.

70. Winter, C. Priapism treated by a modification of creation of fistulas between glans penis and corpora cavernosa. *J. Urol.* 121:743, 1978.

71. Winter, C. Cure of idiopathic priapism. *Urology* 8:389, 1976.

10

Drug-Related Male Sexual Dysfunction

HARRIS M. NAGLER AND
CARL A. OLSSON

Much of the literature dealing with drug-related male sexual dysfunction is anecdotal in nature. We will review drugs that exert an adverse effect on any of the factors associated with normal male sexual function. Use of the term *sexual dysfunction* therefore should not be limited to erectile dysfunction, since abnormalities of ejaculation and depressed libido are similarly disturbing to the normal male.

DRUGS OF ABUSE

In the category of *drugs of abuse* we include a variety of compounds employed in an addictive or recreational fashion. These agents have wide-ranging physiologic and psychologic effects and represent a significant cause of sexual dysfunction in modern society. The discussion of the effects of these agents on potency can be oriented toward various classes of compounds, including (1) alcohol, (2) marijuana, (3) stimulants, (4) sedatives, and (5) narcotics.

Alcohol Abuse

Alcohol consumption exerts effects on sexual function that vary according to the amount consumed. Furthermore, chronic overconsumption results in physiologic changes that also affect sexual performance. Ingestion of small quantities of alcohol may have a disinhibiting effect and actually lead to improved sexual performance in some individuals. Acute alcohol intoxication, however, impairs erectile capability because of its sedating influence as well as its vasodilatory properties. Since there is often a fine line between disinhibition and intoxication, patients often will describe an increased desire for sexual activity after consumption of alcohol, but ability to perform adequately is diminished.

Chronic alcohol abuse results in a multitude of physiologic and psychologic sequelae affecting sexual performance. Both a central and peripheral neuropathy may develop, as well as endocrine abnormalities. Libido may be maintained in chronic alcoholics, and this offers further evidence of the contribution of peripheral neuropathy as an etiologic factor in alcohol-induced impotence [29].

The effect of chronic alcohol consumption on endocrine homeostasis has been well documented. Gordon and co-workers demonstrated that alcohol has a direct effect on testosterone metabolism, even in the absence of cirrhosis and/or associated nutritional factors [30]. Plasma testosterone levels were decreased in subjects in this study, related, in part to suppression of luteinizing hormone. In additional animals and in in-vitro studies conducted by the same workers, Leydig cells were demonstrated to be refractory to gonadotropins, and increased peripheral conversion of testosterone was demonstrated [31].

There is good evidence of increased hepatic clearance of testosterone in patients subjected to alcohol administration [71]. In part, this is a result of increase of hepatic aromatization of testosterone; additionally, there is an apparent increase in the metabolic activity of liver microsomal 5-α-reductase.

Historically, feminization accompanying cirrhosis has been explained by increases in the total plasma estradiol as a result of increased peripheral aromatization of testosterone to estrogen. There is an apparent increase in sex steroid–binding globulin seen in cirrhosis; this increase, however, is not sufficient to bind all of the increased plasma estradiol; as a result there is an overall increase in free estradiol in cirrhotics [79]. Another proposed mechanism for abnormal steroidogenesis is the excessively high concentration of testicular reduced nicotinamide adenine dinucleotide seen in chronic alcoholism [79].

Van Thiel offers the hypothesis that altered sexual function associated with alcoholism occurs on an organic basis secondarily to a hypoandrogenic state. A vicious cycle ensues, in which the sexually dysfunctional alcoholic is driven to seek solace in further alcohol consumption [78].

Therefore, although there is much controversy concerning the mechanism by which alcohol exerts effects on steroid metabolism, there is no doubt that hypogonadism, decreased fertility, and impotence are real sequelae of alcohol abuse. In 1971, there were 9 million alcohol abusers in the United States. Van Thiel has stated, "In view of the frequency of disturbances of sexual function in chronic alcoholics, alcoholism is certainly the most common cause of nonfunctional impotence and sterility in the United States."

Marijuana

There are conflicting reports as to the effect of cannabis compounds on serum testosterone levels. Initial reports by Kolodny suggested that chronic use of marijuana led to suppression of plasma testosterone [48]. Subsequent reports by Mendelson and associates as well as Hembree and co-workers did not substantiate these findings, however [39,59]. Recently, it has been shown that chronic administration of marijuana leads to a mild elevation of serum gonadotropins [27].

Kolodny has reported impotence secondary to long-term marijuana use [48]. Other authors suggest that marijuana exerts a mildly aphrodisiac effect, resulting in improved sexual performance [26]. In summary, it does appear that short-term marijuana use may result in improved sexual performance in some individuals (perhaps related to its disinhibiting properties). In contrast, long-term use of marijuana may lead to impotence, based on organic and psychogenic changes.

Stimulants

Amitriptyline (Elavil) is a tricyclic antidepressant known to have strong anticholinergic effects [29]. If acetylcholine were the final neurotransmitter responsible for penile erection, one might expect a high rate of impotence in patients administered these compounds; but this has not been shown by clinical reviews. Inhibition of ejaculation has been reported with amitriptyline, however [73].

Imipramine (Tofranil) rarely has been reported as a cause of erectile dysfunction. An incidence of 0.5 percent impotence was noted in over 1000 cases treated with this agent [73].

Monoamine oxidase (MAO) inhibitors block the oxidative deamination of neural monoamines [29]. Wyatt employed phenelzine in the management of narcolepsy. He reported three males who, during initial therapy with phenelzine, developed erectile dysfunction that later resolved without cessation of the drug [84]. Further, ejaculatory difficulty has been reported with the use of MAO inhibitors [29].

By far, the stimulants most subject to abuse in our society are the amphetamines and cocaine. Amphetamines have been associated with an increase in libido [29]. Further, Kramer reported that the sexual act could be prolonged by delay of orgasm with the use of amphetamines, and the intensity of orgasm was apparently increased in subjects studied [50]. Cocaine has psychogenic properties similar to those of amphetamines [21]. Although it is not well documented in the medical literature, individuals using cocaine in a recreational fashion claim to experience increased libido and delay in orgasm as well as an increase in intensity of orgasm. In our own experience, however, there have been some circumstances in which patients report orgasmic failure with the recreational use of amphetamines and/or cocaine. Furthermore, some men report erectile failure, despite experiencing increased libido, with the use of these agents.

Sedating Agents
Phenothiazines are a group of compounds that exert peripheral cholinergic blocking activity. In addition, they exert an alpha-adrenergic antagonist activity and an adrenergic effect related to block of peripheral reuptake of amines [29]. These various neurologic actions make the prediction of response to a particular drug unreliable.

Because of the complicated neurologic actions of the phenothiazines, various effects on sexuality may result. The major side effect attributed to these compounds is ejaculatory impotence [32]. The mechanism by which ejaculatory failure is produced is thought to be related to the sympatholytic effects of phenothiazines. The anticholinergic effects of these compounds may provide an explanation for the impotence associated with their use [49]. Kotin found a 50 percent incidence of sexual dysfunction in men administered thioridazine (Mellaril) [49]. Forty-four percent of patients in this study had experienced diffi-

culty attaining or maintaining an erection. Forty-nine percent of men complained of ejaculatory difficulty. Kotin compared the effects of thioridazine with other major tranquilizers studied in the series. Overall, patients administered sedating agents experienced a 19 percent incidence of erectile dysfunction and generally reported no ejaculatory difficulties. Thus, the incidence of sexual dysfunction with thioridazine (one of the most widely prescribed major tranquilizers in the United States) was significantly higher than that reported with other tranquilizing agents.

An additional mechanism by which phenothiazines interfere with sexual function may be related to the elevation of serum prolactin levels noted with use of these agents [42]. Franks has clearly established the relationship between hyperprolactinemia and impotence [24].

Chlordiazepoxide (Librium) is a widely used anxiolytic agent. Isolated reports of ejaculatory and erectile failure have appeared in the literature [45]. Ejaculatory difficulties also have been noted in patients administered trifluoperazine, butaperazine, and the butyrophenones as well [7]. Chlorprazine and chlorprothixine are other phenothiazinelike drugs that have been reported to cause ejaculatory failure [66].

Narcotic Agents
Addiction to heroin, methadone, or other narcotics may lead to loss of potency by several mechanisms. The most obvious mechanism is the sedative-depressant effect of these drugs. However, an addiction process leads to social disruption, and social factors interfering with sexual performance are difficult to assess.

Hanbury found that one-third of patients in a methadone maintenance program experienced some form of sexual dysfunction [38]. Of this one-third, 50 percent experienced erectile impotence and 88 percent complained of orgasmic failure. Overall, more than one-third of patients on methadone maintenance complain of a loss of libido. Polydrug abuse or polydrug dosage was not correlated with the degree of sexual dysfunction. Similar sexual dysfunction was experienced with heroin.

In contrast to this experience, animal studies have demonstrated no alteration in sexual behavior with methadone administration [18]. Furthermore, Mintz found sexual dysfunction in 50 percent of drug-free, previously addicted veterans [62]. These findings raise the real question of the "horse before the cart" [16, 19, 58, 60]. Is sexual dysfunction resulting from heroin and methadone use based on psychologic factors associated with the addictive personality, so that sexual dysfunction becomes "unmasked" by the addiction?

There have been many studies of the effects of heroin and methadone on endocrine function. Cicero demonstrated a reduction in secondary sex organ and gonadal function subsequent to methadone or heroin addiction [16]. Nearly all heroin addicts and methadone maintenance patients report decreased libido. Mendelson reported a decrease in plasma testosterone levels in both heroin addiction and methadone maintenance patients, with an even more significant reduction in serum testosterone in the latter [60].

Decreased testosterone levels may indeed affect sexual function, but, since it has been well established that some castrated patients are capable of normal sexual function, there may be a great psychosocial or psychosexual contribution to the sexual dysfunction seen in patients receiving heroin or methadone.

ANTIHYPERTENSIVES

The drugs most often implicated as causing erectile impotence are the antihypertensives. "All drugs used for the treatment of hypertension can cause adverse sexual effects" [77]. Antihypertensive agents of each class work by a different mechanism of action, and not all classes cause impotence; ejaculatory disturbances occur with some of the drugs used to control hypertension. This section will deal with the various classes of drugs employed in the management of hypertension; prototype agents in each class will be addressed specifically regarding effects on sexual activity.

Methyldopa

Methyldopa (Aldomet) initially was thought to exert its antihypertensive effect as a peripheral adrenergic blocking agent. However, it is now thought to act on the central nervous system [29]. This belief is supported by the major side effect seen with this drug (drowsiness and/or depression).

Alexander and Evans reported a 53 percent incidence of erectile failure with Aldomet [4]. Bulpitt and Dollery also observed sexual dysfunction with methyldopa, recording impotence and ejaculatory failure in 35.7 and 18.5 percent of men, respectively [12]. These figures must, of course, be compared to control groups to substantiate the influence of methyldopa on sexual function.

Bulpitt stated that 17 percent of untreated hypertensive males complain of erectile failure [12]. If this observation is correct, one can easily conclude that methyldopa does indeed lead to sexual dysfunction. Gibb did not report any alterations in libido in 17 patients treated with methyldopa [28], but no direct questions regarding sexual function were posed in this study. It is well established that, unless specific questions regarding sexual function are asked, many patients will not volunteer information about dysfunction. In contrast, Newman and Salerno reported that more than 25 percent of patients treated with methyldopa experienced decreased libido, as well as erectile and ejaculatory difficulties [65]. Furthermore, when this medication was discontinued, sexual dysfunction resolved.

The mechanism by which methyldopa causes sexual dysfunction is unknown. It may cause central nervous system depression, which may result in altered libido. In addition, prolactin levels have been reported to be elevated secondarily to administration of methyldopa. Regardless of the mechanism by which sexual dysfunction results from methyldopa use, the high incidence of this complication has resulted in a general avoidance of this drug in the management of hypertension in the sexually active male.

Rauwolfia Alkaloids

The rauwolfia alkaloids are agents that exert

their major pharmacologic effect by means of central depletion of catecholamines and 5-hydroxytyramine [29]. A significant degree of psychologic depression is associated with these compounds, so they largely have fallen into disfavor as primary agents in the management of the hypertensive patient.

The most common rauwolfia alkaloid employed is *reserpine*. This compound is associated with impotence in 33 percent of patients, and ejaculatory failure in 14 percent [11]. A recent report by Boyden and co-workers suggested that only 1 of 27 patients administered reserpine developed impotence [9]. Thus it would seem that, in doses of less than 0.3 mg daily, reserpine does not appear to alter sexual function. The U.S. Veterans Administration cooperative study of hypertensive agents showed no difference in sexual dysfunction in hypertensive patients regardless of the treatment regimen employed [80]. For example, the impotence rate with reserpine was 3.6 percent (8 of 220 patients). Thus, it is not clear that reserpine is associated with increased sexual dysfunction if dosage is minimized and central depression avoided, but it should be recalled that in doses higher than 0.25 mg, reserpine can cause elevation of plasma prolactin levels, and this may be a mechanism whereby sexual dysfunction occurs [53].

Propranolol

Propranolol is an effective beta-adrenergic blocking agent used in the treatment of hypertension. The proposed mechanism whereby hypertension is alleviated is the reduction of plasma renin, with decreased arterial resistance [29]. The U.S. Veterans Administration Cooperative Study Group on Antihypertensive Agents did not find that propranolol use resulted in any higher incidence of impotence in hypertensive patients than did the use of any other treatment regimen. In fact only 6 of 229 patients receiving propranolol experienced erectile impotence [80]. Warren and Warren, in contrast, reported impotence occurring in slightly more than 5 percent of men treated with propranolol in dosage exceeding 120 mg daily

[82]. It should be recalled, however, that untreated patients with hypertension may experience impotence in a much higher percentage. Therefore the influence of propranolol, even in high doses, on sexual function is still not known.

Forsberg found an alteration in the penile-brachial artery flow acceleration ratio in patients who reportedly became impotent after propranolol administration [22]. Furthermore, they demonstrated the restoration of normal penile-brachial acceleration ratios and return of potency with the cessation of this drug. They hypothesized an alpha-adrenergic predominance in "vulnerable persons," with a release of dominant penile vascular constriction and consequent impotence in some men. This is consistent with the observation that a Raynaud-like phenomenon has been observed in up to 5 percent of patients treated with propanolol [34, 56].

Ganglionic Blocking Agents

Guanethidine is the prototype of the class of drugs that depress the function of postganglionic adrenergic nerves. Both alpha- and beta-adrenergic receptors are equally suppressed by guanethidine administration [29]. The sympatholytic effects of guanethidine should not produce erectile impotence, but may indeed cause ejaculatory failure. It has been our experience, as well as that of others, that erectile impotence may follow closely ejaculatory failure because of psychogenic concerns.

Hollander reported ejaculatory impotence in 60 percent of patients treated with guanethidine [41]. Bulpitt and Dollery also reported a 60 percent ejaculatory failure rate in patients treated with this drug; a 41 percent rate of ejaculatory disturbance was seen with a similar agent, *bethanidine* [11]. In addition, the Bulpitt and Dollery survey demonstrated erectile difficulties in 54 percent of patients receiving guanethidine and 67 patients on bethanidine.

Thus, there is a definite relationship between ejaculatory dysfunction and the use of ganglionic blocking agents. There was also an apparent increase in erectile dysfunction as well. The mechanism by which this drug causes impotence is not clear, and it may be merely a secondary phenomenon arising from psychologic concern about ejaculatory failure. Unfortunately, it is not possible to assess this factor retrospectively at this time.

Clonidine

Clonidine (*Catapres*), like guanethidine, is a sympatholytic agent. Its activity is primarily central, as opposed to peripheral, although there is a definite peripheral alpha-adrenolytic effect as well [29].

Onesti and co-workers reported a 22 percent rate of impotence in 59 patients treated with clonidine [67]. The erectile dysfunction occurring with clonidine is apparently dose related. The mechanism of clonidine-induced impotence may be its central depressive effects as well as a more complex means by which presynaptic alpha-adrenergic stimulation results [29]. That clonidine is rarely used as a single antihypertensive agent makes the assessment of the sexual dysfunction associated with this drug a difficult task.

Hydralazine

Vasodilating agents have not been linked clearly with erectile difficulties in man [43]. Hydralazine, however, preferentially causes dilatation of arterioles, with extensive peripheral vasodilatation [29]. Coronary, splanchnic, cerebral, and renal vascular perfusion are augmented, whereas cutaneous and muscular blood flow is decreased [47].

There have been a few case reports of erectile dysfunction in men undergoing therapy with hydralazine [3, 46] but hydralazine is infrequently used alone, and its role in altering sexual function is therefore clouded. There is, in fact, no clear mechanism by which impotence secondary to hydralazine use can be explained; the association of hydralazine and impotence is not well established.

DIURETIC AGENTS

Spironolactone

Spironolactone is a diuretic agent similar to the thiazides, which leads to a reduction in plasma volume when used in the treatment of hypertension [29]. A well-known side effect of this drug is the estrogenlike effects it has in men; these are manifested by loss of libido, impotence, and gynecomastia [55].

Experimental evidence shows that spironolactone inhibits testosterone production in children, although alterations in plasma testosterone are difficult to document in adults treated with this drug. Moreover, spironolactone acts as an antiandrogen and binds competitively for androgen receptors [17, 69]. This antiandrogen effect may be the mechanism whereby sexual dysfunction occurs in men receiving this medication. Although there has been much work elucidating the mechanisms of sexual dysfunction secondary to spironolactone use, there is great controversy regarding the incidence of impotence resulting from use of this drug [35]. For example, Castro and associates found that only 1 in 17 patients treated with spironolactone developed impotence on the treatment regimen [15]. Zarren and Black reported one case of impotence and four instances of decreased libido in seven men treated with spironolactone [85]. Spark and Melby in using spironolactone in the diagnosis of aldosteronism, found that 39 percent of patients so treated had relative impotence on a spironolactone dosage of 3 mg daily [74].

Chlorthalidone

Reports of impotence secondary to use of chlorthalidone (a diuretic) are scarce. However, Stessman and Ben-Ishay have clearly documented cases of impotence and decreased libido who recovered after decreasing or discontinuing this drug [75].

Carbonic Anhydrase Inhibitors

Acetazolamide is a carbonic anhydrase inhibitor that has limited diuretic properties but that is of great clinical value in the management of glaucoma and conditions requiring urine alkalinization [29]. Wallace and associates reported 39 patients with glaucoma who developed erectile dysfunction when treated with carbonic anhydrase inhibitors [81]. Drug cessation and reexposure confirmed that diminished libido and erectile dysfunction were directly related to use of the drug. Lichter conducted a crossover study employing both placebo and carbonic anhydrase inhibitors [54]. This study demonstrated decreased libido with the diuretic agent, but not with placebo. The mechanism by which acetazolamide produces erectile dysfunction is unknown. It may be related to the resultant systemic acidosis or it may be a direct depressive effect of the agent on the central nervous system [63].

CARDIAC DRUGS
Digitalis Compounds
Digitalis is believed to exert an effect on endocrine metabolism because of its chemical similarity to the sex steroid hormones [29]. Neri and associates demonstrated a subjective deterioration of sexual function in patients administered long-term digitalis therapy [64]. In addition, they documented an increase in serum estradiol, a decrease in serum testosterone, and decreased erectile capability in men. The cardiac glycosides, digitoxin and digoxin (which do not occur naturally) exert estrogenic effects as well [13, 70, 76]. Gynecomastia, a well-documented side effect of digitalis therapy, is further supportive evidence of a strong estrogenic effect of these compounds [40].

In addition to the alterations in endocrine status secondary to use of digitalis, patients requiring this medication may experience many other physiologic and psychologic changes contributing to sexual dysfunction. This tends to obscure the precise contribution of the medication to sexual dysfunction.

Disopyramide
Disopyramide (Norpace) is used to prevent arrhythmias following myocardial infarction [29]. It has strong anticholinergic properties and has been reported to cause erectile impotence in high plasma concentrations [57].

Perhexiline Maleate
Perhexiline (Texid) is used in the management of angina [29]. Howard and Reese reported the onset of impotence in 9 of 16 men treated over a long period with this agent [44]. Withdrawal of the drug for a period of 1 month did not restore potency in these men, however. As with digitalis preparations, persons requiring treatment for angina are difficult to assess because of associated changes in physiology and psychologic status common in angina sufferers.

PROLACTIN-ALTERING DRUGS
Many drugs have been reported to alter serum prolactin concentration. Some of these agents are discussed in other sections of this chapter. Both alpha-sympatholytic and -sympathomimetic agents have been implicated in producing hyperprolactinemia. Beta-adrenergic blockers, dopaminergic blockers, and seratoninlike agents also have been responsible for elevations of serum prolactin [52].

The influence of hyperprolactinemia on sexual function is well documented. Franks and associates reported 20 patients with elevated prolactin levels, of whom 17 experienced decreased libido and only six had no sexual dysfunction [23]. Treatment of the hyperprolactinemia with normalization of prolactin led to return of normal sexual function in those patients affected. Carter also reported on 22 men with abnormal prolactin levels, of whom 20 had decreased libido or impotence [14]. Here again, patients experiencing sexual dysfunction improved after bromocriptine therapy. There is experimental evidence suggesting that prolactin may alter the conversion of testosterone to dihydrotestosterone. This is a potential mechanism by which hyperprolactinemia results in sexual dysfunction. It should be emphasized that in both the Franks and Carter reports, a number of men had low normal levels of serum testosterone that generally returned to normal range after correction of the hyperprolactinemia. In summary, it can be stated that various agents produce the side effect of hyperprolactinemia; the condition usually is associated with some degree of sexual dysfunction in men.

HORMONES
This section will not discuss the known influences of estrogenic agents on sexual function in the male. Erectile potency has been as-

sumed to be androgen-dependent since male sex hormones were isolated in the 1930s, but potency can be maintained for long periods after castration, despite the associated lowering of plasma testosterone. Brenner documented this variable response to castration [10]. As is mentioned in the section of this chapter dealing with hyperprolactinemia, more importance must be attributed to the interrelationship between testosterone and other endocrine events in modulating sexual function.

Agents acting as antiandrogens, such as cyproterone acetate and spironolactone have been associated with sexual dysfunction, and such abnormalities are usually correlated with decreasing plasma testosterone levels [51]. Similarly, progestational agents exert an antiandrogenic effect and also are associated with sexual dysfunction [61].

"While there is a strong clinical impression of the importance of androgens in restoring sexual function to men with postpubertal primary hypogonadism, evidence of a systematic and detailed kind is hard to find"[5]. Hypogonadism always should be searched for in evaluating the impotent patient and, if it is documented, replacement therapy should be attempted. Empiric use of androgens has met with repeated failure in the treatment of the impotent male, however.

ANTICHOLINERGIC DRUGS

Any drug exerting anticholinergic activity may cause erectile impotence [29]. There are a multitude of such agents, some of which have been discussed in previous sections of this chapter. The categories of agents that exert anticholinergic effects include the tricyclic antidepressants; antiparkinsonian drugs such as trihexylphenidyl and benztropine; agents used in the management of vertigo and nausea; antihistamines; antidepressants; and various other psychoactive agents.

Propantheline and other smooth muscle relaxants exerting an antinicotinic effect also have been associated with erectile impotence. Finally, some skeletal muscle relaxants have been associated with erectile dysfunction [29].

The mechanism of penile erection is poorly understood. Undoubtedly, it is a more complicated phenomenon than one of simple mediation by parasympathetic innervation. Thus, although anticholinergic agents are associated with erectile dysfunction in some men, it is also clear that one cannot predict the occurrence or incidence or erectile dysfunction resulting from treatment with these drugs.

MISCELLANEOUS AGENTS
Cimetidine
Cimetidine (Tagamet) is a histamine- (H2) receptor antagonist employed in the treatment of peptic ulcer [29]. Several observations of erectile impotence associated with cimetidine therapy have been published, and many more cases have been reported to the Committee on Safety of Medicines (England) [1, 6, 36, 68, 82]. Cimetidine has been shown to cause an endocrinopathy, leading to gynecomastia in men [6, 36]. Elevated gonadotropin levels have been reported in patients who became impotent after administration of this drug [8]. Cimetidine has been demonstrated in laboratory studies to compete at dihydrotestosterone-binding sites; this may be one mechanism in which the antiandrogenic effect of cimetidine is revealed [25]. Hyperprolactinemia also has been seen after cimetidine administration, although this has not been a constant observation [1, 6, 8, 36, 68]. Other workers have postulated that histamine may be a neurotransmitter of importance in penile erection and that cimetidine prevents erection by blocking H2 receptors in the penis [1, 2, 6, 8, 25, 36].

Thus, several endocrinologic abnormalities have been associated with cimetidine treatment, although these have not been documented consistently. The mechanism whereby impotence results from cimetidine use remains elusive, but the overall incidence of erectile dysfunction with cimetidine therapy is apparently low [61].

Levodopa
L-Dopa is an agent useful in the management both of Parkinson's disease and depression

[29]. This drug also has been used in metastatic prostate cancer to reduce serum prolactin, which is thought to have a facilitative effect on prostate growth. Erectile dysfunction has not been reported with this agent, but Hallstrom and Persson have noted ejaculatory failure in some individuals [37]. The mechanism by which L-dopa results in nonemission on orgasm is probably related to its adrenolytic properties.

Clofibrate

Clofibrate has become one of the most widely used hypolipidemic drugs [29]. It has been reported that impotence that occurred while the patient was on medication improved after discontinuance (returning again after reexposure) [72].

ε-Aminocaproic Acid

ε-Aminocaproic acid (Amicar) is an antifibrinolytic agent employed in various coagulopathies as well as in the management of urinary tract bleeding [29]. The agent has been shown to cause loss of ejaculation without inhibition of orgasm or erection in 5 of 26 patients receiving prophylactic medication after tooth extraction [20]. With cessation of the medication, ejaculatory difficulty was short-lived and normal ejaculation was restored.

CONCLUSIONS

This chapter discusses some of the many drugs that can alter male sexual function. In some instances, the mechanism by which an agent causes sexual dysfunction has been evaluated; with most drugs, however, the mechanism of action causing dysfunction remains obscure. The reason for this obscurity is that normal sexual function is a synthesis of complicated events, so it is nearly impossible unequivocally to ascribe abnormal sexual function to use of particular drug. Before we can further clarify drug actions that are deleterious to sexual function, a greater understanding of endocrinologic, neurologic, and vascular contributions to normal sexual function is required.

Meanwhile, the physician continues to administer to men agents that interfere with their normal sexual activity. It is important for the practitioner to become especially familiar with agents that are known to cause sexual dysfunction. Patients should be questioned directly regarding sexual functioning before one prescribes these medications; after initiation of therapy, another evaluation should be carried out. In this fashion, we should be able to further clarify the effects of treatment regimens (as opposed to the disease processes for which they are prescribed) on sexual functioning in the male.

REFERENCES

1. Adaikan, P. G., and Karim, S. M. Male sexual dysfunction during treatment with cimetidine. *Br. Med. J.* 1:1282, 1979.
2. Adaikan, P. G., and Karim, S. M. Effects of histamine on the human penis muscle in vitro. *Eur. J. Pharmacol.* 45:261, 1977.
3. Ahmad, S. Hydralazine and male impotence. *Chest* 78:359, 1980.
4. Alexander, W. D., and Evan, J. I. Side effects of methyldopa. *Br. Med. J.* 2:501, 1975.
5. Bancroft, J. Hormones and sexual behavior. *Psychol. Med.* 7:553, 1977.
6. Barber, S. G. Male sexual dysfunction and cimetidine. *Br. Med. J.* 1:1147, 1979.
7. Blair, J. H., and Simpson, G. M. Effect of antipsychotic drugs on reproductive function. *Dis. Nerv. Syst.* 27:645, 1966.
8. Bohnet, H. G., et al. Effects of cimetidine on prolactin, LH, and sex steroid secretion in male and female volunteers. *Acta Endocrinol. (Copenh.)* 88:428, 1978.
9. Boyden, T. W., et al. Reserpine, hydrochlorothiazide, and pituitary gonadal hormones in hypertensive patients. *Eur. J. Clin. Pharmacol.* 17:329, 1980.
10. Brenner, J. *Asexualization: A Follow-up Study of 244 Cases.* New York: Macmillan, 1959.
11. Bulpitt, C. J., and Dollery, C. T. Side effects of hypotensive agents evaluated by self-administered questionnaire. *Br. Med. J.* 3:485, 1973.
12. Bulpitt, C. J., Dollery, C. T., and Carne, S. A symptom questionnaire for hypertensive patients. *J. Chronic Dis.* 27:309, 1974.
13. Burkhardt, D., Verra, C. A., and LaDue, Y. S. Effects of digitalis on urinary pituitary gonadotropin excretion: A study of postmenopausal women. *Ann. Intern. Med.* 68:1069, 1968.
14. Carter, J. N., Tyson, J. E., and Tolis, G. Prolactin-secreting pituitary tumors and hypogonadism in 22 men. *N. Engl. J. Med.* 299:852, 1978.

15. Castro, J. E., Griffiths, H. J. L., and Edwards, D. E. A double blind controlled clinical trial of spironolactone for benign prostatic hypertrophy. *Br. J. Surg.* 58:485, 1971.

16. Cicero, T. J., et al. Function of the male sex organs in heroin and methadone users. *N. Engl. J. Med.* 292:882, 1975.

17. Corvol, P., et al. Antiandrogenic effect of spironolactones mechanism of action. *Endocrinology* 97:52, 1975.

18. Crowley, T. J., et al. Monkey motor stimulation and altered social behavior during chronic methadone administration. *Psychopharmacologia* 43:135, 1975.

19. Cushman, P. Sexual behavior in heroin addiction and methadone maintenance. *N. Y. State J. Med.* 72:1261, 1972.

20. Evans, B., and Aledorf, L. M. Inhibition of ejaculation due to ε-aminocaproic acid. *N. Engl. J. Med.* 298:166, 1978.

21. Fishman, M. W., et al. Cardiovascular and subjective effects of intravenous cocaine administration in humans. *Arch. Gen. Psychiatry* 33:983, 1976.

22. Forsberg, L., et al. Impotence, smoking, and β-blocking drugs. *Fertil. Steril.* 31:589, 1979.

23. Franks, S., et al. Hyperprolactinaemia and impotence. *Clin. Endocrinol.* 8:277, 1978.

24. Franks, S., et al. Hyperprolactinaemia and impotence. *Clin. Endocrinol. (Oxf.)* 8:277, 1978.

25. Funder, J. W., and Mercer, J. E. Cimetidine, a histamine H_2-receptor antagonist, occupies androgen receptors. *J. Clin. Endocrinol. Metab.* 48:189, 1979.

26. Gag, G., and Sheppard, C. Sex in the "drug culture." *Med. Hum. Sex.* 6:28, 1972.

27. Garnick, M. B. Spurious rise in human chorionic gonadotropin induced by marijuana in patients with testicular cancer. *N. Engl. J. Med.* 303:1177, 1980.

28. Gibb, W. E. et al. Comparison of bethanidine, α-methyldopa, and reserpine in essential hypertension. *Lancet* 2:275, 1970.

29. Gilman, A. G., and Goodman, L. S. (eds.), *The Pharmacologic Basis of Therapeutics.* New York: MacMillan, 1980.

30. Gordon, G. G., et al. Effect of alcohol (ethanol) administration on sex hormone metabolism in normal men. *N. Engl. J. Med.* 295:793, 1976.

31. Gordon, G. G., et al. The effect of alcohol ingestion on hepatic aromatase activity and plasma steroid hormones in the rat metabolism. *Metabolism* 28:20, 1979.

32. Green, M. Inhibition of ejaculation as a side-effect of Mellaril. *Am. J. Psychiatry* 118:172, 1961.

33. Greenberg, H. R. Erectile impotence during the course of Tofranil therapy. *Am. J. Psychiatry* 121:1021, 1965.

34. Greenblatt, D. J., and Koch-Weser, J. Adverse reactions to beta-adrenergic receptor blocking drugs: A report from the Boston Collaborative Drug Surveillance Program. *Drugs* 7:118, 1974.

35. Greenblatt, D. J., and Koch-Weser, J. Gynecomastia and impotence: Complications of spironolactone therapy. *J.A.M.A.* 223:82, 1973.

36. Hall, W. H. Breast changes in males on cimetidine. *N. Engl. J. Med.* 295:841, 1976.

37. Hällström, T., and Persson, T. L-Dopa and non-emission of semen. *Lancet* 1:1231, 1970.

38. Hanbury, R., Cohen, M., and Stimmel, B. Adequacy of sexual performance in men maintained on methadone. *Am. J. Drug Alcohol Abuse* 41:13, 1977.

39. Hembree, W. C., Zeidenberg, P., and Naboa, G. Marihuana's Effect on Human Genital Function. In G. G. Nahas (ed.), *Marihuana: Chemistry, Biochemistry, and Cellular Effects.* New York: Springer, 1976.

40. Hoffman, B., and Bigger, J. T. Digitalis. In *The Pharmacologic Basis of Therapeutics.* A. G. Gilman, L. S. Goodman, and A. Gilman, (eds.), New York: Macmillan, 1980.

41. Hollander, W. Rauwolfia compounds: Pharmacological and Clinical Use. In A. M. Brest and J. H. Moyer (eds.), *The Second Hahneman Symposium on Hypertensive Disease.* Philadelphia: Lea & Febiger, 1961.

42. Horowitz, J. D., and Goble, A. J. Drugs and impaired male sexual function. *Drugs* 18:206, 1979.

43. Horowitz, J. D., and Goble, A. J. Drugs and impaired sexual function. *Drugs* 18:207, 1979.

44. Howard, D. J., and Rees, J. R. Long-term perhexiline maleate and liver function. *Br. Med. J.* 1:133, 1976.

45. Hughes, J. M. Failure to ejaculate with chlordiazepoxide. *Am. J. Psychiatry* 121:610, 1964.

46. Keidan, H. Impotence during antihypertensive treatment. *J. Can. Med. Assoc.* 114:974, 1970.

47. Koch-Weser, J. Vasodilator drugs in the treatment of hypertension. *Arch. Intern. Med.* 133:1017, 1974.

48. Kolodny, R. C., et al. Depression of plasma testosterone levels after chronic intensive marihuana use. *N. Engl. J. Med.* 290:872, 1974.

49. Kotin, J., et al. Thioridazine and sexual dysfunction. *Am. J. Psychiatry* 133:1, 1976.

50. Kramer, J. C., Fischman, V. S., and Littlefield, D. C. Amphetamine abuse. *J.A.M.A.* 201:305, 1967.

51. Laschet, U., and Laschet, L. Antiandrogens in the treatment of sexual deviations of men. *J. Steroid Biochem.* 6:821, 1975.

52. Lawson, D. M., and Gala, R. R. The influence of adrenergic, dopaminergic, cholinergic, and serotinergic drugs on plasma prolactin levels

in ovariectomized estrogen-treated rats. *Endocrinology* 96:313, 1975.

53. Lee, P. A., Kelly, M. R., and Wallin, J. D. Increased prolactin levels during reserpine therapy of hypertensive patients. *J.A.M.A.* 235:2316, 1976.

54. Lichter, P. R., et al. Patient tolerance to carbonic anhydrase inhibitors. *Am. J. Ophthalmol.* 85:495, 1978.

55. Loicaux, D. L. Spironolactone and endocrine dysfunction. *Ann. Intern. Med.* 85:630, 1976.

56. Marshall, A. J., Roberts, C. J. C., and Barritt, D. W. Raynaud's phenomenon as a side effect of beta blockers in hypertension. *Br. Med. J.* 1:1498, 1976.

57. McHaffie, D. J., Guz, A., and Johnston, A. Impotence in patients on disopyramide. *Lancet* 1:859, 1977.

58. Mendelson, J. H., and Mello, N. K. Plasma testosterone level during chronic heroin use and protracted abstinence. *Clin. Pharmacol. Ther.* 17:529, 1975.

59. Mendelson, J. H., et al. Plasma testosterone levels before, during, and after chronic marihuana smoking. *N. Engl. J. Med.* 291:1051, 1974.

60. Mendelson, J. H., Mendelson, J. E., and Patch, V. Plasma testosterone levels in heroin addiction and during methadone maintenance. *J. Pharmacol. Exp. Ther.* 192:211, 1975.

61. Millar, J. G. B. Drug-induced impotence. *Practitioner* 223:634, 1979.

62. Mintz, J. Sexual problems of heroin addicts. *Arch. Gen. Psychiatry* 31:700, 1974.

63. Mudge, G. H. Diuretics and Other Agents Employed in Mobilization of Edema Fluid. In A. G. Gillman, L. S. Goodman, and A. Gillman (eds.), *The Pharmacologic Basis of Therapeutics.* New York: Macmillan, 1980.

64. Neri, A., et al. Subjective assessment of sexual dysfunction of patients on long-term administration of digoxin. *Arch. Sex Behav.* 9:343, 1980.

65. Newman, R. J., and Salerno, H. R. Sexual dysfunction. *Br. Med. J.* 4:106, 1974.

66. Nininger, J. E. Inhibition of ejaculation by amitriptyline. *Am. J. Psychiatry* 135:750, 1978.

67. Onesti, G., et al. Clonidine: New antihypertensive agent. *Am. J. Cardiol.* 28:74, 1971.

68. Peden, N. R., et al. Male sexual dysfunction during treatment with cimetidine. *Br. Med. J.* 1:659, 1979.

69. Pita, J. C., et al. Interaction of spironolactone and digitalis with dihydrotesterone (DHT) receptor of rat central prostate. *Endocrinology (Suppl.)* 96:176, 1975.

70. Rifka, S. M., Pita, J. C., and Loriaux, D. L. Mechanism of interaction of digitalis in the estradiol-binding sites in rat uterus. *Endocrinology* 99:1091, 1976.

71. Rubin, E., et al. Prolonged ethanol consumption increases testosterone metabolism in the liver. *Science* 191:563, 1976.

72. Schneider, J., and Kaffarnik, H. Impotence in patients treated with Clofibrate. *Atherosclerosis* 21:455, 1975.

73. Simpson, G. M., Blair, J. H., and Amuso, D. Effects of antidepressants on genitourinary function. *Dis. Nerv. Syst.* 26:787, 1965.

74. Spark, R. F., and Melby, J. C. Aldosteronism in hypertension. The spironolactone response test. *Ann. Intern. Med.* 69:685, 1968.

75. Stessman, J., and Ben-Ishay, D. Chlorthalidone-induced impotence. *Br. Med. J.* 281:714, 1980.

76. Stoffer, S. S., et al. Digoxin and abnormal serum hormone levels. *J.A.M.A.* 225:1643, 1973.

77. The Medical Letter. Drugs that cause sexual dysfunction. 22:25, 1980.

78. Van Thiel, D. H., and Lester, R. Sex and alcohol. *N. Engl. J. Med.* 291:251, 1974.

79. Van Thiel, D. H., Sherin, R. J., and Lester, R. Mechanism of hypogonadism in alcoholic liver disease. *Gastroenterology* 65:574, 1977.

80. Veterans Administration Cooperative Study Group on Antihypertensive Agents. Propranolol in the treatment of essential hypertension. *J.A.M.A.* 237:2303, 1977.

81. Wallace, T. R., et al. Decreased libido. A side effect of carbonic anhydrase activity. *Ann. Ophthalmol.* 11:1563, 1979.

82. Warren, S. C., and Warren, S. G. Propranolol and sexual impotence. *Ann. Int. Med.* 86:112, 1977.

83. Wolfe, M. M. Impotence on cimetidine treatment. *N. Engl. J. Med.* 300:94, 1979.

84. Wyatt, R. J., et al. Treatment of intractable narcolepsy with a monoamine oxidase inhibitor. *N. Engl. J. Med.* 285:987, 1971.

85. Zarren, H. S., and Black, P. M. Unilateral gynecomastia with impotence during low-dose spironolactone administration in men. *Milit. Med.* 140:417, 1975.

11

Iatrogenic Impotence

IRWIN GOLDSTEIN
MIKE B. SIROKY
ROBERT J. KRANE

The term *iatrogenic impotence* is used to describe conditions of abnormal erectile function occurring in a patient as a side effect of therapy. Impotence induced by either surgical manipulation or radiation therapy will be reviewed in this chapter. In most cases, however, the exact mechanisms of the erectile dysfunction are not known. New research in this area, especially in vascular and neurologic testing, may help unlock these mysteries. This chapter will attempt to classify iatrogenic impotence by probable mechanism of action (Table 11-1).

ARTERIAL VASCULAR MECHANISMS

A therapeutic activity that reduces arterial inflow into the hypogastricocavernous arterial bed may result in iatrogenic arterial vasculogenic impotence. This topic may best be discussed by separating adverse iatrogenic effects into those on large and those on small vessels.

Large Vessels (Internal Iliac Artery Inflow)

AORTOILIAC RECONSTRUCTION. In 1923, Leriche noted that occlusive arterial disease within the abdominal aortic bifurcation adversely affected erectile capacity [46]. Since then, this association between aortoiliac occlusive arterial disease and erectile impotence has been confirmed by numerous studies [53, 57, 71]. Recent emphasis, however, has been on the recognition of iatrogenic arterial vasculogenic impotence that is the direct result of a vascular reconstructive procedure [16, 31, 53, 64, 69, 77, 81]. Internal iliac artery blood flow reduction and subsequent drops in Doppler-derived penile blood pressure [21, 37, 64] have been identified in these cases. This has occurred especially after aortofemoral graft replacements with end-to-end proximal aortic anastomoses in the presence of external iliac artery occlusive disease [64]. In this condition, the aorta is transected, and blood flow in the internal iliac artery is derived from the aortofemoral graft anastomosis retrograde through the femoral and external iliac arteries. If the latter vessels are severely occluded, internal iliac blood flow may be compromised inadvertently.

Table 11-1. Non-pharmacologic
iatrogenic impotence

Mechanism	After therapy or treatment
Arterial vascular	
Large vessel	Aortoiliac reconstruction
	Renal transplantation
	Pelvic surgery
	Uncontrolled pelvic
	hemorrhage
	treatment
Small vessel	Pelvic radiation therapy
Venous vascular	Priapism treatment
Neurologic	
Central	Bilateral ansotomy
Suprasacral	Lumbar laminectomy
or sacral	
Peripheral	Sacral rhizotomy
Infrasacral	Abdominoperineal
Autonomic	resection
	Radical cystectomy
	Radical prostatectomy
Somatic	Pudendal neurectomy
Endocrinologic	
Hypergonadotropic	Bilateral orchiectomy
Hypogonadism	
Hypogonadotropic	Pituitary resection
Hypogonadism	Hemodialysis
Mechanical	Partial penectomy
	Hypospadias repair
Psychologic	Transurethral resection
	of the prostate

Maintaining blood flow in the internal iliac artery during vascular reconstruction is the key to preserving erectile function. In patients with aortic bifurcation occlusion and external iliac artery atherosclerotic disease preventing retrograde flow, reconstructive procedures such as end-to-side proximal aortic anastomoses should be considered [64]. In this fashion, anterograde flow to the internal iliac artery will be permitted. Alternatively, performing internal iliac endarterectomies, femorofemoral grafting, or internal iliac artery grafting to one arm of an aortobifemoral graft [64] might, in the particular situation, sustain flow in the hypogastricocavernous arterial bed and ensure adequate erectile function.

RENAL TRANSPLANTATION. Any procedure that involves the internal iliac artery and has the potential for subsequent compromise may affect penile blood flow adversely. *Renal allograft transplantation,* as performed in most transplant centers, is such a procedure. During this operation, the internal iliac artery is classically transected, ligated distally, and anastomosed proximally end-to-end to the donor kidney. In Burns' review [9] of 16 renal transplant recipients, the penile blood pressure of seven unilateral transplants was 64 mm Hg and lay in the range of abnormal pelvic hemodynamics as determined by Queral [64] and others [21, 37].

The problem appears greater if the patient requires a second renal transplant. In this situation, *both* internal iliac arteries may be sequentially ligated distally. Burns [9] and Gittes [25] have found a marked increase in impotence after the second renal transplant. Nine of nine patients and 13 of 20 patients, respectively, were impotent after the second transplant, as compared to three of seven and 2 of 20 patients, respectively, who were impotent after the first transplant.

Preservation of internal iliac blood flow again appears to be a major consideration in these patients. The maintenance of erectile function might be better protected if the allograft renal artery were anastomosed end-to-side to the external iliac artery. In this procedure, internal iliac artery blood flow would not be compromised. Alternatively, the possibility of end-to-side internal iliac artery anastomoses might be explored. Theoretically, this latter procedure could be evaluated both for adequate allograft renal artery blood flow and distal cavernous body blood flow. A further aspect of this procedure would be the lack of involvement of the external iliac artery, thus the ipsilateral lower extremities would not be endangered.

PELVIC SURGERY—RADICAL CYSTECTOMY. During radical cystectomy for carcinoma of the bladder, the internal iliac artery is exposed to the superior vesical artery. After clamping, division, and ligation of the latter vessel, the dissection is continued with the division of all arterial branches to the bladder and prostate [44]. If selective arteries are not individually divided, but rather the distal internal iliac and internal pudendal artery are divided (as often happens), arterial vasculogenic impotence may result. Clearly, numerous other factors in radical cystectomy surgery may account for erectile dysfunction, including neurologic damage and psychologic trauma [76]. Nevertheless, altered penile blood pressure secondary to compromised internal iliac blood flow is a likely contributing factor.

UNCONTROLLED PELVIC HEMORRHAGE. If severe bleeding is encountered after prostatic enucleation or pelvic trauma, or arises from pelvic malignancies, some authors recommend surgically ligating the internal iliac arteries bilaterally. One author has reported on the use of routine prophylactic bilateral internal iliac artery ligation in 110 cases of prostatectomy [2]. With this procedure he noted a lower volume of intraoperative and postoperative blood loss.

Occlusion of the internal iliac arteries bilaterally for uncontrolled pelvic hemorrhage also can be performed in a percutaneous, nonoperative manner [12, 30, 73]. The radiologic procedure transcatheter embolization recently has come into widespread use. Arterial occlusion is achieved by the selective injection of solid material (clots, Gelfoam, barium, cyanoacrylates) into the vessel [11]. Theoretically, this procedure might be more effective than surgical ligation, because arterial occlusion through embolization can occur not only in the larger branches but also in the smaller distal vessels. These procedures have been used mainly for uncontrolled hemorrhage; however, a recent report [12] suggests that unilateral internal iliac embolization be used for treating priapism.

Small Vessels (Internal Pudendal and Penile Artery)

PELVIC IRRADIATION. Pelvic external beam radiation therapy is used for patients with pelvic malignancies (bladder, prostate, colon) in an effort either to cure the disease or to gain local-regional control of it. For example, in patients with appropriately staged prostate cancer, a radiation dose of 6000 to 7000 rad

has been widely used instead of radical prostatectomy. In fact, since impotence is strongly associated with radical surgery, it is often this fear of erectile dysfunction that motivates patients to choose pelvic irradiation treatment over radical surgery. Radiation also can be used an an adjunct to surgery. In appropriately staged colon cancer, 5500 rad may be given after surgical resection.

Impotence after pelvic external beam radiation has been documented best in studies of patients with prostate cancer. One reason may be that the prostate gland itself is involved in normal sexual function. Other more probable reasons may be that prostate cancer patients tend to live longer than patients with bladder or colon cancer. Because a 5- to 10-year survival time is common after radiation treatment for prostate cancer, the development of sexual dysfunction may have additional significance.

Reported incidence of impotence after external beam radiation therapy for prostate cancer has varied from 22 to 84 percent [1, 29, 58, 59, 61, 65, 66, 78] with an average of 35 to 40 percent. Bagshaw initially reported a 30 percent incidence of impotence [65]; however, in a later report he noted a 41 percent incidence [1]. Rhamy's [66] group described a 47 percent incidence, whereas Hafermann's group [29] demonstrated 69 percent impotency prior to radiation and only a 27 percent change in potency after radiation.

A recent clinical study performed at Boston University may help to clarify the etiology of radiation-induced impotence. Erectile function tests were performed on prostate cancer patients undergoing either definitive or adjunctive external beam radiation therapy. Sixty-three percent of patients had changed erectile capacity after radiation therapy. No change in erectile function was noted after ^{125}I interstitial implantation or pelvic lymphadenectomy. This latter observation accords with Herr's review [34] of 41 similar patients.

Of the patients whose erectile capacity changed after radiotherapy, neurologic and endocrinologic testing were within normal limits. Vascular testing, however, was abnormal in all cases in which erectile function changed. In addition, these patients had a higher incidence of hypertension (50% versus 17%) and of smoking (75% versus 17%) as compared to patients whose erectile capacity did not change during radiation treatment.

The possibility that radiation-induced impotence is vasculogenic is strongly supported by animal [70] and clinical studies. Lindsay [47] (1962) demonstrated the sequence of large-vessel injury to dogs subjected to localized aortic radiation (i.e., internal elastic membrane fragmentation), mucopolysaccharide and ground substance deposition in the intima, fibroelastic proliferation in the intima, and subsequent development of atheromatous plaques in the intima. Gold [26], Kirkpatrick [38], and Lamberts [43] demonstrated the synergistic atheromatous response in animals receiving both radiation and hypercholesterolemic diets. Clinically well-documented cases of cerebrovascular accidents [13], myocardial infarcts [45], renovascular hypertension [23] subclavian steal syndrome [8, 48] and lower-extremity claudication [10, 33] have resulted from radiation therapy.

The conclusions of the clinical radiation study are as follows: Radiation-induced erectile dysfunction may well be vasculogenic in etiology, vascular risk factors such as hypertension and smoking appear to predispose the patient to radiation-induced impotence.

VENOUS VASCULAR MECHANISMS

Impotence may result when appropriate intracavernous pressures cannot either be generated or sustained [55] because of abnormal venous outflow [19].

Iatrogenic impotence therefore may result as a long-term complication of *priapism therapy*. Established procedures for treating priapism involve (1) the anastomosis of the saphenous vein to one corpus cavernosum [27], (2) the creation of surgical windows between one corpus cavernosum and the corpus spongiosum [63], or (3) the percutaneous "coring" of the septum separating the glans from the corpus cavernosum [83]. These interventions share one common problem, that is, the possibility of creating a per-

manently abnormal venous outflow.

Since priapism itself may induce cavernous fibrosis and, possibly, mechanical impotence, an infusion cavernosogram [19] made during artificial erection may be used to differentiate between abnormal venous drainage impotence and inadequate corporal mechanical capacity secondary to fibrosis.

It is intriguing to consider this mechanism as the possible cause of impotence in patients who have undergone resection of Peyronie's plaque. The "flail penis" that often results may be related to anatomic weakness in the tunica albuginea of the cavernous bodies and subsequent abnormal venous outflow.

NEUROLOGIC MECHANISMS

Iatrogenic impotence may be caused by surgical interference with the normal function of the central or peripheral nervous system.

Central-Suprasacral-Sacral Mechanisms

The exact anatomic pathways in the central nervous system that control penile erection are not known. Nevertheless, treatment for neurologic disease, especially neurosurgical treatment, has caused well-documented cases of impotence.

The most publicized report on this subject in the cerebral region has been by Meyers [56] (1962). To control disabling myoclonus, the ansa lenticularis was severed bilaterally in two patients (ages 35 and 44), and unilaterally in one patient (age 18). In addition, lesions were induced in the dorsomedial hypothalamic nucleus, the posterior septum pellucidium, and the posterior-inferior aspect of the anterior commissure. Postoperatively, the two patients with bilaterial ansotomy complained of new inability to achieve erection, whereas the one patient with a unilateral ansotomy had normal erections. Meyers [56] concluded that human neural mechanisms in the erectile pathway were located near the above locations and that bilateral destruction in these areas represented the highest risk in erectile dysfunction.

Neurosurgical procedures designed to treat cervical spondylosis, cervical or lumbar disk degeneration, and central nervous system tumors occasionally have been associated with impotence. Several of these cases have been documented in our institution with genito-cerebral-evoked response testing. In lesions involving the sacral cord, sacral latency testing is abnormal [74].

Another cause of iatrogenic neurogenic impotence may be a rare and unfortunate result of postoperative spinal cord infarction after retroperitoneal lymphadenectomy for cancer of the testis, or after repair of aortic aneurysm [75].

Peripheral-Infrasacral (Autonomic) Mechanisms

The prevailing opinion on the pathways of peripheral neurologic control of penile erection is that nerve impulses reach the cavernous bodies by way of pelvic parasympathetic nerves. Although these nerves may not be directly responsible for vasomotor control in the corpora, their function and integrity is essential [42]. Anatomically, these pelvic parasympathetic nerves originate in the intermediolateral region of the gray matter of sacral segments S2–S4. These preganglionic fibers travel at first with the somatic pudendal plexus but later separate to become the pelvic nerve. This pelvic nerve courses to the pelvic plexus lateral to the rectal ampulla, to the vesical plexus at the bladder base, to the prostatic plexus on the lateral surface of the prostate, and to the cavernous plexus at the base of the corpus cavernosum [80]. Injury to these parasympathetic nerves may occur (1) at their roots, (2) along the rectum at the pelvic plexus, (3) at the vesical plexus, (4) at the prostatic plexus, and (5) at the cavernous plexus. Note that objective testing through cystometrography and bethanechol testing is useful only for parasympathetic nerve injuries involving (1) the sacral roots, (2) the parapelvic-pararectal plexus, and (3) the paravesical plexus. Distal parasympathetic lesions involving the prostatic or corporal plexuses are not readily confirmed by direct, objective testing. This may explain in part why the etiology of impotence in the distal locations remains questionable.

SACRAL ROOT SECTION. Sacral rhizotomy is a procedure resulting in complete bilateral section of the anterior and posterior roots of S2–S4 [5]. It is usually performed on the patient with a hyperreflexic, contracted bladder in whom anticholinergic medication has failed. Obviously, nerve interruption of the sacral roots involves a high incidence of impotence. Differential sacral rhizotomy procedures [67], by not completely sectioning all roots, may possibly entail a lower incidence of erectile dysfunction.

PARARECTAL SURGERY. The incidence of impotence after abdominoperineal resection has been reported as 0 to 20 percent for benign disease, and 30 to 100 percent for malignant disease [5, 17, 18, 82, 84]. During this surgery, the pelvic parasympathetic plexus, in its pararectal location, either may be removed or injured, and this may be true especially if the surgical resection is wide and involves lymph node removal. This may explain the higher association of impotence with surgical resection for malignant disease in contrast to treatment for benign disease [5, 17, 18, 82, 84]. Alternatively, other features such as patient age and vascular risk factors may play a more significant role in the genesis of postoperative impotence after rectal surgery. Older patients tend to have cancer surgery, whereas younger ones tend to have noncancer surgery.

Detrusor areflexia and positive bethanechol supersensitivity tests have been identified at our institution in several patients after abdominoperineal resection. These objective studies help confirm the contribution of parasympathetic denervation to the dysfunction.

PARAVESICAL SURGERY. Radical cystectomy for bladder cancer also may involve either injury to or removal of both the vesical and pelvic plexuses and thus cause neurogenic impotence [4]. As in other radical cancer surgical procedures, additional factors may contribute to erectile dysfunction, especially vascular factors, as were previously discussed (bilateral internal pudendal artery ligation during surgery).

PARAPROSTATIC SURGERY. Radical prostatectomy has been incriminated as the cause of impotency in 85 to 100 percent [35, 36, 41, 62] of patients treated. A recent study [22], however, showed that only 57 percent of patients who were potent preoperatively developed erectile dysfunction after radical prostatectomy. The most likely cause of erectile disturbance in these patients is injury to the prostatic autonomic plexus during total prostatectomy [76], although direct, objective evidence of this is lacking.

Perineal incisions and the open perineal prostatic biopsy have been incriminated by some [15] as impairing potency. The data, however, are conflicting, and there may be in fact no organic neurologic basis for impotence arising from this confined surgery.

CAVERNOUS PLEXUS INJURY DURING SURGERY. Surgery in the urethra, such as transurethral external sphincterotomy [14, 39, 68, 72] and transurethral direct-vision internal urethrotomy [54] may be associated with impotence. Some authors speculate that penile vessels coagulated during external sphincterotomy account for the dysfunction [39]. Another possible mechanism is neurologic injury to the autonomic nerves alongside the corpora cavernosa during extravasation of the corpus spongiosum. Just as the pathophysiology is unclear, the method of reducing the incidence of this iatrogenic impotence is controversial. It has been reported by several authors that during external sphincterotomy 3- and 9-o'clock incisions [39, 72] increase the rate of erectile dysfunction, whereas others [14, 68] find no adverse effect on erections with these incisions.

Peripheral-Infrasacral (Somatic) Mechanisms

Pudendal neurectomy [40] may be indicated in cases of severe vesicosphincter dyssynergia. In most cases, best results from neurectomy (relief of neurologic obstruction) follow bilateral procedures. As is expected, however, erectile dysfunction is inevitable. This procedure is seldom indicated, however, because external sphincterotomy apparently reduces external sphincter resistance better and more reliably [28].

ENDOCRINE CAUSES

Dysfunction arising from interference with the hypothalamic-pituitary-gonadal axis during treatment may be termed *iatrogenic endocrinologic impotence.*

Hypergonadotropic Hypogonadism

A low serum testosterone level that is the result of an iatrogenic primary testicular problem is most commonly the consequence of either bilateral orchiectomy or exogenous estrogen administration for prostate cancer palliation. The mechanism of castration-testosterone level impotence is not known. It even has been shown that erectile dysfunction is not an inevitable sequel to castration. In one prostate cancer series [20], there existed a 54 percent incidence of impotence prior to endocrine manipulation, and an 80 percent incidence after therapy. It is unclear how much of the increase in impotence was related to therapy, and how much to the effects of continued chronic illness from metastatic prostate cancer. It is clear, however, that some patients who underwent bilateral orchiectomy remained potent [20]. This fact was further emphasized by the observation that prepubertal males subjected to bilateral orchiectomy for nonmedical reasons [49] could be potent. In summary, iatrogenically castrate testosterone levels may cause impotence; however, the pathophysiology is poorly appreciated.

Hypogonadotropic Hypogonadism

Neurosurgical injury to the hypothalamus or the pituitary may cause insufficient secretion of pituitary gonadotropin luteinizing hormone. Low testosterone levels result, and erectile dysfunction may become manifest. This form of impotence generally responds either to testosterone, human chorionic gonadotropin, or, in appropriate circumstances, gonadotropin-releasing hormone [79].

Hemodialysis patients in one series had low-normal levels of gonadotropins and low levels of testosterone. A hypothalamic origin of this potentially iatrogenic abnormality has been suggested because it was determined that serum testosterone levels normalized with the use of gonadotropin-releasing hormone [52].

MECHANICAL CAUSES

Iatrogenic impotence may be the result of a partial penectomy for cancer of the penis. In these cases, there may be insufficient residual penile length for successful mechanical vaginal penetration. In cases when sufficient length remains, however, it is not unusual for patients to achieve frequent and satisfactory intercourse [7].

Mechanical iatrogenic impotence may occur after corrective hypospadiac surgery as a result of shortening or angulation of the penis. Most hypospadiac surgery is performed in children, and only recently has a follow-up study been done of sexual adjustment in these patients. Berg [3] has shown that even severer cases of hypospadiac men have an excellent chance of maintaining normal erectile function.

PSYCHOLOGIC CAUSES

Psychologic factors play a major role in iatrogenic erectile dysfunction, even when it is obviously secondary to an organic abnormality. In radical surgery, for example, after abdominoperineal resection or radical cystectomy, an external appliance is necessary to collect body excretions. In these cases altered self-esteem and self-image may play a major role in the genesis of sexual dysfunction [6].

Iatrogenic impotence after transurethral resection of the prostate appears to have no obvious organic basis, and, as several studies suggest, it most likely has a strong psychologic basis. Classifying impotence after this form of transurethral surgery as psychologic while not classifying impotence after other forms of such surgery (e.g., external sphincterotomy or direct-vision urethrotomy) may be, in fact, arbitrary and incorrect. There are few objective data and therefore no obvious organic basis for the latter two forms of iatrogenic impotence.

The incidence of impotence after transurethral prostatectomy varies from 0 to 40 percent of cases in reported series [32, 50, 85]. When patients were studied prospectively [85], those who were provided with a detailed explanation of the procedure and its potential side effects had a much lower incidence of postoperative impotence. Furthermore, in another series, no patient demonstrated any objective changes when studied prospectively with a battery of organic tests [5].

In summary, the etiologies and mechanisms of iatrogenic erectile dysfunction are only beginning to be appreciated. Further research and more direct objective testing ultimately will result in the recognition of the various pathophysiologic observations. A more rational plan of treatment in each specific case can follow only when the mechanism is understood. For example, the vascular abnormalities of radiation-induced impotence may be best avoided by radiating the prostatic field only and not including the entire pelvic field. Radiation patients with strong vascular risk factors may also have the total radiation dose reduced by 10 percent [60]. This practice is standard for surgical patients who have had multiple laparotomies and require postoperative radiation therapy.

REFERENCES

1. Bagshaw, M. A., et al. External beam radiation therapy of primary carcinoma of the prostate. *Cancer* 36:723, 1975.
2. Bao, Z. M. Ligation of internal iliac arteries in 110 cases as hemostatic procedure during suprapubic prostatecotomy. *J. Urol.* 124:578, 1980.
3. Berg, R., Svensson, J., and Astrom, G. Social and sexual adjustment of men operated for hypospadias during childhood: A controlled study. *J. Urol.* 125:313, 1981.
4. Bergman, B., Nilson, S., and Petersen, I. The effect on erection and orgasm of cystectomy, prostatectomy and vesiculectomy for cancer of the bladder: A clinical and electromyographic study. *Br. J. Urol.* 51:114, 1979.
5. Bernstein, W. C., and Bernstein, E. F. Sexual dysfunction following radical surgery for cancer of the rectum. *Dis. Colon Rectum* 9:328, 1966.

6. Beutler, L. E. Psychological Evaluation: Its Importance in Treatment Decisions. In A. C. Von Eschenbach, and D. B. Rodriguez, (eds.), *Sexual Rehabilitation of the Urologic Cancer Patient.* Boston: G. K. Hall, 1981. Pp. 175–190.

7. Bracken, R. B. Cancer of the Testis, Penis, and Urethra: The Impact of Therapy on Sexual Function. In A.C. Van Eschenbach and D. B. Rodiguez (eds.), *Sexual Rehabilitation of the Urologic Cancer Patient.* Boston: G. K. Hall, 1981. Pp. 109–127.

8. Budin, J. A., et al. Vascular-induced erectile impotence in renal transplant recipients. *J. Urol.* 121:721, 1979.

9. Burns, J. R., Cassarella, W., and Harisiadis, L. Subclavian artery occlusion following radiotherapy for carcinoma of the breast. *Radiology* 118:169, 1976.

10. Butler, M. J., Lane, R. H. S., and Webster, J. H. H. Irradiation injury to large arteries. *Br. J. Surg.* 67:341, 1980.

11. Carmignani, G., et al. Clots, Oxycel, Gelfoam, barium, and cyanoacrylates in transcatheter embolization of rat kidney. *Invest. Urol.* 16:9, 1978.

12. Carmignani, G., et al. Idiopathic priapism successfully treated by unilateral embolization of internal pudendal artery. *J. Urol.* 124:553, 1980.

13. Conomy, J. P., and Kellermeyer, R. W. Delayed cerebrovascular consequences of therapeutic radiation. *Cancer* 36:1702, 1975.

14. Crane, D. B., and Hackler, R. H. External sphincterotomy: Its effect on erections. *J. Urol.* 116:316, 1976.

15. Dahlen, C. P., and Goodwin, W. E. Sexual potency after perineal biopsy. *J. Urol.* 77:660, 1957.

16. DePalma, R. G., Levine, S. B., and Feldman, S. Preservation of erectile function after aortoiliac reconstruction. *Arch. Surg.* 113:988, 1978.

17. Devlin, H. B., Plant, J. A., and Griffin, M. Aftermath of surgery of anorectal cancer. *Br. Med. J.* 3:413, 1971.

18. Dwight, R. W., Higgins, G. A., and Keehn, R. J. Factors influencing survival after resection in cancer of the colon and rectum. *Am. J. Surg.* 117:512, 1969.

19. Ebbehoj, J., and Wagner, G. Insufficient penile erection due to abnormal drainage of cavernous bodies. *Urology* 13:507, 1979.

20. Ellis, W. J., and Grayhack, J. T. Sexual functioning in aging males after orchiectomy and estrogen therapy. *J. Urol.* 89:895, 1963.

21. Engel, G., Burnham, S., and Carter, M. F. Penile blood pressure in the evaluation of erectile impotence. *Fertil. Steril.* 30:687, 1978.

22. Finkle, A. L., and Taylor, S. P. Sexual potency after radical prostatectomy. *J. Urol.* 125:350, 1981.

23. Gerlock, A. J., Jr., Goncharenko, V. A., and Ekelund, L. Radiation-induced stenosis of the renal artery causing hypertension: Case report. *J. Urol.* 118:1064, 1977.

24. Gibbon, N. O. K. Neurogenic bladder in spinal cord injury. *Urol. Clin. North Am.* 1:147, 1974.

25. Gittes, R. F., and Waters, W. B. Sexual impotence: The overlooked complication of a second renal transplant. *J. Urol.* 121:719, 1979.

26. Gold, H. Atherosclerosis in the rat: Effect of x-ray and a high fat diet. *Soc. Exo. Biol. Med. Proc.* 111:593, 1962.

27. Grayhack, J. T., et al. Venous bypass to control priapism. *Invest. Urol.* 1:509, 1964.

28. Hackler, R. Surgical treatment of the adult neurogenic bladder dysfunction. In R. J. Krane, and M. B. Siroky (eds.), *Clinical Neuro-Urology* Boston: Little, Brown, 1979. Pp. 197–212.

29. Hafermann, M. D. External radiotherapy. *Urology* [Suppl.] 17:15, 1981.

30. Hald, T., and Mygind, T. Control of life-threatening vesical hemorrhage by unilateral hypogastric artery muscle embolization. *J. Urol.* 112:60, 1974.

31. Hallbook, T., and Holmquist, B. Sexual disturbance following dissection of the aorta and the common iliac arteries. *J. Cardiovas. Surg.* 11:255, 1970.

32. Hargreave, J. B., and Stephenson, T. P. Potency and prostatectomy. *Br. J. Urol.* 49:683, 1977.

33. Hayward, R. H. Arteriosclerosis induced by radiation. *Surg. Clin. North Am.* 52:359, 1972.

34. Herr, H. W. Preservation of sexual potency in prostatic cancer patients after I^{125} implantation. *J. Am. Geriatr. Soc.* 27:17, 1979.

35. Jewett, H. J. Treatment of early cancer of the prostate. *J.A.M.A.* 183:373, 1963.

36. Jewett, H. J. The present status of radical prostatectomy for stage A and B prostatic cancer. *Urol. Clin. North Am.* 2:105, 1975.

37. Kempczinski, R. F. Role of the vascular diagnostic laboratory in the evaluation of male impotence. *Am. J. Surg.* 138:278, 1979.

38. Kirkpatrick, J. B. Pathogenesis of foam cell lesions in irradiated arteries. *Am. J. Pathol.* 50:291, 1967.

39. Kiviat, M. D. Transurethral sphincterotomy: Relationship of site of incision to postoperative potency and delayed hemorrhage. *J. Urol.* 114:399, 1975.

40. Kleeman, F. J., and Chute, R. A plan for the evaluation of patients with bladder dysfunction and the use of pudendal neurectomy. *J. Urol.* 97:1029, 1967.

41. Kopecky, A. A., Laskowski, T. Z., and Scott, R., Jr. Radical retropubic prostatectomy in the treatment of prostatic carcinoma. *J. Urol.* 103:641, 1970.

42. Krane, R. J., and Siroky, M. B. Neurophysiology of erection. *Urol. Clin. North Am.* 8:91, 1981.

43. Lamberts, H. B., and de Boer, W. G. R. M. Contributions to the study of immediate and early x-ray reactions with regard to chemoprotection: IX. X-ray–induced coronary occlusion leading to heart damage in rabbits. *Int. J. Radiat. Biol.* 8:359, 1964.

44. Leadbetter, W. F. Bladder malignancies. In J. F. Glenn (ed.), *Urologic Surgery.* Hagerstown, Md.: Harper & Row, 1975. Pp. 323–347.

45. Leong, A. S. Y., Forbes, I. J., and Ruzic, T. Radiation-related coronary artery disease in Hodgkin's disease. *Aust. N.Z. J. Med.* 9:423, 1979.

46. Leriche, R. Des obliterations arterielles hautes obliteration de la terminaison de l'aorte comme cause d'insuffisance circulatoire des membres inferieures. *Bull. Soc. Chir. (Paris)* 49:1404, 1923.

47. Lindsay, S., Kohn, H. I., and Dakin, R. L. Aortic arteriosclerosis in the dog after localized aortic x-irradiation. *Circ. Res.* 10:51, 1962.

48. Loeffler, R. K. Subclavian artery occlusion following radiation therapy: A case history. *Invest. Radiol.* 10:391, 1975.

49. Mack, W. S. Ruminations on the testis. *Proc. R. Soc. Med. (London)* 57:47, 1964.

50. Madorsky, M. L., et al. Post-prostatectomy impotence. *J. Urol.* 115:401, 1976.

51. Manfredi, R. A., and Leal, J. F. Elective sacral rhizotomy for the spastic bladder syndrome in patients with spinal cord injuries. *J. Urol.* 100:17, 1968.

52. Massey, S. G., et al. Impotence in patients with uremia: A possible role of parathyroid hormone. *Nephron* 19:305, 1977.

53. May, A. G., DeWeese, J. A., and Rob, C. E. Changes in sexual function following operation on the abdominal aorta. *Surgery* 65:41, 1969.

54. McDermott, D. W., et al. Erectile impotence as complication of direct-vision cold-knife urethrotomy. *Urology* 18:467, 1981.

55. Metz, P., and Wagner, G. Penile circumference and erection. *Urology* 18:268, 1981.

56. Meyers, R. Three cases of myoclonus alleviated by bilateral ansotomy, with a note on postoperative alibido and impotence. *J. Neurosurg.* 19:71, 1962.

57. Michal, V., Kramar, R., and Bartak, V. Femoro-pudendal bypass in the treatment of sexual impotence. *J. Cardiovasc. Surg.* 15:356, 1974.

58. Mollenkamp, J. S., Cooper, J. F., and Kagen, A. R. Clinical experience with supervoltage radiotherapy in carcinoma of the prostate. Preliminary report. *J. Urol.* 113:374, 1975.

59. Perez, C. A., et al. Radiation therapy in the treatment of localized carcinoma of the prostate. *Cancer* 34:1059, 1974.

60. Phillips, T. L., and Fu, K. K. Acute and late effects of multimodal therapy on normal tissues. *Cancer* 40:489, 1977.

61. Pistenma, E. A., Ray, G. R., and Bagshaw, M. A. The role of megavoltage radiation therapy in the treatment of prostatic carcinoma. *Semin. Oncol.* 3:115, 1976.

62. Pond, H. S., et al. Defense of the radical perineal prostatectomy. *South. Med. J.* 7:541, 1978.

63. Quackles, R. Cure of a patient suffering from priapism by cavernospongiosa anastomosis. *Acta Urol. Belg.* 32:5, 1964.

64. Queral, L. A., et al. Pelvic hemodynamics after aortoiliac reconstruction. *Surgery* 86:799, 1979.

65. Ray, G. R., Cassady, J. R., and Bagshaw, M. A. Definitive radiation therapy of carcinoma of the prostate: A report on 15 years' experience. *Radiology* 106:409, 1973.

66. Rhamy, R. K., Wilson, S. K., and Caldwell, W. L. Biopsy-proved tumor following definitive irradiation for resectable carcinoma of the prostate. *J. Urol.* 107:627, 1972.

67. Rochswold, G. L., Bradley, W. E., and Chou, S. N. Differential sacral rhizotomy in the treatment of neurogenic bladder dysfunction: Preliminary report of six cases. *J. Neurosurg.* 38:748, 1973.

68. Ross, J. C., Gibbon, N. O. K., and Sunder, G. S. Division of the external urethral sphincter in the neuropathic bladder: A twenty-year review. *Br. J. Urol.* 48:649, 1976.

69. Sabri, S., and Cotton, L. T. Sexual function following aortoiliac reconstruction. *Lancet* 2:1218, 1971.

70. Sarns, A. Histological changes in the larger blood vessels of the hind limb of the mouse after x-irradiation. *Int. J. Radiat. Biol.* 9:165, 1965.

71. Scheer, A. Impotence as a symptom of arterial vascular disorder in the pelvic region. *Munch. Med. Wschr.* 102–1713, 1960.

72. Schoenfeld, L., Canion, H. M., and Politano, V. A. Erectile impotence: Complications of external sphincterotomy. *Urology* 4:681, 1974.

73. Schuhrke, T. D., and Barr, J. W. Intractable bladder hemorrhage: Therapeutic angiographic embolization of the hypogastric arteries. *J. Urol.* 116:523, 1976.

74. Siroky, M. B., Krane, R. J., and Sax, D. S. Sacral signal tracing: The electrophysiology of the bulbocavernosus reflex. *J. Urol.* 122:661, 1979.

75. Skinner, D. G. Complications of Lymph Node Dissection. In R. B. Smith and D. G. Skinner (eds.), *Complications of Urologic Surgery.* Philadelphia: Saunders, 1976. Pp. 422–435.

76. Swanson, D. A. Cancer of the Bladder and

Prostate: The Impact of Therapy on Sexual Function. In A. C. Von Eschenbach and D. Rodriguez (eds.), *Sexual Rehabilitation of the Urologic Cancer Patient*. Boston: G. K. Hall, 1981. Pp. 89–107.

77. Van Vroonhoven, T. J. M. V. Sexual dysfunction after aortoiliac surgery. *Vasa* 6:226, 1977.

78. Von Eschenbach, A. C. Sexual dysfunction following therapy for cancer of the prostate, testis, and penis. In J. M. Vaeth (ed.), *Frontiers of Radiation Therapy and Oncology: Proceedings of the 14th Annual Symposium* (vol. 14). Basel: S. Karger, 1980. Pp. 42–50.

79. Weidman, C. L., and Northcutt, R. C. Endocrine aspects of impotence. *Urol. Clin. North Am.* 8:143, 1981.

80. Wein, A. J., and Raezer, D. M. Physiology of Micturition. In R. J. Krane and M. B. Siroky (eds.), *Clinical Neruo-Urology*. Boston: Little, Brown, 1979. Pp. 1–33.

81. Weinstein, M. H., and Machleder, H. I. Sexual function after aortoiliac surgery. *Ann. Surg.* 181:787, 1975.

82. Weinstein, M., and Roberts, M. Sexual potency following surgery for rectal carcinoma. *Ann. Surg.* 185:295, 1977.

83. Winter, C. C. Cure of idiopathic priapism: New procedure for creating fistula between glans penis and corpora cavernosa. *Urology* 8:389, 1976.

84. Yeager, E. S., and Van Heerden, J. A. Sexual dysfunction following proctocolectomy and abdominoperineal resection. *Ann. Surg.* 191:169, 1980.

85. Zohar, J., et al. Factors influencing sexual activity after prostatectomy: A prospective study. *J. Urol.* 116:332, 1976.

History and Physical Examination of the Impotent Male

MIKE B. SIROKY
ROBERT J. KRANE

The history and, to a lesser extent, the physical examination can provide a very accurate assessment of the etiology of impotence. With refinements in behavioral and surgical therapy, etiologic considerations have become increasingly important in the selection of appropriate therapy and in predicting the patient's response to that therapy.

It is commonly stated that erectile impotence is either organic or psychogenic. With improvements in diagnostic techniques, it is increasingly clear that this is an oversimplification. The identification of psychologic conflicts does not imply that they are the cause of erectile impotence, because many organically impotent men are understandably anxious about their situation. Similarly, physical abnormalities, e.g., low serum testosterone levels, should not lead one to conclude that organic impotence is present.

Therefore, the history and physical examination serve several purposes: (1) characterization of the functional disability, (2) identification of possible etiologic factors, (3) assessment of physical findings, and (4) formulation of a diagnostic approach based on points 1, 2, and 3.

CHARACTERIZATION OF THE PROBLEM

The term *impotence* has various meanings; the physician therefore must determine what the patient understands by this term. In this discussion, *impotence* is defined as the persistent inability to obtain or maintain penile erection suitable for vaginal penetration and completion of intercourse. Confusion most commonly arises from situations involving decreased libido and ejaculatory dysfunction.

Occasionally, a patient will complain of "impotence" because he has noted a gradually decreased frequency of coitus with aging. Sexual function is completely normal when intercourse does take place. Libido is present but is less persistent than during youth. Such a patient is not, strictly speaking, impotent; nevertheless, reassurance and counseling should be offered if this is a source of anxiety.

Loss of libido is characterized by a nearly complete lack of sexual interest. This may be noted by the patient himself, but, more often, he seeks medical advice at the insistence of his spouse. Such a situation is most often psychologic in origin, especially due to clinical depression, but it may be caused by androgen deprivation.

The patient who has satisfactory erections but is unable to achieve intravaginal ejaculation suffers from *retarded ejaculation* or *anorgasmia*. Almost without exception, this is a manifestation of sexual conflict and requires psychotherapy or behavorial therapy. It should be distinguished from organic causes of loss of ejaculation, which include drug therapy (alpha-adrenergic blocking agents) and retroperitoneal surgery. In contrast, many patients complain of losing their erections because of *premature ejaculation*. This symptom has no known organic cause and is successfully treated with psychologic techniques.

If none of the above situations pertain, the nature of the erectile dysfunction should be assessed by history as follows:

1. Has the patient noted inability to achieve erection, inability to maintain erection, or both? What is the time course of this change in erectile function? Does the patient lose penile rigidity with pelvic movement?
2. What is the patient's assessment of the maximum rigidity obtained as a percentage of his situation prior to the onset of impotence?
3. Are there situations in which erections are normal or nearly normal, e.g., during masturbation, with new partners, on awakening, spontaneously?
4. What change, if any, has occurred in ejaculatory function and libido during this period of erectile insufficiency?

By using this approach, one can make a preliminary assessment of etiology (Table 12-1). Patients with vasculogenic impotence generally report a gradual decline in erectile function over a period of months or years. They first note decreased firmness and frequency of erections. With further progres-

Table 12-1. Preliminary assessment of impotence etiology

History	Psychologic aspects	Organic aspects
Time course	Sudden change	Gradual
Persistence	Situational	Persistent
Libido	Usually decreased	Slight decrease or unchanged
Ejaculation	Decreased	Preserved (absent in some cases of neurogenic impotence)

sion, there may be inability to sustain the erection, especially with pelvic movement. Finally, the patient notes that his erections are always partial at best. In time, he finds that the erections are insufficiently rigid for penetration.

In contrast, patients with psychogenic impotence report a rather sudden onset of impotence that is characterized by difficulty in attaining erection in some situations but not in others. When the patient is successful in achieving erection, it is described as being normal or nearly normal in rigidity. Libido often is decreased in patients with psychogenic impotence, but unchanged in those with vasculogenic or neurogenic sexual dysfunction. Of course, decreased libido is also characteristic of androgen deprivation or hyperprolactinemia.

In particular, it has been our experience that ejaculatory function is a useful discriminant of nonvascular as opposed to vascular etiology. Almost without exception, patients with hypogastric arterial insufficiency are able to ejaculate, despite the complete absence of erection, this often is not the case in psychogenic, neurogenic, and endocrine impotence.

ASSESSMENT OF ETIOLOGIC FACTORS

A wide variety of conditions may be pertinent to the complaint of impotence and should be sought in the history. Table 12-2 provides a

Table 12-2. Causative factors in impotence

Category	Examples
Pharmacologic	Antihypertensives, pheno-thiazines, estrogens
Vascular	Claudication, priapism
Neurologic	Peripheral neuropathies, herniated disk, multiple sclerosis
Endocrine	Hypogonadism, thyroid dysfunction, obesity, diabetes mellitus
Surgical	Radical pelvic surgery
Miscellaneous	Renal failure, hepatic cirrhosis

Table 12-3. Vasculogenic versus nonvasculogenic impotence

	Control group ($n = 68$)	Nonvasculogenic impotent patients ($n = 178$)	Vasculogenic impotent patients ($n = 231$)
Age	49	48	53
Hypertension	24%	32%	47%
Claudication or PVD	0	34%	41%
Smoking	47%	56%	72%
Diabetes	6%	20%	30%

Source: New England Male Reproductive Center, University Hospital, Boston.

partial list of the more common factors in approximate order of incidence.

Pharmacologic Causes

A wide variety of commonly used drugs have been reported to cause impotence [3]. The most common by far are the antihypertensive agents, especially α-methyldopa and propranolol. However, even diuretic agents may worsen erectile function. Thus, it seems that antihypertensives may act nonspecifically to reduce perfusion of an already compromised hypogastric vascular bed. This is supported by the fact that discontinuing these medications, rarely, if ever, completely restores erectile function.

Vascular Causes

The well-known *Leriche syndrome* describes aortoiliac occlusion and erectile impotence [2]. However, the majority of patients with vasculogenic impotence have little or no history of peripheral vascular disease (PVD). Nevertheless, the incidence of PVD is higher than in age-matched controls or in unselected patients complaining of impotence (Table 12-3). Furthermore, the incidence of risk factors for PVD such as hypertension, smoking, and diabetes is also higher than in controls or unselected impotent patients (Table 12-3).

Thus, it is extremely pertinent to inquire carefully regarding vascular symptoms such as claudication, leg atrophy, and rest pain. In addition, the presence, duration, and degree of systemic hypertension should be noted. The number of pack-years of cigarette smoking should be estimated. In this regard, we should note that some patients will relate that they do not smoke currently but neglect to mention a past history of 40 pack-years. Finally, the degree and duration of diabetes mellitus, if present, should be assessed, as well as any resulting complications such as nephropathy, neuropathy, and retinopathy.

Neurologic Causes

In our experience, approximately 10 percent of cases of impotence are due to neurologic causes [1]. The patient should be questioned regarding a history of numbness, weakness, visual difficulties, back problems, and urinary or bowel dysfunction. In patients with spinal cord injury (SCI), the level and completeness of the injury should be determined. In SCI, it is not uncommon to have poorly sustained erections that are inadequate for intercourse, rather than to have complete impotence.

Endocrine Causes

Endocrine impotence is rare, and it is even more uncommon as an initial manifestation of a previously undiagnosed endocrinopathy. Hypogonadism, hyperprolactinemia, and thyroid dysfunction, in that order, constitute the vast majority of cases of endocrine impotence.

Hypogonadism may be manifested by diminished libido and diminished sense of well-being as well as decreased beard growth. Hyperprolactinemia may manifest itself with decreased libido with or without gynecomastia. Thyroid dysfunction is extremely rare as a cause of impotence.

Miscellaneous
Hepatic cirrhosis may cause impotence due to abnormal metabolism of estrogens. The patient should be questioned regarding alcohol intake and history of hepatitis or jaundice.

PHYSICAL EXAMINATION
A systemic physical examination (Table 12-4) may corroborate the impression gained from the history. In addition, the physical examination is useful in ascertaining the presence of anatomic factors that may help in determining the surgical approach should a penile prosthesis be required (e.g., previous scars, excess adipose tissue).

General Findings
The development of secondary sexual characteristics is a gross index of androgen stimulation. Specifically, one can note the body and facial hair pattern, muscular development, and presence of gynecomastia. The size and consistency of the testes correlate well with the testosterone level when this is markedly depressed. Bilateral or unilateral cryptorchidism may be present.

Vascular and Neurologic Findings
The dorsal penile arterial pulse is rather easily palpated in normal males, and its absence should be noted. Sensation in the sacral dermatomes may be tested with a pinprick. The bulbocavernosus reflex is clinically present in almost all normal males. This reflex is evoked by squeezing the glans penis and digitally assessing the resultant contraction of the anal

Table 12-4. Examination of the impotent male

General findings
    Secondary sex characteristics
    Gynecomastia
Vascular-neurologic findings
    Dorsal penile pulse
    Sacral sensation
    Bulbocavernosus reflex
Genital findings
    Penile development
    Corporal fibrosis
    Phimosis
    Meatal stenosis
    Scrotal masses

sphincter. Assessment of the bulbocavernosus reflex is most conveniently carried out in conjunction with rectal examination of the prostate gland.

Genitalia
The corpora cavernosa should be palpated to assess their bulk and detect possible Peyronie's plaques. Fibrosis of the corpora may significantly increase the difficulty of placing an intracorporal prosthesis. Phimosis may rarely cause impotence by causing pain on erection. Furthermore, a foreskin that does not retract easily may cause problems after implantation of a penile prosthesis, which increases the circumference of the glans. The presence of meatal stenosis should be noted, since voiding difficulty may occur after surgery.

The scrotum should be examined for masses. A significant hydrocele may interfere with sexual function by virtue simply of its size.

REFERENCES
1. Goldstein, I. Personal communication, 1982.
2. Leriche, R. Des obliterations arterielles hautes comme cause d'insuffisance circulatoire des membres inferieures. *Bull. Soc. Chir. (Paris)* 49:1404, 1923.
3. Lipman, A. G. Drugs associated with impotence. *Mod. Med.* 45:81, 1977.

13

Vascular Noninvasive Diagnostic Techniques

MILORAD J. JEVTICH

The life of the flesh is in the blood.
Leviticus 17:11

Chapter 12 discussed the medical and sexual history, physical examination, and laboratory investigation in the assessment of the impotent patient. However, clinical methods such as these do not permit detection of many of the causes of impotence. This is particularly true regarding the detection of vascular disease causing erectile dysfunction.

Little progress in urologic evaluation or therapy has been made until recently. There are three reasons for this: (1) patients tend to be subjective and inaccurate about the history; (2) there is a lack of reliable methods for objective evaluation, and (3) there is a tendency on the part of physicians to categorize most impotence as psychologic in origin. Thus, studies of the hemodynamic aspects of erection, for the most part, have been neglected. Except for a few suggestions linking vascular disease and erectile failure (such as the Leriche syndrome, postulated in 1923), vascular diagnostic methods were not introduced until the early 1970s.

Recently, these procedures have come into more common use, particularly since the concept of vascular impotence has gained acceptance [25].

The advantages of noninvasive vascular procedures to be described are as follows:

1. Objective data is gained to support the always important history and clinical data.
2. Screening impotent patients is facilitated.
3. The accuracy of diagnosis is increased.
4. Selection of therapeutic options is refined.
5. Patients can be offered a concrete explanation of their impotence, based on solid diagnostic findings.
6. By and large, these techniques are simple and easy to perform, without incurring large costs.

With the above in mind, this chapter has several goals. The first is to evaluate different noninvasive methods of penile hemodynamic investigation with an emphasis on understanding of basic principles, techniques, and interpretation of their results. The second intention is to encourage clinicians to use their offices as diagnostic noninvasive laboratories. Techniques will be presented and explored in order of their sensitivity. They range from simple, inexpensive procedures to the more elaborate ones available in large medical centers. New practical suggestions will be introduced to complement clinically proved methods.

The notion that impotence is "all in one's mind" is a misconception. A clinician should approach "psychogenic impotence" as a *diagnosis by exclusion*. For this to take place, he must search for, and then accurately rule out, possible underlying vascular (or other organic) causes of impotence.

This does not mean that it is necessary to use each of the presently available noninvasive methods to diagnose penile vascular insufficiency. In fact, clinical judgment in an obvious case may indicate use only of an invasive method for arriving at a diagnosis. Such cases are infrequent, however. Most often a clinician sees patients without significant clinical findings, healthy men of all ages, or men with well-controlled associated diseases, yet their main complaint is erectile failure. For those, vascular noninvasive tests are of prime interest to a clinician.

HISTORY AND EXAMINATION

Prior to a discussion of noninvasive vascular investigation of impotent patients, however, let us look at some of the symptoms and signs that may lead one to suspect penile vascular insufficiency:

Cold fingers and feet
Cold penis
Penis "bends in the middle"
Color changes in the penis
Shrinking, or diminished size, of the penis
Minor complaints of claudication

In many instances, these will be only additional, or secondary, complaints offered by the patient. The clinician also may obtain information by asking about certain signs of erectile failure. Unsustained, semirigid, or poor erection are the most common complaints. Infrequent coitus, interrupted by the loss of a nonfirm erection is also pathognomonic. Attention should be paid to complaints of losing the erection while moving the legs, losing the erection while changing position during intercourse, or only achieving a firm erection while in an upright position. An erection achieved only while the body is at complete rest is a rare but significant clue. Penile deviation to one side, in primary or secondary impotence, is yet another clue.

During routine initial penile examination the physician should carefully palpate the consistency of the corpora cavernosa. In some instances of scleroderma, the corpora may feel firm and fibrotic similar to the way it feels following priapism, according to Scott [34]. Significant arteriosclerotic changes may cause the shaft of the penis to appear atrophied, while the glans penis appears larger than normal.

Finally, all diagnostic methods are best performed in an unhurried atmosphere. Clinicians should set aside time, perhaps one day a week for diagnostic screening, so that they might best serve their patients.

PENILE PULSE PALPATION

Pulse palpation has been recognized since ancient times as a method of observing the state of general health in humans, yet this classic method has seldom been used to evaluate the sexual function of the penis.

Penile arteries are delicate, and arterial pulses are sometimes difficult to detect. However, the clinician should master the technique of *penile arterial pulse palpation*. This is a natural first step in the procedure of noninvasive vascular screening for causes of impotence.

History

Canning and co-workers [8] palpated the penile pulses of 451 patients. They observed that 31 of this group, who complained of diminished sexual potency, had no palpable pulses. Abelson [1] reviewed the importance of penile pulse examination through palpation in studying impotent diabetics. Furlow [13] suggested that penile pulse palpation is an important aspect of the clinical examination given any impotent man.

Although Michal and co-workers [5] conducted their study of the penile dorsal arteries while the patients were anesthetized, they nevertheless found total consistency between the absence of pulsation in the dorsal arteries and angiographic findings of penile arterial occlusion.

Technique
To obtain the maximum diagnostic benefit from penile pulse palpation, the following method is suggested.

The paired dorsal arteries of the penis are the only ones that can be palpated. The clinician should bear in mind the need for a fine and sensitive touch. By placing the index finger at the base of the flaccid penis at a 12- to 1-o'clock position, while simultaneously pressing on the base of the left corpus cavernosum with the thumb, the index finger comes in contact with the left dorsal artery. The usual qualities of any pulse should be observed during this palpation (Fig. 13-1).

The right dorsal artery can be examined in one of two ways. The first is by moving the same finger and thumb across the midline of the penile base. The second involves the finger and thumb of the opposite hand being placed on the dorsal base of the penis and the ventral base of the corpus cavernosum, respectively.

If pulses are not easily detected in either of the paired dorsal arteries, the examining finger and thumb can be moved distally along the penile shaft. If a distal pulse is detected, another attempt should be made to locate a pulse at the base of the penis. Occasionally, the examiner may notice a small fibrotic cord. This represents a remnant of a once patent artery. Also, some patients may not have noticed a small fibrotic plaque (Peyronie's

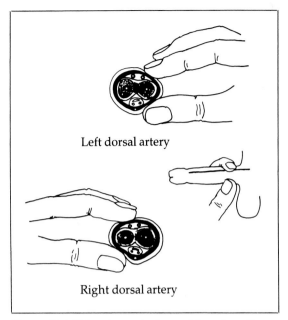

Left dorsal artery

Right dorsal artery

Figure 13-1. Palpation technique of dorsal penile arteries.

disease) in the path of the dorsal artery. The clinician should be alert to this because the patient may not have noticed its presence.

Comments
In the flaccid state, bilateral dorsal pulsations were detected by us in almost every sexually normal man. Abelson [1] stated that penile pulses were palpated in all of 29 normal men.

Among impotent men, especially the middle-aged and older group, we frequently found uneven or weak pulses either unilaterally or bilaterally. (In some cases penile pulses were completely undetectable.) Such abnormalities in penile pulses are even more noticeable in diabetics and patients with peripheral vascular disease. Abelson found that 6 of 15 diabetics had no discernible penile pulse [1].

Abnormal penile pulses, as detected by palpation, serve as a "first alert" to a clinician that vascular causes of impotence may be present. In addition, since the cavernous arteries are the first of the penile arteries to show vascular pathology [15] discovery of some irregularity in the dorsal arterial pulse usually will be indicative of coexisting pathology in the cavernous arteries.

PENILE TEMPERATURE

Recording the temperature of the human body has long been one of the tools used to determine diagnosis, prognosis, and treatment.

Production of heat is accomplished by metabolic processes. The circulatory system distributes heat from the sites of its production to cooler tissue. Temperature of a limb at rest is largely maintained by heat transferred into it by its blood supply [6]. Thus, the temperature of an extremity has been used as an assessment of the integrity of its circulation.

The same principle can be applied in assessing the blood supply of the penis. There are three pairs of small striated muscles attached to the perineal base of the penis. The penile shaft, however, contains only smooth muscle. Since there is no significant heat generated by the penis itself, the temperature of the penis is chiefly controlled and maintained by its arterial blood flow. Therefore, the measurement of penile temperature can be used as a noninvasive index of penile circulation.

History

There do not seem to be records of penile temperature available in the literature. The closest studies are those done by Moore [28], Badenoch [2], and Morales [29] each of whom measured scrotal and testicular temperatures.

In 1977, Ishii [18] reported a thermographic study of penile skin temperature changes during erection produced by drugs and visual stimulation. Six normal control subjects had an average temperature rise during erection of 1.28°C. Six psychogenically impotent patients had an average temperature rise of 1.58°C. In 13 organically impotent patients the temperature rise was only 0.77°C. The authors concluded that the rise of surface penile temperature, as recorded by this rather complicated method, could be used to differentiate between psychogenic and organic impotence.

Casey, reporting in 1979 [9], used thermography to record the temperature of the penis in his workup of some impotent men.

Penile Temperature

Penile temperature can be measured in two ways: externally, from the penile skin, and internally, through the inner body of the organ.

PENILE SKIN SURFACE TEMPERATURE. Large-skin-surface temperature currently is measured by thermography [37]. The general principle of thermography was applied to evaluation of penile surface temperature by Ishii [18], Tordjman [35], and Casey [97]. Thermography of the penis, however, is an expensive and somewhat complicated technique. A graphic picture of the penile surface temperature is produced by a scanning radiometer. The necessary equipment is found only in a few medical centers and is not readily available to the practicing urologist. Moreover, the temperature ascertained is not a reliable measurement of the total volume of blood flowing to the penis itself but is rather an index only of the blood flow to the skin of the organ.

INTERNAL PENILE TEMPERATURE. Measuring the penile temperature internally, however, will give a more accurate indication of penile arterial blood supply. To date, no methodology for such a measurement has been described. In early 1979, I developed the following examination procedure, which is easy to do on the flaccid penis.

Technique

In a room of average warmth (72–76°F), the patient, supine on an examining table, is checked first for arm blood pressure and pulse. Sublingual temperature is then recorded. A standard, battery-operated electronic thermometer with a heat sensor mounted in the tip of the probe is used. Accuracy of the thermometer is ± 0.02°F. The meatus of the urethra is cleaned with aqueous Zephiran and lubricated with 1% Xylocaine (lidocaine) jelly. As soon as the sublingual temperature is taken, the probe, covered with a new sterile plastic sheath, is inserted into the meatus. While holding the glans penis with two fingers, the examiner inserts the probe into the urethra to a depth approximately 1 in. from the level of the pubic surface. By bending the distal shaft of the

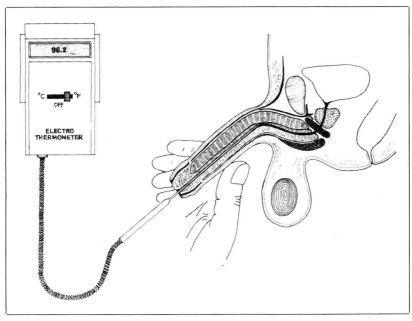

Figure 13-2. Technique of penile intraurethral temperature recording.

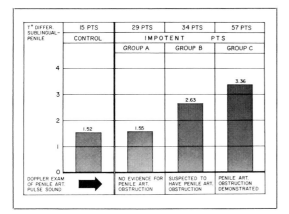

T° DIFFER. SUBLINGUAL– PENILE	15 PTS	29 PTS	34 PTS	57 PTS
	CONTROL	IMPOTENT	P T S	
		GROUP A	GROUP B	GROUP C
4				3.36
3			2.63	
2	1.52	1.55		
1				
0				
DOPPLER EXAM OF PENILE ART. PULSE SOUND	→	NO EVIDENCE FOR PENILE ART. OBSTRUCTION	SUSPECTED TO HAVE PENILE ART. OBSTRUCTION	PENILE ART. OBSTRUCTION DEMONSTRATED

Figure 13-3. These are the results of penile intraurethral temperature recording in 15 control and 120 impotent patients as compared to Doppler PAPS exam.

penis downward at the point of the probe's tip, the sensor can make maximum contact with the midportion of the corpora cavernosa, through the thin roof of the urethra (Fig. 13-2). (This is practical because the temperature sensor mainly records heat in the corpora cavernosa.) The temperature is registered in 30 to 40 seconds, and the probe is then removed. The procedure causes minimal discomfort and has no aftereffects.

Material and Results

The internal penile temperature was measured in 120 consecutive impotent patients. Gradients between sublinqual and flaccid penile temperatures were calculated easily.

As a control, 15 nonsymptomatic urologic patients with normal erectile function also were measured for the differential gradient.

Group A; 29 patients (24.1%), had an average penile temperature of 96.3°F. The median temperature difference was 1.55°F.

Group B; 34 patients (28.1%), had a median difference of 2.6°F.

Group C; 57 patients (47.5%) had an average penile temperature of 94.6°F with a median difference of 3.3°F. The difference was 2.2 to 9.3°F.

The control group showed an average penile temperature of 96.6°F and a median difference of 1.52°F.

Figure 13-3 illustrates the results obtained in this study.

Comments

To further assess the status of the penile arterial flow in these patients and controls, our method of Doppler ultrasound examination of penile arteries was used [19] (see under Method at the end of this chapter).

The patients in the control group and group A, with similar internal penile temperature (96.6 and 96.3°F, respectively) showed normal circulation of the penile arteries on Doppler examination.

Patients in group C, who showed an average internal penile temperature substantially lower, and a median difference between sublingual and penile temperature of 3.3°F, indicated positive signs of obstructed arterial flow on Doppler examination. It was assumed that their impotence was caused by vascular deficiency.

In group B, the penile arterial pulse sound (PAPS) Doppler examination suggested possible penile arterial flow impairment in some instances. Most of group B appeared to have mixed etiologic causes of impotence.

By use of other diagnostic criteria, the patients in group A were found to have nonorganic causes of impotence.

Later, most of patients in group C having positive signs of obstruction of penile arteries were classified as vasculogenically impotent by other evaluations.

Discussion

Too often, routine clinical examinations in the past did not suggest an organic cause of impotence. There are two reasons for this:

1. There were no objective methods for evaluation of a patient's complaint.
2. Past medical focus favored the psychogenic approach as an explanation of impotence.

Intraurethral measurement of penile temperature can yield results that suggest the need for further study of a man affected by impotence. An awareness of possible physical impairment that could cause erectile difficulties was gained through a simple clinical procedure. This, in turn, suggested that further noninvasive investigations could lead to a more definite diagnosis. Any of the other noninvasive tests for evaluation of penile arterial circulation can further demonstrate possible impaired arterial flow in the penis. We, however, prefer verification by our method of Doppler ultrasound examination of penile arterial pulse sound [19]. This method has proved to be reliable and specific in our hands.

Possible errors in this intraurethral measurement of penile temperature are negligible, since the sensor of the thermometer is in contact with the voluminous mass of the corpora cavernosa through the thin roof of the corpus spongiosum.

Cavernosal cylinders are the most voluminous part of the penile body, even in the flaccid state. They are also the main reservoirs of penile blood that deliver heat to the organ.

In our experience, patients having more than 3°F difference between sublingual and internal penile temperature are most likely to have significant penile arterial obstruction. For this reason, we recommend obtaining internal penile temperature as a part of an initial clinical examination of any patient complaining of impotence. Since vascular causes of impotence were discovered in recent years to be high on etiologic lists, the physician should consider the use of a simple, inexpensive screening test, as is done with any other diagnostic problem in medicine. Only in this way can we hope to make progress in the diagnosis and treatment of impotence.

PENILE PLETHYSMOGRAPHY

Plethysmography is one of the oldest methods used for measuring volume changes in the extremities [16]. The volume changes of an organ or limb relate directly to the amount of blood flowing to that organ or limb. Many current vascular principles deal with the study of blood volume changes. The most common relates to the volume changes produced by each pulse beat. These are recorded by a pulse plethysmograph [4].

Two plethysmographic methods frequently are employed in urologic investigations of impotence.

The first uses a mercury strain gauge plethysmograph for monitoring the slowly developing periodic volume changes that should occur during nocturnal penile tumescence (NPT) cycle.

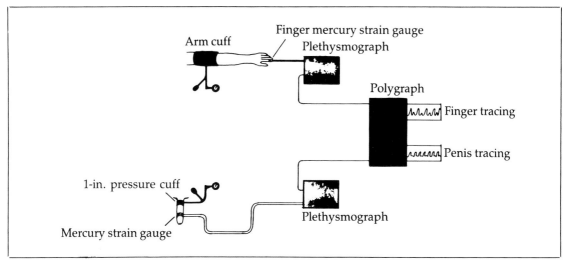

Figure 13-4. Scheme of penile plethysmography.

The second method, which employs a pulse-type mercury strain gauge plethysmograph will be discussed in this section. This method is designed to record the volume of each pulse-produced expansion of the penis.

History
Whitney [38] introduced the mercury strain gauge in 1953 to register volume changes. His method has been refined and improved in the past 20 years and is currently used in many vascular laboratories.

Canning [8] was probably the first to apply plethysmography to evaluation of penile circulation in impotence. His study was published in 1963.

Eight years later, in 1971, Britt and coworkers [7] revived the pulse-type mercury strain gauge method. They used it to determine the penile blood flow in impotent patients suspected of obstructed penile circulation.

This method continues to be used as one of the noninvasive studies for the evaluation of possible vascular causes of impotence.

Method and Technique
The *strain gauge* is a small-caliber tube, made of elastic rubber and filled with mercury. When the gauge is placed around the distal part of the flaccid penis, pulse volume changes in the organ produce a corresponding stretching of the mercury in the elastic band. This, in turn, increases the electrical resistance of the mercury. The gauge is connected to a plethysmograph, which is hooked to an amplifier-recorder. The recorder produces the pulse curve [7].

The simplicity of this method is deceptive. In addition to the mercury strain gauge many examiners place a 1-in. pediatric blood pressure cuff around the base of the penis.

Moreover, it is recommended that the examiner obtain a simultaneous study of the arm and index finger for comparison. This requires two plethysmographs and a dual-channel recorder (Fig. 13-4). The examiner may choose to record the pulse volume changes in the finger first and then use the same equipment for penile recording, but this is less desirable.

The examination should be conducted in a warm room, with the patient relaxed and resting horizontally. It is suggested that the baseline pulse curve, systolic blood pressure, and postocclusive reactive hyperemia tests all be evaluated. In addition, it is further recommended that the pulse curve be identified at the 40 mm Hg pressure point in the cuff. (Penile systolic blood pressure reading is obtained at the exact point where the pulse curve reappears while one is slowly deflating the cuff.)

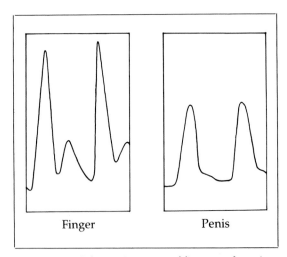

Figure 13-5. Schematic curves of finger and penis. Plethysmographic normal findings.

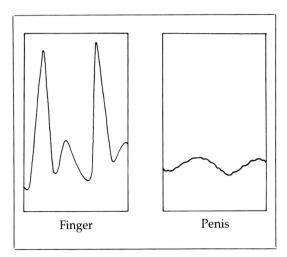

Figure 13-6. Schematic curves of finger and penis. Abnormal plethysmographic findings.

Interpretation

According to Britt [7], and, more recently, Montague [27], a normal penile pulse curve is similar to that of the index finger. Figure 13-5 illustrates the digital and penile pulse curve in a normal person. The ascending limb of a systolic peak is sharp; it is followed by a slower downslope limb.

The minute dicrotic notch is not always present on the penile pulse curve [7]. Moreover, the appearance of the penile pulse curve can be modified by changes in local temperature and autonomic nervous activity. The mercury strain gauge must be filled properly because mercury has a high frequency response [4]. It should be noted that this method registers only a total pulse volume.

If there is penile arterial obstruction, the general shape of the curve is more rounded and of less amplitude. There is a delay in the occurrence of the systolic peak, and no diastolic notch is found (Fig. 13-6).

In severely obstructed arterial flow, the penile pulse curve is markedly reduced, or even absent [7].

Penile systolic blood pressure (PBP) will be discussed in the next section. It is suggested that PBP readings be added to the interpretation of the plethysmographic recordings.

Postocclusive reactive hyperemia is also needed for further assessment of the functional capacity of penile arterial circulation [7]. After the blood pressure cuff has totally occluded the penile blood flow for 3 to 5 min, the pressure in the cuff is swiftly released, and the pulse curve recording is repeated.

In a normal penis, the postocclusive pulse wave is almost doubled. If there is impaired arterial flow, the pulse curve shows little change after occlusion. There may even be a decrease in pulse amplitude (Fig. 13-7).

Results

Canning and co-workers [8] presented results showing that of 41 impotent patients, 26 had a flattening of the plethysmographic curve. In 18 of the 26, abnormal plethysmographic recordings were confirmed by aortograms showing obstructive changes in the pelvic vessels.

In a study performed by Britt [7] 25 healthy, sexually normal males were examined as controls. None of them showed abnormalities in penile circulation. Of 40 vascular patients complaining of impotence, only 10 were considered to have definitely abnormal penile blood flow. It is interesting that four of his patients were clinically diagnosed as having vascular causes of impotence, yet their plethysmographic studies were normal. The author concluded that this discrepancy could have resulted either from the use of an insufficiently sensitive method to detect penile vascular obstruction, or a possible mis-

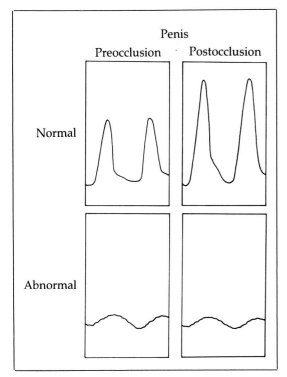

Figure 13-7. Schematic curves of normal and abnormal penile postocclusive reactive hyperemia.

diagnosis as to the cause of impotence.

Also of interest is a recent study by Montague and co-workers [27]. Out of 165 patients studied, penile plethysmography reported significant abnormalities of the penile systolic blood pressure and pulse volume in only 13 men (16.8%).

Discussion

It is generally recognized that pulse volume fluctuations are produced by passive expansion or contraction of the vascular channels in an organ or limb. It is not clear, however, as to which type of vessels are involved in the pulse volume changes of an organ. Since the venous system is larger in volume than the arterial, more significant volume changes may take place in the venous vessels [31].

If, in fact, the reported results deal with the venous system, one then gets the impression that penile pulse plethysmography may not be the most sensitive or accurate of the more sophisticated noninvasive methods used to determine vascular causes of impotence. One of the reasons for this may be the possibility, as mentioned, that plethysmography records the penile venous mass rather than the arterial. Second, no matter what vessels it measures, it records information of the total blood volume to the penis. It does not give any specific information about which of the particular vessels of the complex circulatory system of the penis is being measured. Third, and most important, the complex nature of the penile arterial system itself may give rise to further confusion in plethysmographic measurement. The penis not only has a completely paired arterial inflow, but arterial circulation is divided into nutritive and functional (erectile) capabilities. Therefore, for example, arterial flow to the corpora spongiosa and superficial penile tissue could be completely normal, yet the blood supply to the corpora cavernosa itself, severely impaired. This has been documented recently in some angiographic and histologic studies of the penile arteries [32].

Therefore, some pathologic changes in the penile arteries very well may go undetected by the mercury strain gauge. Plethysmographic recordings may indicate normal or not sufficiently altered penile pulse curves, that in fact could disguise an existing pathology.

In contrast to the above, recent reports [19, 20, 24] based on Doppler ultrasound studies of all the penile arteries gave much higher indications for possible arterial obstructions.

PENILE BLOOD PRESSURE

Blood pressure measurement in the extremities of the body is a standard procedure for the assessment of their circulatory process.

Penile blood pressure measurement is not yet standard. The method was not introduced and suggested as a test for evaluation of impotence until 10 years ago.

History

In May, 1971, Britt and co-workers [7] published a study on penile plethysmography. One of the reported measurements was systolic penile blood pressure. Assuming that the sexually normal person has similar blood pressure in the arm and the penis, they concluded that if the PBP was 20 mm Hg below the arm pressure, there was evidence of impaired penile circulation.*

More than a year after Britt's paper was accepted, Gaskell [14] published findings in November, 1971, that dealt exclusively with PBP. He is generally credited as the first to show the importance of PBP in an objective evaluation of impotence.

Nevertheless, the diagnostic value of penile pulse and blood pressure measurements did not really come to the attention of urologists until Abelson's paper [1] in 1975.

In the last 5 years, other authors [11, 13, 26] also have presented their experience with penile blood pressure measurement. Consequently, PBP is now considered one of the basic tests for vasculogenic evaluation of the penis.

Methods and Techniques

According to the literature, there are four methods for recording PBP.

The *plethysmographic method*, as introduced by Britt and co-workers [7], gives a systolic reading of the pressure in the penis. A 1-in. pneumatic cuff is placed around the base of the penis while the strain-gauge band is placed distally to the cuff. The band is attached to a plethysmograph recorder. The baseline plethysmographic curve is first recorded. The pressure cuff is then inflated above the systolic pressure and slowly deflated until the pulse curve reappears on the recorder, at which point the PBP is measured.

Gaskell's [14] method of obtaining a PBP reading employed a *spectroscope*. This had been used in the past to measure the systolic pressure in the fingers. Because it is a technically complicated method, it has been replaced in recent years by the Doppler ultrasound method.

Abelson [1] introduced the *Doppler ultrasound method* of obtaining PBP in 1975. His original technique made use of an ultrasound transducer recessed in a narrow ½-in. cuff. It

*I consider this article to be the first objective evaluation of vasculogenic impotence, because the paper was accepted for publication in September, 1970.

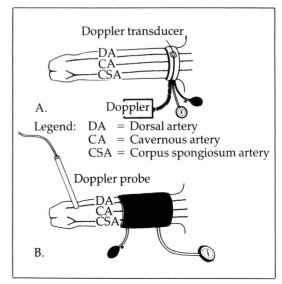

Figure 13-8. Techniques of penile blood pressure examination. A. Preferred method. B. "Simplified" method.

had been developed to measure the arm blood pressure in infants. In his PBP measurements, the cuff is placed around the base of the penis. The cuff, containing the transducer, is moved to either side of the penis until the dorsal artery is located on the ipsilateral side. The systolic pressure of the dorsal artery is determined by the pulsating sound heard between inflation and deflation of the cuff. Abelson determined separate values for both right and left dorsal arteries. Although he also recorded diastolic pressures he questioned the validity of his diastolic findings, and used only the systolic readings to establish a normal criterion for PBP [3, 12, 23, 26].

Since 1975, others have used a "simplified" Doppler evaluation of PBP (Fig. 13-8).

A standard 1-in. cuff attached to a manometer is wrapped around the proximal part of the penile shaft. The pencil probe of the Doppler is placed distally to the penis at the dorsum, glans, or frenulum. The first arterial sound detected by the probe during deflation of the cuff is used to record the systolic pressure of the penis.

Although they used different methods of obtaining PBP, all authors agreed that a penile systolic pressure measuring 20 to 30 mm Hg, lower than brachial systolic pressure could be a sign of impaired penile blood flow. Moreover, there was also agreement that such a lowered pressure and possible arterial obstruction could be capable of causing impotence.

Penile Brachial Indices

Abelson [1] derived normal measurements by comparing brachial, popliteal, and penile pressures. He found that normal penile systolic pressure was between arm and leg pressures. Popliteal was slightly higher, and brachial slightly lower, than penile pressure. In addition, he established the penile mean pressure in sexually active males as being significantly higher than either popliteal or brachial.

Zorgniotti [26, 39] and Engel and co-workers [12] continued work on penile-brachial indices as measures of normal-abnormal penile arterial circulation.

According to Zorgniotti, the penile-brachial mean pressure (PBMP) is calculated by the formula:

Penile systolic pressure (mm Hg)

$$\pm \left[\frac{\text{Brachial pulse pressure}}{3} + \text{Brachial diastolic pressure} \right] = \text{PBMP}$$

In his studies, normal subjects showed a lower PBMP (+14) than that calculated in Abelson's data (PBMP = +43). He concluded that his parameter for abnormal PBMP would be any measurement below +14.

Engel [12], however, came up with still another calculation for penile-brachial index.

$$\frac{\text{Penile systolic BP}}{\text{Brachial systolic BP}} = \text{PB index}$$

According to his studies, the PB index was not altered by minor changes in systemic blood pressure, by general anesthesia, or by the pressure of a urethral catheter.

He found that normally potent patients had a PB index of >0.961 (±0.053). Impotent patients without any symptoms of vascular dis-

ease were found to have a PB index of >0.593 (±0.114). (Patients with documented psychogenic impotence were found to have a PBI in the normal range.)

Although these authors differ in calculating their penile-brachial indices, their conclusions nevertheless should be considered in the diagnostic evaluation of penile arterial blood flow.

Comments

PBP evaluation is a more sensitive measurement than palpation of penile arteries. However, to maximize the evaluation, the examiner must be knowledgeable about the arterial anatomic differences that exist between the penis and other extremities.

Arms or thighs have only one major artery, so there can be only one pressure reading. Thus, a brachial index is determined from only one artery.

The penis, however, has a dual arterial blood supply with three arteries on each side. Of these six arteries, the two cavernosa, and to a lesser extent, the two dorsal are responsible for erection. The two arteries of the corpus spongiosum have no significant erectile function. Therefore, the most accurate evaluation of PBP would be accomplished by a separate determination of the pressure in each of the four erectally functional arteries. Such a method gives more objective data about PBP than the previously mentioned penile-brachial mean pressures or the penile-brachial index because one deals with four separate data rather than total data.

Of the different PBP methods cited at the beginning of this section, it appears that Abelson's technique is the most reliable. This method yields the most objective measurement of the pressure in the functional arteries of the penis. A plethysmograph, in addition to being complicated, can measure only the estimated total flow at a distal location of the organ.

There are several reasons for reaching this conclusion. The "simplified" Doppler method, in which the Doppler probe is placed over the distal portion of the penile body, may produce misleading results because it measures only the terminal arterial pressure of the corpus spongiosum arteries or the distal dorsal arterial branches.

Moreover, the histologic studies of penile arteries, done by Ružbarsky and Michal [32] suggest that pathologic changes are seldom found in intima or in the muscle walls of the corpus spongiosum arteries. Fibrosis, atherosclerotic obliteration, or thrombosis resulting in obstructive penile arterial flow were found only in the four functional arteries.

In addition, angiographic recordings indicate that significant arterial lesions are located most often in the distal pudendal or proximal parts of penile arteries at the level of the pubis and base of the penis. These are areas where the penile blood pressure is not checked when one is using the simplified Doppler method. Since the cuff is placed at the base of the penis in the simplified method, the probe has room only to search over the distal areas of the organ. (Casey [10] also has commented on the possibility of error when one is measuring single-point PBP at the level of the glans.)

Zorgniotti stated in May, 1980 [40], "Blood pressure determination only gives a rough idea of the presence of vascular disease. It is possible that penile blood pressure measurements, ultimately, will be judged of little value . . ."

The preceding facts suggest that the simplified Doppler method of PBP examination is less sensitive and less accurate. Our preference therefore has been to utilize the Abelson Doppler ultrasound method.

DOPPLER EXAMINATION OF PENILE ARTERIAL PULSES

The discovery of Doppler ultrasound and its subsequent use in medicine has been recognized as a most valuable adjunct to clinical work with patients. Doppler ultrasound has been used in an assessment of arterial and venous circulation. The measurements of the flowmeter have become the most simple, accurate, and versatile test for detection of peripheral vascular disease [22].

It therefore is logical to consider the use of Doppler ultrasound in the diagnosis of penile arterial obstruction. It would be expected that in a man with normal erectile capabilities it would indicate intact penile arterial flow. Conversely, altered flow, which might be a cause of impotence, also could be determined.

Doppler Principle and Signal Processing
Detailed information about the "shift principle," which is the basis of ultrasound examination, can be found in references 5 and 22.

Briefly, the Doppler instrument produces an ultrasound beam that is directed toward a blood vessel. The motion of the red blood cells provides a frequency shift, a backscattering signal. This returns to the instrument, where it is amplified by the audio component into a pulsating sound proportional to the blood flow velocity [17].

For most clinicians, an audible output is the simplest and cheapest method of producing a sound satisfactory for interpretation. Accurate interpretation of the Doppler audio signals does require experience, but, with practice, the examiner soon can learn to recognize the difference between normal and abnormal sounds.

If a more accurate and objective evaluation of the signals is desired, however, the use of a permanent chart tape recording is recommended when recording a pulse waveform. The audio output is connected to a DC amplifier with a strip chart recorder.

Many new clinical applications of Doppler ultrasound have been introduced recently into various branches of medicine, including urology.

History
Satomura [33] introduced the use of the Doppler flowmeter in 1959 as a diagnostic tool for peripheral vascular diseases.

In 1973, Malvar and co-workers [24] used the Doppler flowmeter to study the penile blood flow of three penile arteries in 36 volunteers. They used radial arterial flow as a control standard. The right and left cavernous arteries were reportedly recorded separately, although the flow of the two dorsal arteries was calculated as a single entity. Earlier studies [8, 30] were corroborated by their conclusions that a normal flow rate coexists with potency, whereas a low flow rate is often found with impotency.

Abelson used the Doppler method in 1975 [1] mainly to evaluate the PBP in volunteers and in diabetics. His method and results are described in the preceding section on PBP.

In 1978, three papers were presented that studied penile arterial flow by Doppler ultrasound.

Casey and Kaufman [11] measured the blood pressure and penile arterial flow of all six arteries in 19 patients. They suggested that ultrasound studies of penile arterial pulses is a valid method for assessing vascular impotency.

Jevtich [19] evaluated the penile arterial pulse in all penile arteries of 42 impotent patients. Doppler signals were interpreted aurally and also processed by quantitative evaluation of tape recordings. Positive findings of penile arterial obstruction were elicited in 17 patients (40.4%). Of these, obstruction was further confirmed in 9 out of 10 cases (90%) by penile angiography. The Doppler examination thus assumes an important role as part of the screening test that should be administered to any impotent patient.

Juhan [21] also used Doppler velocimetry of penile arteries as a method of selecting patients for arteriography. In a study of 55 patients, 50 showed obstructive signs during the Doppler examination. These signs were confirmed in 49 of the 50 patients. He used five normal subjects as controls. Both the Doppler examination and subsequent arteriography showed normal penile arteries in the control subjects.

Velcek, in a recent article [36], used a method similar to that of Jevtich but included a complicated and time-consuming penile blood flow index, theoretically to improve the qualitative judgment of penile circulation. However, there was only a 50 percent correlation in his findings between his method and further penile angiographic studies in 26 patients. This may be explained by the fact that Velcek calculates the flow of only one dorsal artery as being representative of both dorsal arteries.

Having performed the Doppler method in over 250 patients, we believe that vasculogenic impotence is more easily identified by the following technique.

Method

We use a 9.3 MHz Doppler instrument with nondirectional, continuous-wave, zero-crossing frequency. The Doppler has a small pencil probe. The built-in speaker is connected to the DC amplifier chart recorder of a single-channel ECG machine. Our unit also has input-output levels as well as an output filter that improves sensitivity and reduces accessory noises. The recording speed is 2.5 cm/sec.

The patient is placed in a supine position. Blood pressure and pulse are determined. The pulse sound at the base of the second or third left finger is recorded for a comparative control. (In a few patients, radial pulse was used for this purpose.)

A coupling gel is applied to the penile skin near its base, and the pencil probe is placed over the area of the right dorsal artery. The position of the probe should be at a 35- to 40-degree angle to the direction of the blood flow. Pressure applied while examining the dorsal or other superficial arteries should be *very light*. However, when one is examining the corpora cavernosa arteries, increased pressure from the probe will not alter the sound or wave.

After ultrasounding of the right dorsal artery, the other penile arteries are examined in a clockwise direction. Both dorsal arteries are examined easily at the level of the base. The probe is then moved distally to the penile shaft, proximal to the corona glans, where examination of the distal branches of the penile arteries is done in the same manner.

Sound over the corpus cavernosum represents blood flow in the corporal artery or its branches, but it is not always easy to detect.

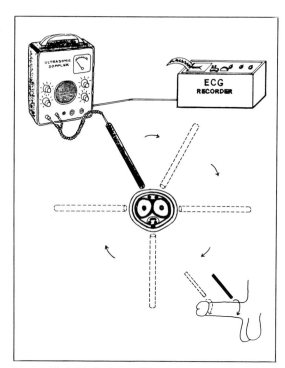

Figure 13-9. Technique of Doppler penile arterial pulse sound (PAPS) examination.

Table 13-1. Penile arteries pulse sound criteria

Normal	Good sound (2 DA)
	Good to poor sound (2 CB and FA)
Positive	No sound (2 DA)
	No sound (1 DA and 2 CB)
	Poor sound (2 DA) and no sound (2 CB)
Suspect	Fair to poor sound (2 DA and 2 CB)
	Poor sound (1 DA) and no sound (2 CB)

Note: These are the criteria for analysis of Doppler penile arteries pulse sound exam.
Key: DA = dorsal penile arteries; CB = cavernous body of penis; FA = frenular artery.

evaluated by making a recording of each individual artery. A standardized chart is used for this purpose.

Table 13-1 illustrates the criteria for analysis of penile arterial pulse sound. Waveforms of normal PAPS show larger waves, rapid upstroke, a small dicrotic notch at the end of the down stroke, and, very rarely, a smaller third notch in younger patients.

Figures 13-10 and 13-11 illustrate the PAPS recording of a 19-year-old and an 88-year-old control subject.

An obstructed penile artery shows a slow upstroke, smaller waveforms, and lack of the dicrotic notch. (Complete occlusion produces no waves at all during recording.)

Figures 13-12 and 13-13 show the PAPS of a 36- and a 50-year-old nondiabetic patient.

Figures 13-14 and 13-15 illustrate waveform analysis of a 41- and a 49-year-old diabetic.

Figures 13-16 and 13-17 show PAPS recording of a 31-year-old postpriapism patient and a 45-year-old past alcoholic.

The PAPS Doppler examinations in Figures 13-11 through 13-16 were confirmed by subsequent penile angiography.

Some patients have penile pulses that contain both normal features and waveform shapes indicating obstruction. There is a somewhat slower upstroke. The downstroke has a very small, less noticeable dicrotic notch, which usually appears in the upper portion of the down slope curve. There is a small, irregular notch at the peak of the wave. This finding suggests some disturbance in the penile artery that we are classifying at present as WNL.

With experience, however, sound detection will become more frequent. Occasionally, this sound may be confused with the flow in the branches of the dorsal arteries (Fig. 13-9).

Normally, Doppler penile flow velocity signals are biphasic. There is a prominent, high-pitched sound of the systolic, with a less prominent, softer, diastolic sound. Sometimes, in younger patients, a third very soft sound can be heard.

In conjunction with the ultrasound examination and, as a further check we apply a squeezing maneuver to the distal shaft of the penis. After a few seconds of compression, normal penile arteries produce an improved Doppler signal sound that lasts for several seconds. Obstructed or functionally impaired arteries show no improvement in sound or recorded waves as a result of compression.

Usually, sound analysis is sufficient for rapid screening of penile circulation. If an experienced examiner detects normal flow, no recording is necessary, but a positive sound analysis suggesting impaired flow is further

Results
For 3 years we examined over 250 patients of ages 19 to 78, who had complaints of erectile impotence. In addition, 21 sexually normal patients, ages 14 to 88 were examined. A total of 319 studies were performed. Table 13-2 indicates the past history of the last 170 patients.

CONTROLS. Of the 21 sexually normal patients who were examined for PAPS, 20, or 95.2 percent, were found to have normal penile arterial flow.

One was classified as suspect. As a double control, we later reexamined 33 of the impotent patients (1–4 months later). All but one showed findings identical to the first PAPS examination.

IMPOTENT. As is shown in Table 13-3 positive ultrasound examination for penile arterial obstruction was elicited in 104 of 250 impotent males (41.6%). Of the group, 66 showed normal PAPS (26.4%). (They were later classified by other diagnostic methods as having psychogenically related impotence.) There were also 77 patients who were suspected to have some degree of diminished arterial flow. Most of the patients in this latter group had associated abnormalities of testosterone levels, neural changes, or other associated diseases.

Our data agree with some findings [24], but they are not corroborated by another series [27]. In the latter, the simplified Doppler technique and/or plethysmography were the methods of evaluation. These authors found only 16.8 percent vascular insufficiency. A possible explanation of this difference is given in the section on penile blood pressure.

Comments
There were 40 patients of the 104 showing positive signs of penile arterial obstruction who required further evaluation. Consequently, these 40 patients were examined by penile angiography.

Penile angiography confirmed not only an obstruction of the blood flow to the penis in 36 patients (97.3%), but in a majority of cases, confirmed the site and severity of the obstructive process (89.3%).

In three patients, penile angiography was not technically satisfactory for a final diagnosis.

Further findings in these 40 patients will be discussed in Chapter 14.

Michal and Pospichal [25] recently stated, "on the basis of phalloarteriographic findings and histological investigation of the arterial bed of the penis, we believe that most impotence is the symptomatic and functional result of arterial disease."

It appears that severe stenosis and obstructed penile arterial flow are not accidental findings but are closely related to the presence of impotence. Finding 41.6 percent of patients to have penile arterial obstruction as a possible cause of impotence seems to confirm this statement.

Our study and methods once again indicate the value of objective testing in the workup of the impotent man. In particular, the method we use appears to be more specific and sensitive than noninvasive vascular evaluations of impotence described in prior sections. There are four reasons for this belief:

1. Each functional artery of the penis is examined separately, first, by sound analysis; then, if necessary, a quantitative recording is made and further evaluated.
2. We examine the arteries of the penile base, where pathologic changes often occur, and then compare this to an examination of the distal arteries.
3. The squeezing maneuver is added during the Doppler examination for further functional evaluation.
4. We employ the most precise angle of the Doppler probe, while maintaining the lightest pressure.

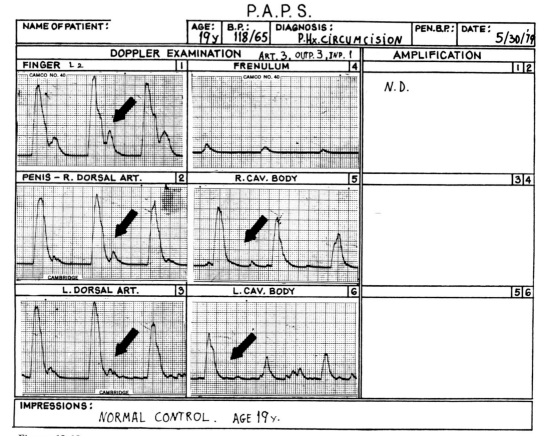

Figure 13-10

Figures 13-10 and 13-11. PAPS waveform analysis of 19- and 88-year-old control subjects. Both patients showed normal appearance of the waveforms.

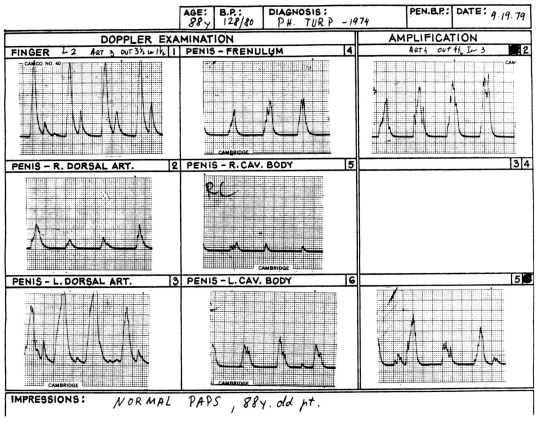

Figure 13-11

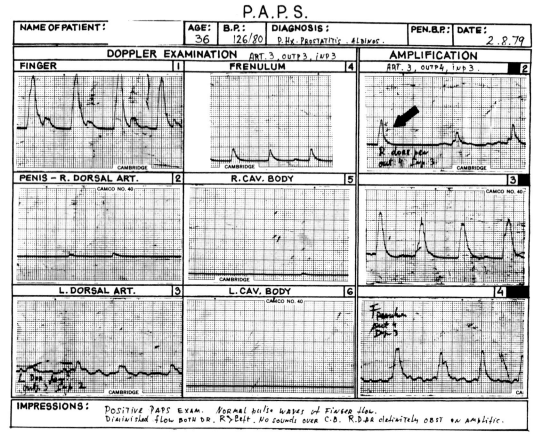

Figure 13-12

Figures 13-12 and 13-13. These figures indicate the PAPS of 36- and 50-year-old nondiabetic patients. Both examinations were positive. The first patient illustrates absent waves of the cavernosa arteries and the right dorsal artery. The second patient shows early changes in the right dorsal artery and an obstructed flow in the arteries of the left side.

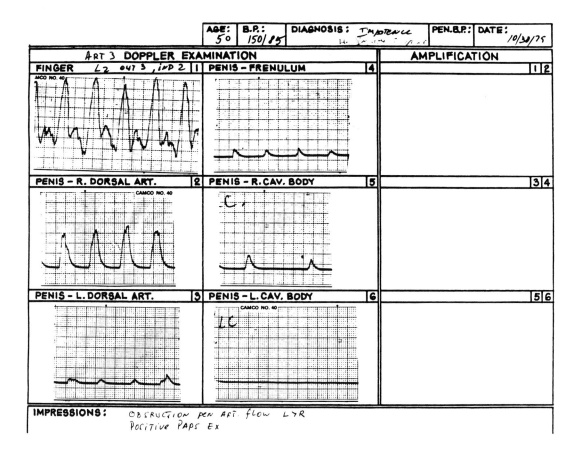

Figure 13-13

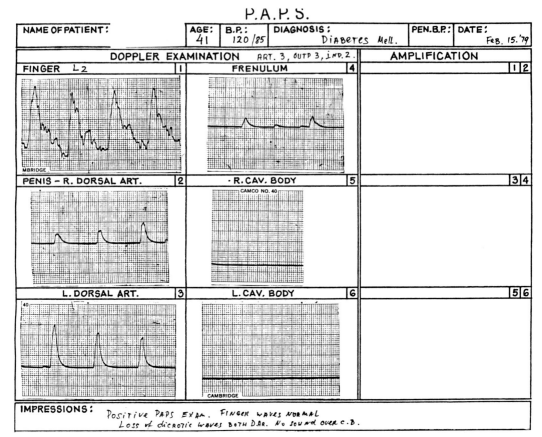

P.A.P.S.

NAME OF PATIENT:	AGE: 41	B.P.: 120/85	DIAGNOSIS: Diabetes Mell.	PEN.B.P.:	DATE: Feb. 15.'79

DOPPLER EXAMINATION	ART. 3, OUTP 3, IND.2.	AMPLIFICATION

FINGER L2 |1| FRENULUM |4| |1|2|

PENIS - R. DORSAL ART. |2| R. CAV. BODY |5| |3|4|
CAMCO NO. 40

L. DORSAL ART. |3| L. CAV. BODY |6| |5|6|
CAMBRIDGE

IMPRESSIONS: Positive PAPS Exam. Finger waves normal
Loss of dicrotic waves both D.Ar. No sound over C.B.

Figure 13-14

Figures 13-14 and 13-15. These figures illustrate the waveform analysis of 41- and 49-year-old diabetics. Both examinations were positive. There is an obstructed flow of the right arteries in both patients. There is also an early impairment of the left dorsal artery, and no flow in the left deep artery.

P.A.P.S.

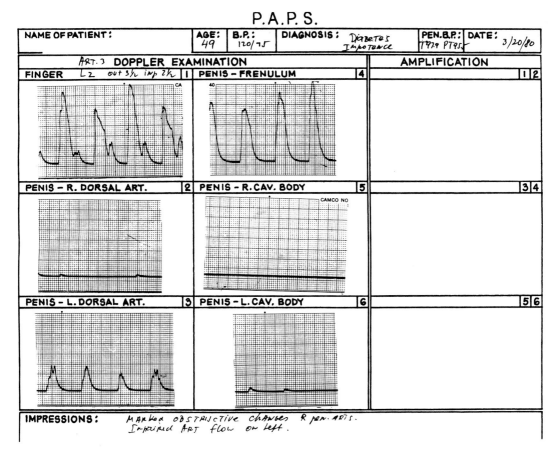

| NAME OF PATIENT: | AGE: 49 | B.P.: 120/75 | DIAGNOSIS: Diabetes Impotence | PEN.B.P.: T929 PT95 | DATE: 3/20/80 |

ART. 3 DOPPLER EXAMINATION — **AMPLIFICATION**

FINGER L2 out 3k imp 2k | 1 PENIS – FRENULUM | 4 — 1 | 2

PENIS – R. DORSAL ART. | 2 PENIS – R. CAV. BODY | 5 — 3 | 4

PENIS – L. DORSAL ART. | 3 PENIS – L. CAV. BODY | 6 — 5 | 6

IMPRESSIONS: Marked obstructive changes R pen. arts. Impaired Art flow on left.

Figure 13-15

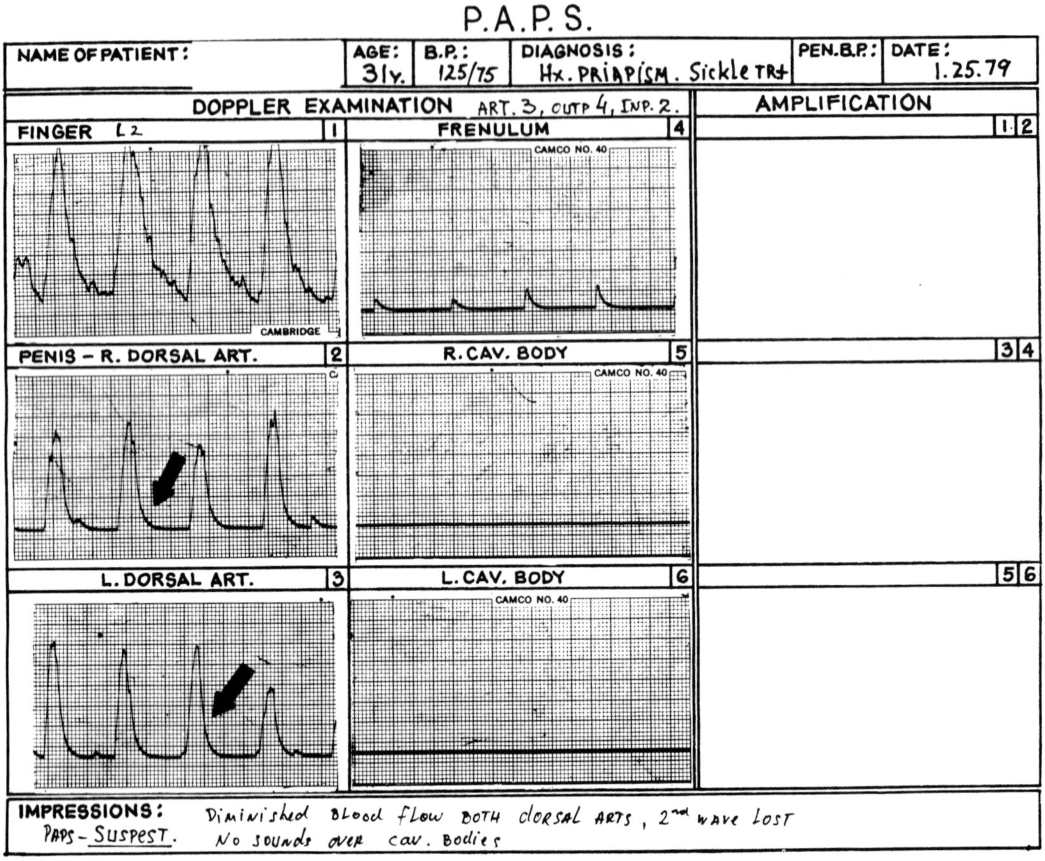

P.A.P.S.

NAME OF PATIENT:	AGE: 31y.	B.P.: 125/75	DIAGNOSIS: Hx. PRIAPISM. Sickle TR+		PEN.B.P.:	DATE: 1.25.79

DOPPLER EXAMINATION ART. 3, OUTP 4, INP. 2.	AMPLIFICATION

FINGER L2	1	FRENULUM	4		1 2

CAMBRIDGE / CAMCO NO. 40

PENIS – R. DORSAL ART.	2	R. CAV. BODY	5		3 4

CAMCO NO. 40

L. DORSAL ART.	3	L. CAV. BODY	6		5 6

CAMCO NO. 40

IMPRESSIONS: Diminished blood flow both dorsal arts, 2nd wave lost
PAPS - SUSPECT. No sounds over cav. bodies

Figure 13-16

Figures 13-16 and 13-17. These figures show the PAPS recording of a 31-year-old postpriapism patient and a 45-year-old past alcoholic. Both examinations were positive. In the first case, note the early changes of the dorsal arteries. There is no flow in the deep arteries. In the second patient, there is obstructed flow of the left arteries and impaired circulation in the arteries of the right side.

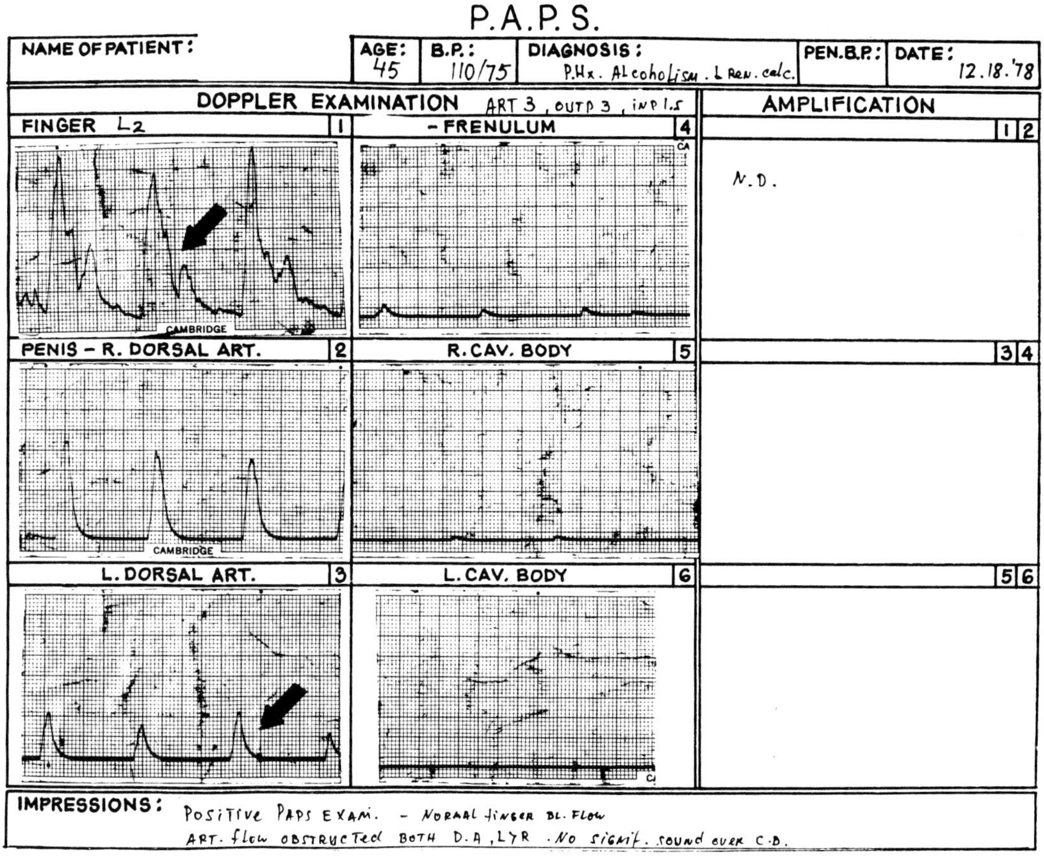
P.A.P.S.
NAME OF PATIENT:
AGE: 45
B.P.: 110/75
DIAGNOSIS: P.Hx. Alcoholism. L Ren. calc.
PEN.B.P.:
DATE: 12.18.'78
DOPPLER EXAMINATION ART 3, OUTP 3, INP 1.5
AMPLIFICATION
FINGER L2 1
- FRENULUM 4
1 2
N.D.
CAMBRIDGE
PENIS - R. DORSAL ART. 2
R. CAV. BODY 5
3 4
CAMBRIDGE
L. DORSAL ART. 3
L. CAV. BODY 6
5 6
IMPRESSIONS: Positive PAPS exam. - Normal finger bl. flow
ART. flow obstructed both D.A, L>R. No signif. sound over C.B.

Figure 13-17

Table 13-2. Part history of 170 patients

No significant history	35
Prostatitis	33
Diabetes	26
Hypertension	22
Trauma, disk, back pain	12
Benign prostatic hypertrophy	8
Alcoholism	6
Primary impotence	6
Myocardial infarction	4
Peyronie's disease	4
Cancer of prostate	2
Miscellaneous	13

Note: These are the past histories of the last 170 impotent patients examined by Doppler PAPS method.

Table 13-3. Results of PAPS examination of 250 consecutive impotent males

Normal	66 (26.4%)
Positive	104 (41.6%)
Suspect	77 (30.8%)

Note: These are the results of Doppler PAPS exam in 250 consecutive impotent patients.

CONCLUSIONS

The mystery of impotence can be explored, and possibly solved. It is the author's strong belief that the initial investigation in non-invasive screening of impotent patients can take place in the physician's office.

In choosing the method or methods necessary to result in intelligent diagnostic solutions to the problems of sexual dysfunction, one should consider cost, amount of time needed, simplicity, availability, objectivity, and accuracy.

A few large medical centers use penile blood pressure measurement alone, or in conjunction with plethysmography, to determine the need for a further search for possible vascular causes of impotence. Often, they are successful.

Our own preference, however, is represented by the following order: palpation of penile arteries; evaluation of internal penile temperature; and individual Doppler ultrasound examination of penile arteries.

In our experience, we have found the methods described to have the following order of sensitivity (from most to least):

1. Individual Doppler pulse examination of penile arteries by sound and waveform analysis (PAPS)
2. Penile blood pressure measurement as described by Abelson
3. Plethysmography
4. Penile internal temperature (this still needs to be confirmed by others)
5. Finger palpation of penile dorsal arteries

Following the completion of necessary noninvasive vascular testing, the clinician should make a judgment based on history, clinical impressions, and objectivity gained through noninvasive testing. This can then lead to recommendations for further invasive vascular procedures.

In our experience, if the noninvasive vascular methods give results that indicate abnormalities, we recommend NPT monitoring prior to subjecting the patient to angiography and/or cavernosography. NPT monitoring can further establish an organic pattern to impotence.

Angiography and cavernosography, their techniques, indications, results, and correlations to noninvasive tests will be discussed in Chapter 14.

REFERENCES
1. Abelson, D. Diagnostic value of the penile pulse and blood pressure: A Doppler study of impotence in diabetics. *J. Urol.* 113:636, 1975.
2. Badenoch, A. W. Descent of the testis in relation to temperature. *Br. Med. J.* 2:601, 1945.
3. Barry, J. M., and Hodges, C. V. Impotence: A diagnostic approach. *J. Urol.* 119:575, 1978.
4. Berstein, E. F. *Noninvasive Diagnostic Technique in Vascular Disease.* St. Louis: Mosby, 1978. Chaps. 8 and 11.
5. Berstein, E. F. *Noninvasive Diagnostic Technique in Vascular Disease.* St. Louis: Mosby, 1978. Sections 1, 2, 26, 30, 32.
6. Brobesk, J. R. (ed.). *Best and Taylor's Physiological Basis of Medical Practice* (10th ed.). Baltimore: Williams & Wilkins, 1979.
7. Britt, D. B., Kemmerer, W. T., and Robinson, J. R. Penile blood flow determination by mer-

cury strain gauge plethysmography. *Invest. Urol.* 8:673, 1971.

8. Canning, J. R., et al. Genital vascular insufficiency and impotence. *Surg. Forum* 14:298, 1963.

9. Casey, W. C. Revascularization of corpus cavernosum for erectile failure. *Urology* 14:135, 1979.

10. Casey, W. C. "Penile blood pressure": A clarification. *Urology* 14:47, 1980.

11. Casey, W. C., and Kaufman, J. J. Doppler ultrasound arterial flow and blood pressure. *Proceedings of the First International Conference on Corpus Cavernosum Revascularization.* 1:7, 1980.

12. Engel, G., Burnham, S. J., and Carter, M. F. Penile blood pressure in the evaluation of erectile impotence. *Fertil. Steril.* 30:687, 1978.

13. Furlow, W. L. Evaluation of the impotent patient. In R. J. Krane and M. B. Siroky (eds.), *Clinical Neuro-Urology.* Boston: Little, Brown, 1979.

14. Gaskell, P. The importance of penile blood pressure in cases of impotence. *Can. Med. Assoc. J.* 105:1047, 1971.

15. Ginestié, J. F., and Romieu, A. *L'exploration radiologique de l'impuissance.* Paris: Maloine, 1976.

16. Hyman, C., and Winsor, T. History of plethysmography. *J. Cardiovasc. Surg.* 2:506, 1961.

17. Hyman, B. N. Doppler sonography. *Am. J. Ophthalmol.* 77:227, 1974.

18. Ishii, N., Mitsukawa, S., and Shirai, M. Studies on male sexual impotence: Differential diagnosis of organic and functional impotence by determining penile skin temperature. *Jpn. J. Urol.* 68:136, 1977.

19. Jevtich, M. J. Experience with penile arterial pulse sounds. *Proceedings of the First International Conference on Corpus Cavernosum Revascularization.* 4:31, 1980.

20. Jevtich, M. J. Importance of penile arterial pulse sound examination in impotence. *J. Urol.* 124:820, 1980.

21. Juhan, C. Doppler velocimetry of penile arteries and diagnosis of arteriogenic impotence. *Proceedings of the First International Conference on Corpus Cavernosum Revascularization.* 3:23, 1980.

22. Keitzer, W. F., and Lichti, E. L. Applications of the Doppler: Common and unusual situations. *Angiology* 26:172, 1975.

23. Kempezinski, R. F. Role of the vascular diagnostic laboratory in the evaluation of male impotence. *Am. J. Surg.* 138:278, 1979.

24. Malvar, T., Baron, T., and Clark, S. S. Assessment of potency with Doppler flowmeter. *Urology* 2:396, 1973.

25. Michal, V., and Pospichal, J. Phalloarteriography in the diagnosis of erectile impotence. *World J. Surg.* 2:239, 1978.

26. Montague, D. K., James, R., and DeWolf, V. Diagnostic screening for vasculogenic impotence. Vasculogenic impotence: Penile blood pressure measurements. *Proceedings of the First International Conference on Corpus Cavernosum Revascularization.* 2:13, 1980.

27. Montague, D. K., et al. Diagnostic evaluation, classification, and treatment of men with sexual dysfunction. *Urology* 14:545, 1979.

28. Moore, C. R., and Quick, W. J. The scrotum as a temperature regulator for the testis. *Am. J. Physiol.* 68:76, 1924.

29. Morales, P. A., and Hardin, J. Scrotal and testicular temperature studies in paraplegics. *J. Urol.* 79:972, 1958.

30. Newman, H. F., Northur, J. D., and Devlin, J. Mechanism of human penile erection. *Invest. Urol.* 1:350, 1964.

31. Parrish, D., et al. Evidence for the venous origin of plethysmographic information. *J. Lab. Clin. Med.* 62:943, 1963.

32. Ružbarsky, V., and Michal, V. Morphologic changes in the arterial bed of the penis with aging. *Invest. Urol.* 15:194, 1977.

33. Satomura, S. Study of flow patterns in peripheral arteries by ultrasonics. *J. Acoust. Science Jpn.* 15:151, 1959.

34. Scott, B. F., et al. Surgical treatment of erectile impotence. *Contemp. Surg.* 16:64, 1980.

35. Tordjman, G., Thierre, R., and Michel, J. R. Nouvelles acquisitions sur pathologie vasculair dans les dysfunctions erectile de l'homme. *Cah. Sex. Clin.* 3:19, 1977.

36. Velcek, D. Penile flow index utilizing a Doppler wave analysis to identify penile vascular insufficiency. *J. Urol.* 123:669, 1980.

37. Whipple, H. E., and Spitzer, M. I. Thermography and its clinical implications. *N. Y. Acad. Sci.* 121:1, 1964.

38. Whitney, R. J. The measurement of volume changes in human limb. *J. Physiol.* (Lond.) 121:1, 1953.

39. Zorgniotti, A. W. Elevated penile blood pressure in patients with premature ejaculation. *Urology* 13:185, 1979.

40. Zorgniotti, A. W., et al. Diagnosis and therapy of vasculogenic impotence. *J. Urol.* 123:647, 1980.

14

Invasive Vascular Procedures

MILORAD J. JEVTICH
DANIEL D. MAXWELL

Two studies used for radiologic evaluation of the penile circulatory system; angiography and cavernosography, are discussed in this chapter. Although corpus cavernosography has been in use for many years [22], its full clinical potential has not yet been realized.

In contrast, penile angiography was developed only recently, yet it is rapidly becoming appreciated as a diagnostic tool in vascular impotence.

When considering invasive studies of penile circulation, one often finds it necessary to determine the radiologic appearance of both the arterial and the venous system.

Penile circulation is unusual and specific. The arterial supply to the penis serves two functions: to bring nutrients to the organ and to create erection. Moreover, this arterial flow takes place in two sets of arteries, left and right. (The chapter dealing with penile anatomy [Chap. 1] has explained this in detail.) So, the fourfold specificity of the penile arterial structure must be taken into account when evaluating penile hemodynamics.

The penile venous system is also unusual. There is one dorsal superficial vein and one deep dorsal vein, which drain the blood from the penis into the pelvic venous plexuses. These veins are interconnected by many circumflex branches that communicate between the deep and superficial systems [11]. These are the veins that play a part in erectile function, i.e., maintenance. There are also veins from the glans and corpus spongiosum that have no function in erectile maintenance. In addition, both the arterial and venous systems of the penis are expanded by the presence of two large cylinders in the corpora cavernosa that serve as blood pools.

Vascular impotence implies a deficiency in penile circulation. As was explained in Chapter 13, a penile arterial pathology could cause erectile dysfunction. However, the term *vascular impotence* refers not only to penile arterial insufficiency but to penile venous insufficiency as well. An abnormally rapid venous drainage also can produce impotence, because the veins remove the blood necessary to sustain an erection.

I would like to express my deep appreciation for the continued support, understanding, and valuable suggestions of Dr. W. Dabney Jarman, for many years Director of the urology department, Washington Hospital Center, Washington, D. C.
I would also like to thank Susan S. McConnell for editorial assistance, Radan Novcic for technical assistance, Sarah Rhodes for secretarial services, my wife Olga Jevtich, for encouragement in this study, and my patients.

As will be discussed in the section on corpus cavernosography, there are a significant number of patients who, in addition to having impaired inflow of blood to the penis also have a significantly increased blood outflow. (Some studies even indicate that rapid venous drainage may be the sole cause of vascular impotence [13, 29].) There are also patients who fall into a middle range. Normal results have been obtained in clinical and noninvasive vascular studies. Yet their sexual histories positively suggest an organic cause for impotence. Moreover, nocturnal penile tumescence (NPT) monitoring suggests abnormal erections or the complete absence of erection.

Such a disparity in facts might suggest that clinicians have not explored penile venous insufficiency as a cause of erectile failure. This diagnostic possibility is challenging and should be examined further. Therefore, angiography and cavernosography will be presented as steps toward a more complete diagnosis.

Correlation between noninvasive vascular studies and penile angiography is important for appreciation of the clinical value of the noninvasive procedures. Studies of penile angiography also can determine whether any circulatory pathology is to be found in the arterial system. Cavernosography will be discussed with relation to possible venous pathologies, and as a method of determining where a vascular problem might be. In addition, there will be a short review covering recent radioactive examinations of penile circulation.

When considering any invasive procedures, the clinician should have clear indications before performing them. They are not to be used as part of a screening test. The indications for each of these procedures are developed as a result of clinical, laboratory, and noninvasive testing.

PENILE ARTERIOGRAPHY

Angiography has long been a proved method of detection and diagnosis of vascular diseases in general.

Penile arteriography (PA) is the ultimate diagnostic procedure for precise detection of pathologic changes in the penile arteries. It is a recently developed technique, currently done in only a few of the world's large medical centers. It is the last procedure to be used for completion of a diagnosis of arterial vascular impotence.

HISTORY
Because PA has been developed and applied as a diagnostic tool for impotence only in the last 7 years, only a few articles have been written on the subject.

There were, however, speculations about this method as long as 30 years ago. Simpson [35], for example, speculated that a diabetic angiopathy involving the small vessels of the erectile tissue could impede the blood flow and lead to impotence.

In 1960, Scheer [32] postulated that relying on the pulse readings of the extremities, in particular the legs, was inadequate for diagnosis of an impotent patient; he recommended the use of aortography as a more definite diagnostic procedure.

Canning [1] studied impotence in 1963. He used 18 aortograms and demonstrated obstructive changes in the pelvic vessels. Lipsky [19] attempted a direct puncture of the penile dorsal artery in 1970. He demonstrated arterial occlusion in a case of priapism.

It is believed that the first report of an internal pudendal arteriography was issued by Evans and co-workers [7] in 1973. The breakthrough in the development of this technique came in mid-1973. Michal [23] put forward the hypothesis that impotence might be related to obstruction in penile arterial flow. In the first case of penile bypass surgery, he used penile arteriography to demonstrate penile arterial obstruction. This historic event opened the field of penile revascularization surgery as a treatment for impotence.

Michal and co-workers [25, 26] next reported their preliminary observations of this method, which they called phalloarteriography.

In 1976, Ginestié and Romieu [14] published

a monograph on the radiologic exploration of impotence. They describe a PA technique and give a detailed radiographic classification of arterial abnormalities and lesions in 250 patients. In all, they did a total of 450 unilateral penile arteriographies. (The book in which these studies are contained is recommended to anyone interested in this new technique.)

Ružbarsky [31] published a report in 1978 that confirmed the presence of pathologic changes in the penile arteries through histologic studies. Cohen and Sharpe [3] also confirmed the presence of penile arterial pathologies.

It appears from the literature cited that PA is a technique discovered and developed in Europe.

The first United States experiences with PA were reported at the First International Conference on Corpus Revascularization, held in October, 1978. Rossi [30] added 20 cases, and Jevtich [18] contributed 14. Both papers, although they did not deal exclusively with PA, did suggest confirmation of the importance of others' findings.

The most recent study is one mentioned by Casey [2] in 1979. In it he reported the use of PA in preoperative evaluation of revascularization of the corpora cavernosa.

PHYSIOLOGIC CONSIDERATIONS

Regulation of blood flow to the penis is controlled by complex neural impulses involving the arterial and venous systems. Conti [4], in 1952, explained the human penile vascular regulatory mechanism as involving the opening and closing of muscular polsters. This action shunts the arterial blood flow into the corpora cavernosa and decreases the blood flow into the venous system of the penis.

Erection is a vascular phenomenon that depends primarily on a normal arterial blood flow to the corpora cavernosa. Therefore, neither intact neural impulses nor the normal functioning of the penile venous system can perform their functions in producing and/or sustaining an erection if the arterial blood flow to the penis is impaired.

To appreciate the amount of blood flow to the penis that is necessary for erectile function, one must also take into consideration the size of the penis, i.e., the volume capacity for full expansion of the corpora cavernosa. Newman [28] did a study on cadavers and 10 live volunteers. He estimated that 20 to 50 ml/min blood flow is necessary to produce an erection and that 12 ml/min is necessary to maintain an erection.

Michal and co-workers [26], however, estimated in 1978 that 45 to 160 ml/min, with a mean volumetric capacity of 90 ml/min (depending on the size of the penis), is the amount of blood flow necessary to create an erection. He calculated the maintenance figure at 60 percent of the initial rate. (Later he revised his figures to 45–180 ml/min, a mean of 119 ml/min, and maintenance at 72 ml/min, respectively [24].

In the past 2 years, Michal's last observations relating to hemodynamics and the capacity of the corpora, as presented above, have been recognized in the United States and are now generally used as guidelines in determining the normal erectile function of the penis.

It seems logical to consider penile arteriography for evaluation of abnormal penile arterial flow after it has been indicated by a noninvasive vascular test.

Penile arteriography can be used for two purposes: (1) in preoperative evaluation for precise study of the penile arterial tree; (2) to rule out penile vascular malformations, such as AV fistulas [38].

In relation to the first point, there is an interesting recent study. Shelling and Maxted [33] reported that in some diabetic patients there might be previously unsuspected significant small vessel disease in the penis. This could present a great postoperative risk since necrosis and infection of the corpora may occur and would complicate the insertion of a penile prosthesis. This situation may be avoided by preoperative use of PA in some diabetics and other patients with severe vascular disease.

Since PA is an invasive procedure, to be

used only as a last, definitive test, certain criteria should be met before the procedure is undertaken.

INDICATIONS

Ginestié [15] emphasizes that although PA is a procedure without any complications, it remains a serious radiologic exploration, and indications must be carefully studied. He recommends that the following conditions be fulfilled prior to the use of PA:

1. There must be a clinical picture of impotence indicating an arterial etiology.
2. Other etiologies for impotence must be ruled out.
3. The therapeutic outlook should be good.

Since early 1978, when we started performing PA, our indications have been:

1. Signs of penile arterial obstruction as detected by the Doppler waveform analysis of penile arteries
2. NPT monitoring showing either no nocturnal erections or significantly abnormal ones
3. Cystometrogram within normal limits
4. Patient in good general health and in need of surgical correction for organically caused impotence

We have since expanded our indications by taking into consideration some abnormal CMG and bulbocavernosum latency readings in selected patients. These patients may also have significant penile arterial obstructive changes.

Casey [2] listed the following indications for PA in 1979:

1. No erection in NPT studies
2. Exclusion of other diseases
3. Doppler ultrasound arterial studies indicating the absence of sound in any of the important penile arteries

METHODS AND TECHNIQUES OF PA

Michal and co-workers [24, 26] employed passive penile erection during penile angiography, reportedly to improve the radiographic utilization of the penile arterial tree. Their studies were done under general anesthesia through bilateral percutaneous catheterization of the femoral arteries. Ginestié [15] also uses general anesthesia and punctures both femoral arteries. (For details of their techniques, see the appropriate literature.)

Since 1978, we have employed the techniques discussed below for PA. The actual studies were performed by Dr. Daniel D. Maxwell, Assistant Clinical Professor of Radiology, George Washington University.

Internal Pudendal Arteriography Technique
Selective arteriography of the penile branches of the internal pudendal arteries is performed by using standard percutaneous arteriographic technique. Bilateral internal iliac artery catheterizations are performed from a single femoral puncture. An 80 cm No. 6 French Cobra catheter is introduced from the femoral artery into the lower abdominal aorta. An arteriogram of the aortic bifurcation and origin of the internal iliac arteries is obtained to rule out aortoiliac disease. The catheter is then advanced across the aortic bifurcation into the contralateral internal iliac artery. Selective internal pudendal arteriography is seldom necessary. The acute angle at the aortic bifurcation frequently causes difficulty in negotiating this turn. If problems are encountered, a Waltman loop [36] is formed in the catheter by using the superior mesenteric artery. The looped catheter can then easily be advanced into the contralateral internal iliac artery. Ipsilateral catheterization of the internal iliac artery is then performed by advancing the looped catheter into the abdominal aorta; the catheter then is withdrawn until its tip is in the ipsilateral common iliac artery. The ipsilateral internal iliac artery is then easily catheterized.

Many angiographers are now familiar with this type of technique because of its use in gastrointestinal angiography. A catheter 80 cm in length is preferred because the additional length allows for formation of a long loop (10–20 cm in length). If problems are encountered with movement of the loop, a guide wire is advanced to the level of the first turn of the catheter for greater stability. If problems are encountered in ipsilateral catheterization of the internal iliac artery, the catheter is exchanged for a narrow-radius simple, hook-shaped catheter. We have not found it necessary to perform the bilateral femoral artery punctures originally described by Ginestié and Romieu [15] and Michal and Pospichal [26].

Radiographic filming is obtained in the oblique projection. Left internal iliac injection is performed with the patient in the right posterior oblique position with the penis over the right thigh. Right internal iliac injection is performed with the patient in the left posterior oblique position with the penis over the left thigh. Contrast injection is performed with Conray 60. The injection is 3 ml/second for a total of 50 ml of contrast. Higher flow rates result in reflux into the external iliac artery. Radiographic filming is obtained with a standard Schoenander 35 × 35 cm changer. A carbon front changer and rare earth screens are used. A focal spot radiographic tube (0.35 mm), is used and filming is obtained in 1.6 to 1 magnification. Exposures are obtained every other second for 20 seconds after a 5-second delay at the beginning of injection.

Normal Radiographic Anatomy of the Internal Iliac Artery

The internal iliac artery arises from the common iliac artery at the level of the L5–S1 interspace. The internal iliac artery has a posterior division and an anterior division. The posterior division has four main branches: the ileolumbar, superior lateral sacral, inferior lateral sacral, and superior gluteal arteries. The anterior division divides into the following branches: obturator, umbilical, inferior gluteal, internal pudendal, inferior vesical, middle rectal, prostatic and deferential arteries. The internal pudendal artery is the artery of the erectile organs. The level of origin of the internal pudendal artery shows great variation, and an accessory internal pudendal artery is present in 6 percent of cases. The penile vessels arise from the obturator artery in 1 percent of cases. The distal internal pudendal artery gives rise to

the superficial perineal artery and the bulbourethral artery, which supply the corpus spongiosum and urethra. The terminal internal pudendal artery then divides into the deep penile artery and the dorsal artery of the penis. The deep penile artery penetrates the center of the corpus cavernosum, and the dorsal artery of the penis sends branches to the prepuce and glans and fascial coverings of the corpora (Fig. 14-1).

Results

Forty-four patients between the ages of 31 and 69 years, having met the requirements, underwent selective arteriography of the internal pudendal vessels over a period of 30 months. A total of 88 individual studies of the internal pudendal arteries were performed. Table 14-1 indicates the past history of these 44 patients.

All x-rays were reviewed by both of us, first separately and then together.

Forty of the 44 patients studied by PA had abnormal angiograms. In three earlier cases, the angiographic demonstrations of penile arteries were not technically satisfactory. These three cases were excluded, leaving 41 cases for interpretation. This represents 97.5 percent abnormal studies. In one patient, the study was considered normal (2.4%).

Of 40 abnormal studies, 28 patients had bilateral involvement of the internal pudendal and penile arteries (70%), and four of these

Table 14-1. Histories of 44 cases selected for pudendal arteriography

Condition	Number of patients
Diabetes	9
No significant history	8
Hypertension	6
Atherosclerotic heat disease	5
Alcoholism	4
Kidney stone	2
Trauma, fracture of the pelvis	1
Peyronie's disease	1
Hypospadias	1
Miscellaneous	5

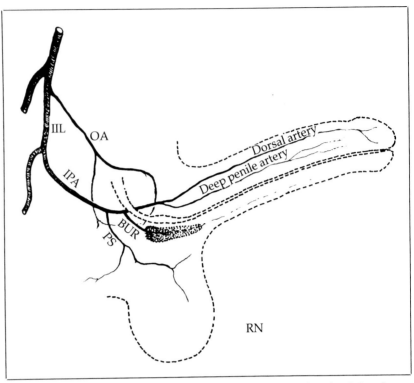

Figure 14-1. Scheme of internal pudendal and penile arteries. Key: IIL = internal iliac artery; OA = obturator artery; IPA = internal pudendal artery; PS = posterior scrotal artery; BUR = bulbourethral artery

also had associated aortoiliac disease. Only 12 patients (30%) had unilateral disease. Left-sided lesions were twice as common as right-sided.

The most common findings involved small-vessel arteriosclerotic lesions resulting in irregular arteriosclerotic plaques or vessel occlusions. Most pathologic lesions were located along the distal internal pudendal artery at the level of origin of the dorsal penile or deep penile arteries (Fig. 14-2). The cavernosa or deep arteries are most frequently involved, and then the dorsal arteries (Fig. 14-3). The urethral arteries were almost always normal in our studies. No morbidity was encountered in this series.

Controls

No participants were used as controls in our series. However, there were 12 patients who showed unilateral penile arterial disease, yet their contralateral pudendal penile arteries were normal. Their studies were used for comparative purposes. In addition, the radiograph of the one patient found to be normal also was used for comparison (Fig. 14-4).

Figure 14-2. Extensive irregular atherosclerotic stenosis of the distal internal pudendal artery and proximal dorsal penile and cavernous artery.

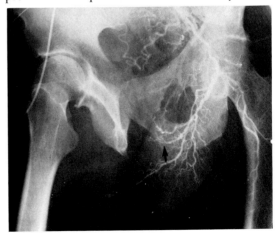

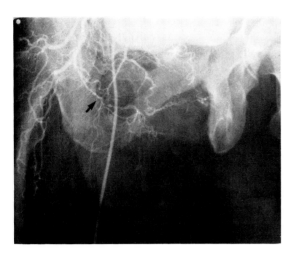

Figure 14-3. Beaded irregular arteriosclerotic stenosis of the distal internal pudendal artery.

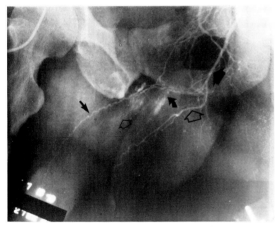

Figure 14-4. Normal penile arteriography. Note: Internal pudendal artery (*large black arrow*), bulbourethral artery (*curved arrow*), dorsal penile artery (*small black arrow*), deep penile artery (cavernosum) (*small white arrow*), and perineal branch (*large white arrow*).

Michal [24] used seven men who did not have a vascular cause of impotence (five were classified as psychogenic and two had multiple sclerosis). All seven had normal arterial appearance.

Ginestié [15] did not address the matter of controls in his monograph, except to describe arteries that appeared normal.

*Case Studies**
Case 1
A 53-year-old black male, impotent for 2 years (Fig. 14-5). PH includes hypertension and alcohol-

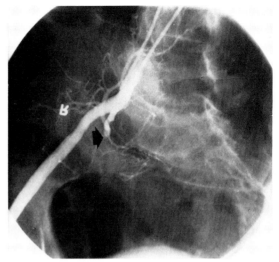

Figure 14-5. Total occlusion of the anterior division of the right internal iliac artery. (There were also abnormalities of the penile arteries of the left side that are not shown.)

ism. Mitral and aortic valves had been replaced. Clinical examination was WNL, with the exception of no palpable penile arteries. BP = 104/75; T = 97.6°F; PT = 93.3°F (difference of 4.3°F). Doppler PAPS indicated bilateral abnormalities. BC reflex latency and CMG both WNL. ST = 445 ng/dl. NPT: No erections recorded. Cavernosogram showed a capacity of 200 cc and less than 50 percent retention at 15 minutes.*
Case 2
A 60-year-old white male (Fig. 14-6). Suffered erectile failure for 1½ years. PH included diabetes, controlled by diet and Peyronie's disease. Clinical examination WNL. Good pulse palpation right dorsal penile artery; no pulses on left. Peyronie's plaque 2 × 3 cm in size at base of penis in a 1- to 2-o'clock position. BP = 120/85; T = 98.2°F; PT = 95.3°F (difference 3.9°F). Doppler PAPS: Bilateral abnormalities, left more than right side. ST = 639 ng/dl. BC reflex latency and CMG: WNL. NPT: one incomplete erection in two nights of monitoring. Cavernosogram: A capacity of 120 cc, which produced only a half erection, and 50 percent retention at 15 minutes.
Case 3
A 51-year-old black male (Fig. 14-7). Suffered impotence for 5 years. PH included hypertension, alcoholism, and pancreatitis. Clinical examination was WNL. In palpation, the right penile pulse was stronger than the left. BP = 110/75. Doppler

*Key: T = body temperature; PT = penile temperature; PH = patient history; CMG = cystometrogram; NPT = nocturnal penile tumescence; WNL = within normal limits; BP = blood pressure; ST = serum testosterone (ng/dl); EMG = electromyogram.

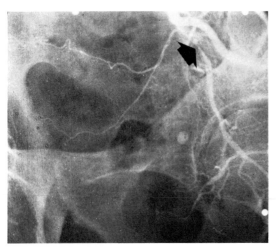

Figure 14-6. High-grade stenosis of the proximal left internal pudendal artery. Discovered, but not shown: occlusion of right deep penile artery; only fair visualization of right dorsal artery.

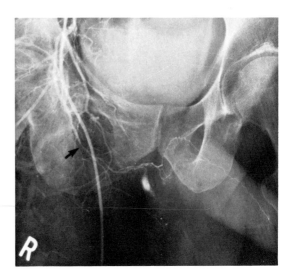

Figure 14-8. Focal atheroschlerotic stenosis of the right distal portion of the internal pudendal artery.

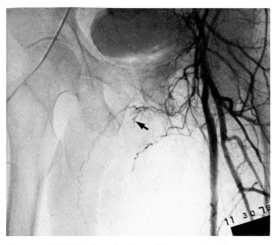

Figure 14-7. Total occlusion of the proximal cavernous artery (deep penile) with normal undulating dorsal penile artery. (The same findings were discovered on the opposite side but are not shown.)

PAPS: Although there was no pulse sound of the cavernous arteries, bilaterally there was fair to good sound of the dorsal arteries. ST = 260 ng/dl. CGM was WNL. NPT monitoring showed no significant erections. Cavernosogram was WNL.
Case 4
A 50-year-old white male (Figs. 14-8 and 14-9). Complained of impotence for 4 years. PH indicated a back injury, alcoholism. Patient had undergone psychotherapy. BP = 150/80; T = 98.1°F; PT = 94°F (with a difference of 4.1°F). Clinical examination was WNL. Weak penile pulse palpation on both right and left sides. Doppler PAPS recorded bilateral abnormalities, greater on the left.

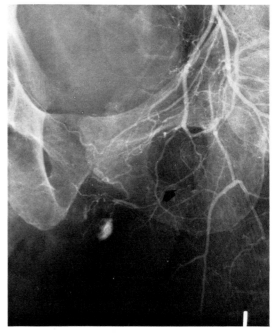

Figure 14-9. (Same patient as in Fig. 14-8.) Long segment high-grade stenosis of the left internal pudendal artery (*black arrow*) with poststenotic dilation of the proximal dorsal penile artery.

ST was WNL. The BC reflex latency, EMG of legs, and CMG tests all were WNL. NPT recording indicated incomplete abnormal erections. Cavernosogram displayed a 180-cc capacity and poor retention at 15 min.

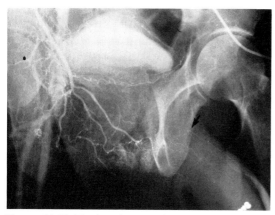

Figure 14-10. Total occlusion of the proximal portion of the right dorsal penile artery with collateral reconstruction of the distal dorsal penile artery from cavernous arterial branches. (Marked abnormalities of the penile arteries of the left side were discovered as well but are not shown.)

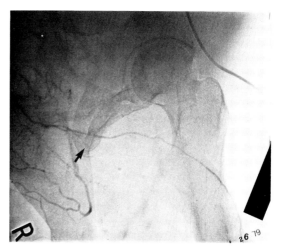

Figure 14-11. Total occlusion of the cavernous artery in a patient post–sickle cell priapism. The dorsal penile artery is well visualized. Biopsy of corpora cavernosa: dense fibrosis with obliteration of vascular spaces.

Case 5

A 52-year-old black male (Fig. 14-10). Impotent for 10 years. PH: Myocardial infarction 7 years ago with no other diseases. Clinical examination was WNL. Penile pulse palpation was weak bilaterally. BP = 140/80; T = 98.5°F; PT = 95.4°F (with a difference of 3.1°F). The Doppler PAPS showed bilateral abnormalities, with greater abnormalities on the left. ST = 430 ng/dl. BC reflex latency and CMG WNL. NPT monitoring showed one incomplete erection and absence of erection during second night. Cavernosogram showed a 95-cc capacity and no retention of dye at 15 minutes.

Case 6

A 31-year-old black male (Fig. 14-11). Impotent for 2 years since sickle cell priapism. PH detailed only a fractured right hip. Clinical examination was WNL. There was a firmness of the corpora cavernosa in the flaccid penis. BP = 120/80. ST was WNL. Doppler PAPS indicated a good pulse sound in both dorsal arteries, but no sound over the corpora cavernosa. The CMG was WNL, but the NPT showed no erections. Cavernosogram indicated marked dense filling defects and an incomplete visualization of both corpora.

Comments

Our experiences with PA corroborate the findings of Michal and Ginestié.

Michal and co-workers [24] performed PA in 134 patients. Seven were used as controls. Of the remaining 127 impotent men, abnormal PA was detected in 105 (82.7%), and normal PA readings appeared in 17.3 percent.

Ginestié reported 93 percent abnormal radiologic findings [15].

In our present series of 41 patients, positive radiologic signs for penile arterial pathology were somewhat higher than in Ginestié's series (97.5%). This could be explained by two factors: We used stricter criteria for indications, and patients were slightly older (average 50 years as compared to Michal's 42.9 years).

The discovery that a majority of the patients had bilateral obstructive lesions (70%) corresponds to findings in other studies. Moreover, we found that the distribution and appearance of the radiographic lesions followed a similar pattern to those of European studies.

One patient, after sickle cell priapism, had bilateral occlusion of the deep penile arteries with no evidence of arteriosclerotic lesions. Another patient had traumatic occlusions of the distal internal pudendal arteries. One patient with Peyronie's disease had a plaque on the same side of the obstructed dorsal and deep arteries. One hypospadic patient showed a thin, hypotrophic appearance of the penile artery corresponding to the dysplasia described by Ginestié. We have not studied patients with primary impotence. They often are reported to have arterial dysplasia and agenesis of the penile arteries [15].

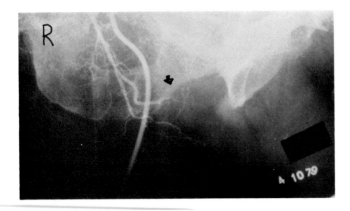

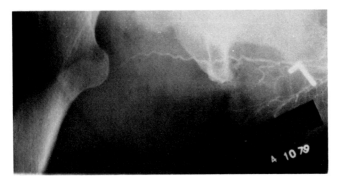

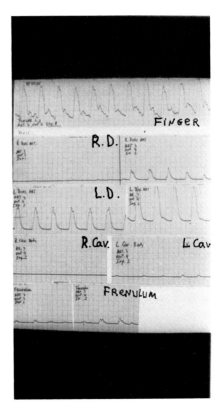

Figure 14-12. Doppler PAPS versus PA correlation: 63-year-old diabetic. Impotence for several years. Patent penile arteries of left side. Total occlusion of right penile arteries.

(One 36-year-old patient had an accessory small pudendal artery and associated bilateral changes of the penile arteries.)

A few cases of collateral reconstruction were seen in the area of the occluded segments of the distal pudendal or penile arteries.

A group of nine diabetics all had lesions of the same angiographic appearance as other patients with arteriosclerotic small-vessel disease.

Correlation between PA and PAPS

Since the majority of patients in our series had a Doppler examination of penile arteries prior to PA, a correlation between a non-invasive vascular study and an invasive one can be made. Juhan and Velcek and co-workers found correlations between non-invasive and invasive studies in 98 percent and 50 percent of cases evaluated, respectively (see Chap. 13) [21, 35].

Of the 44 patients referred to us for PA, 40 had abnormal results on the Doppler PAPS examinations. Four of the 44 were referred by other physicians and had undergone diagnos-

tic testing other than the Doppler examination. They are excluded from the comparison. Also excluded are the three technically unsatisfactory studies.

Thirty-six of the remaining 37 patients had abnormal penile angiographic findings and abnormal Doppler studies (97.3%). One had a normal angiographic study, although he had been classified by the Doppler as suspect, suggesting a Doppler error of 2.7%.

Confirmation of 100 percent as to side and bilateral abnormalities was achieved in 33 studies, representing 89.3 percent of the total number of patients compared (Figs. 14-12, 14-13).

In the other three patients of the 36, PA disclosed more severe pathologic changes than the Doppler study had (8.1%). In the first of these three patients, abnormal waves were present in the penile arteries of the left, but were normal on the right, according to the Doppler. The PA, however, showed bilateral

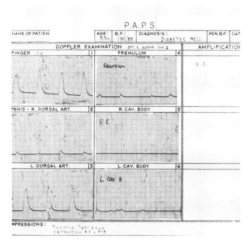

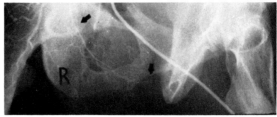

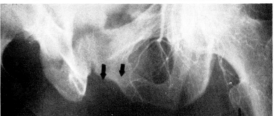

Figure 14-13. Doppler PAPS versus PA correlation: 53-year-old diabetic. Impotence for 7 to 8 years. Stenosis of the right proximal internal pudendal artery and occlusion of penile arteries. Left: stenosis of internal pudendal artery and impaired flow in penile arteries.

abnormalities of penile arteries. The Doppler of the second patient showed normal waveforms in the arteries of the right, and abnormal waveforms on the left. The PA study, however, showed bilateral abnormalities. In the third patient, the Doppler waves were normal on the left and abnormal on the right; yet the PA again showed bilateral abnormalities. We were not surprised by the higher sensitivity of penile arteriography. This may be expected from such a selective and invasive radiologic study.

We earlier reported [17] a 95.7 percent confirmation between the Doppler results and the PA studies in the first 22 cases. The present enlarged series continues to verify an extremely high correlation between these two methods. The Doppler technique of examining penile arteries will probably never be as thorough as PA, but we find it to be a valuable noninvasive test in detecting penile arterial obstruction in impotence; we then recommend PA for a complete study of selected impotent patients.

CONCLUSIONS
Penile arteriography is the definitive diagnostic procedure for assessing obstructive penile arterial flow in impotent patients. Its invasive nature requires strict adherence to complete indications.

The present series of 41 patients had abnormal penile angiographic findings in 97.5 percent. The majority of studies showed bilateral pathological involvement of penile arteries. One hundred percent correlation between penile arteriography and Doppler PAPS exam was achieved in 89.3 percent of the patients.

CAVERNOSOGRAM (CORPUS CAVERNOSOGRAPHY)
Corpus cavernosography is the radiologic visualization of the corpora cavernosa of the penis. It takes place by direct injection of radiopaque contrast material into the corpora. The result is called a *cavernosogram.*

It has been suggested that the venous system of the corpora cavernosa delays venous drainage and, therefore, contributes to erectile maintenance [13, 29]. It is further suggested that rapid drainage occurring from the corpora cavernosa can contribute to erectile failure. Cavernosography allows the visualization of the superficial dorsal and deep dorsal veins, which drain into the pelvic plexuses. This can be accomplished by injection of contrast medium into one of the corpora cavernosa.

History of Methods
May and Hirtl [22] devised the radiographic technique in 1955, to visualize the corpora

cavernosa in connection with Peyronie's disease. In 1963 Fetter and co-workers [8] applied cavernosography in the diagnosis of lesions of the penis. In 1967, Hamilton and Swann [16] described their method, which also is used presently for corpus cavernosography. Between 1973 and 1975 Fitzpatrick [9, 10, 11, 13] used cavernosography (and, in one report, spongiosography) to demonstrate why the corpora cavernosa, but not the glans penis or the corpus spongiosum, are involved in erection.

Clinical and Physiologic Considerations
Penile venous circulation has been studied experimentally as well as clinically, yet there does not seem to be a full appreciation of this system. (The anatomy of the penile venous system is described in Chapter 1.)

Insufficiency of penile veins first came to be thought of as a main factor in poor erection at the turn of the century. At that time Wooten [37] and Lydston [21] both advocated a ligation of the deep dorsal vein as a procedure allowing an impotent man to attain an erection.

The theory regarding malfunction of the penile venous system as a factor in impotence was revived in 1935 when Lowsley and Bray [20] introduced a new operation for the relief of impotence in selected patients. Contrary to the work of Lydston, their clinical procedures were supported by animal laboratory work. Lowsley and Bray performed ligation of deep dorsal veins and associated it with plication and shortening of the ischiocavernosus and bulbocavernosus muscles. Their work was received with great enthusiasm in Great Britain, especially by T. Millin [27].

Conti [4], in his work on vascular polsters of the penis, suggested the theory of a possible inability of the deep dorsal venous system to retain blood within the penis. Newman [28], however, in limited experiments on 10 adults, concluded that erection could occur without a venous closing mechanism.

In 1974 and 1975, studies by Fitzpatrick [10, 11, 13] again suggested the presence of a valvular venous mechanism in the deep dorsal vein of the penis. His study also indicated the presence of circumflex veins. He concluded that the valves of the deep dorsal veins and the presence of the circumflex veins assist in maintaining an erection. He also hypothesized that the destruction of the valves in the deep dorsal vein could be a cause of inability to sustain an erection.

Fitzpatrick [10] and Ney [29] both indicated that rapid drainage of the contrast material injected into the corpora cavernosa suggests a condition of venous insufficiency.

Moreover, Fitzpatrick suggested that in many impotent men, venous return occurs almost totally through the deep dorsal (insufficient) vein, rather than through the circumflex veins. Because, he speculated, there is a rearrangement, or "de-arrangement" in the normally functioning venous system, much less blood can be trapped in the corpora cavernosa. This factor also contributes to the development of a venously caused unsustained erection.

As is apparent, there is currently much controversy over the significance of the penile venous system as a factor in erection. It is hoped that further investigation will resolve and explain fully the role of the penile venous system in impotence.

From the studies performed in the past, it does, however, appear clear that the superficial dorsal vein of the penis and the venous drainage mechanism of the glans and corpus spongiosum have no significant role in the process of erection, even though some degree of venostasis in the deep dorsal venous system is necessary for erection.

It also has been demonstrated to our satisfaction that rapid drainage from the corpora cavernosa [6, 11, 13, 29] can be a factor in impotence. In our estimation, there is great clinical value in corpus cavernosography. We employ the method for the following reasons:

1. To study the drainage of radiopaque contrast material from the corpora cavernosa. (It has been shown [13, 29] that normally functioning corpora cavernosa retain the injected x-ray dye for more than 15–20 minutes.)
2. To evaluate the anatomic appearance of the

corpora and to detect possible filling defects that could affect erectile distention.

3. To evaluate the competency of the penile venous system before consideration of any penile revascularization.

4. To detect any abnormal shunts between the corpora cavernosa and the corpus spongiosum [6].

5. To determine the patency of corporal cylinders prior to insertion of penile prosthesis in some cases.

Since cavernosography is an invasive procedure, it should not be part of the routine investigation of an impotent patient. Our experience has led us to determine the following indications for cavernosography:

1. NPT — abnormal or absent erections.

2. Normal penile arterial circulation as indicated by the Doppler study. Also, in some cases, abnormal Doppler findings when related to possible revascularization surgery.

3. History of unsustained erection in a patient who offers otherwise normal clinical and noninvasive vascular results.

Method and Technique
Four methods will be described.

Hamilton and Swann [16] employ a technique with local anesthesia. A No. 18 to 20 needle is introduced through the anesthetized area into the corpus. Sterile normal saline, 10 ml, is slowly injected. If there is no local reaction, and since the tip of the needle is well inside the corpus, injection is begun with a 20 ml syringe filled with 60% meglumine diatrizoate. Films are obtained after the injection.

Fitzpatrick uses two methods [11, 12, 34].

1. Under local anesthesia, with the patient in a right oblique position, the penis is placed parallel to the femur. A No. 21 butterfly needle is inserted into the distal part of one corpus cavernosum. Meglumine iothalamate, 5 ml, is injected within 30 sec. X-rays are taken every 30 seconds, as needed.

2. The second method, venography, is referred to as the "open" method [10]. Local anesthesia is injected dorsally at the base of the penis. A transverse dorsal incision is made through the skin and Buck's fascia. The deep dorsal vein is identified at midline. A polyethelene radiopaque catheter (int. diam. 0.023 ml) is introduced proximally. Sodium iothalamate, 0.5 to 1.0 ml, is slowly released through the catheter. X-rays are taken before, during, and after injection. The deep dorsal vein is then ligated proximally and distally to the puncture, and the incision is closed. This method is used only for venography of the deep dorsal vein and its vascular system, because the valves usually are located at the base of the deep dorsal vein. (They usually are not found at the level of the lateral plexus of the pelvis or near the root of the internal iliac vein.)

Our method differs somewhat from those described. Because we want to visualize retention of the contrast material in the corpora, as well as to assess the capacity of the corpora to produce an erection, we have not made efforts in our use of the technique to visualize the valves or to assess pathologic overstretching of the deep dorsal vein [10]. We believe that premature emptying of the corpora cavernosa is proof of venous insufficiency irrespective of what causes this.

Under local anesthesia (or after cystoscopy under IV anesthesia), the patient is placed in a left oblique position. The penis is positioned parallel on the flexed left upper thigh. The penile skin is prepped or draped in the usual manner.

In an uncircumcised male, the foreskin is retracted proximally, and, by holding the glans with two fingers, the penis is moderately stretched. A No. 18 butterfly needle is inserted into the distal shaft about 1 in. from the corona glans, usually at a 1- to 2-o'clock position. The needle is inserted in an oblique direction, and the tunica albuginea is punctured. (This gives the typical resistance of a thick fibrotic capsule) (Fig. 14-14). There is usually a reflux of venous blood into the plastic tubing, or blood can appear after injection of a few milliliters of normal saline into the corpus and subsequent aspiration of the syringe. It is only necessary to puncture one

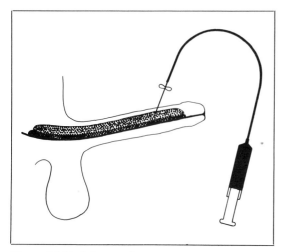

Figure 14-14. Schema of cavernosogram technique.

corpus, because the contrast material passes across to the other corpus. Care must be exercised not to penetrate the full thickness of the corpus cavernosum, so as not to enter the corpus spongiosum or the urethra.

We first rapidly (1 minute) inject normal sterile saline using a 50- to 60-ml syringe to produce a full, passive erection. The capacity of the corpora depends on penile size. The volume needed to achieve full erection in our patients is 80 to 150 ml. Close observation by the examiner is advised during the development of the passive erection. The appearance of the erected penis, any curvature or bending, and the amount of saline needed for full erection should be noted. It is during this time that any deformity of the penis can be examined. (A patient may not have been aware of a deformity because of not having had a full erection for some time.) The time between the development of a passively produced erection and its subsidence also should be noted.

When the erection has subsided completely, 30 to 50 ml of 30% meglumine diatrizoate is injected at the rate of 1 to 2 ml per sec. The first exposure, using 30 × 70 x-ray films is made during the last stage of the injection; the second 15 to 30 sec after the completion of the injection; and a third and fourth film are taken 2 and 7 minutes after the injection, respectively.

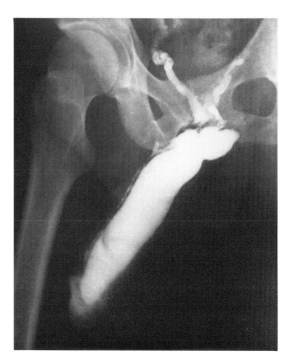

Figure 14-15. Cavernosogram: visualization of corpus cavernosum, the deep dorsal vein of penis, and some pelvic plexuses.

Corporal defects or plaques are best detected by exposure 2 min after injection. The penis is temporarily placed on the mid-lower anterior abdomen for this exposure, because this projection allows both corpora cavernosa to be fully outlined. The last exposure is made at 15 min.

Previously, we had 2 cases of developing penile edema with tenderness that lasted for a few days, subsiding without sequelae. At that time, we were using the recommended [16] 60% solution of radiopaque contrast material. We now use normal saline for production of passive erection and then a subsequent injection of 30% contrast material. Consequently, no local or general reactions have been seen in more than 30 patients studied.

Interpretation and Comments
The first and second radiographs outline most of the anastomosing corpora cavernosa and provide visualization of the deep dorsal vein and some of the pelvic venous plexuses (Fig. 14-15). Some opacification of the glans

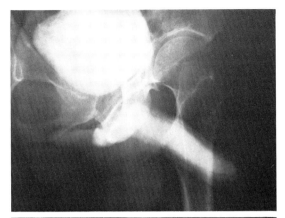

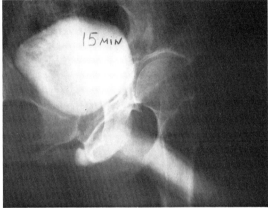

Figure 14-16. Normal cavernosogram in a 36-year-old impotent patient.

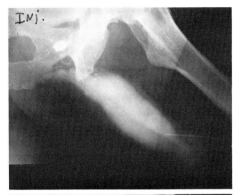

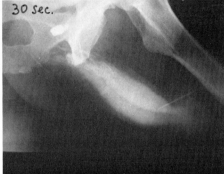

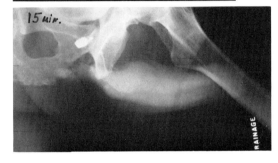

Figure 14-17. Normal cavernosogram in a 57-year-old diabetic having penile arterial obstruction.

penis occasionally shows up on the first x-ray picture, the one taken during the injection. This is seldom seen on the 15- to 30-sec film, and the opacification drains rapidly and is not seen on the remaining films.

The 2- and 7-minute (AP, or lateral) films allow us to evaluate the morphologic appearance of the corpora. The 15-minute film evaluates drainage of corpora.

Figure 14-16 shows a normal cavernosogram, and Figure 14-17, a normal cavernosogram in a diabetic patient with penile arterial obstruction.

Figure 14-18 shows an abnormal cavernosogram. There is rapid drainage at 30 seconds into pelvic veins and complete drainage from corpora at 15 minutes. Figure 14-19 depicts an abnormal cavernosogram. There is rapid run-off of dye at injection and no retention of contrast medium at 15 minutes. Figure 14-20 shows 7- and 15-minute cavernosograms in a 41-year-old patient with penile arterial obstruction.

Recent studies using this procedure, in addition to our own experiences, seem to suggest the need for this invasive radiologic investigation of penile venous circulation [6, 12]. Moreover, cavernosography recently has been suggested [5] as being necessary prior to penile prosthesis insertion in some cases. This theoretically would facilitate insertion and allow one to anticipate technical difficulties in dilating the corpora.

An occasional patient may not respond to the standard technique with adequate visual-

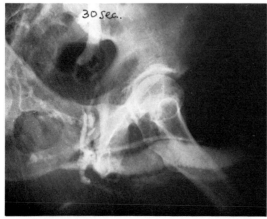

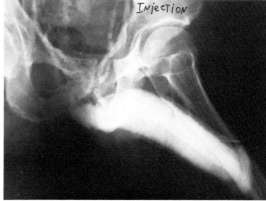

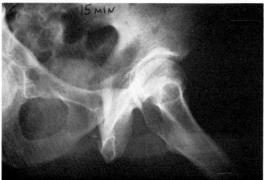

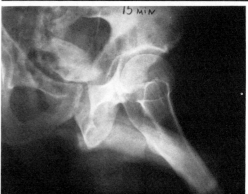

Figure 14-18. Abnormal cavernosogram. Rapid drainage into pelvic veins at 30 sec from injection. Complete drainage from corpora in 15 min. Patient is 52 years old (same patient as in Fig. 14-10).

Figure 14-19. Abnormal cavernosogram. Rapid run-off on injection. No retention of contrast medium in 15-minute film. Patient is 46 years old with no significant past history.

ization. Such a patient may require additional injections of contrast material to the nonvisible parts of the corpora.

In cases in which penile arterial obstruction results in impotence, cavernosography is needed preoperatively. Evaluating the capacity of the corpora cavernosa will disclose valuable information about the blood flow requirement necessary for achieving and maintaining an erection [24]. If the corpora cavernosa have a large capacity, this may indicate the need for a larger, or even double, bypass of the vessels as part of the revascularization procedure. Such foreknowledge, in conjunction with the most correct surgical procedure may, in turn, greatly improve surgical results. On the other hand, revascularization may not be indicated for surgical correction of a penile arterial obstruction if there is also sig-

nificant penile venous insufficiency, as demonstrated by cavernosography.

According to Ebbehoj and Wagner [6], cavernosography also enables detection of abnormal venous communication with the glans and the corpus spongiosum. In that case a different surgical approach to correction of erectile failure will be indicated.

Finally, cavernosography is of value as a method of evaluating impotence. It can be used to study Peyronie's disease, penile trauma, priapism, and metastatic carcinoma of the penis [29]. Figure 14-21 is a cavernosogram after priapism.

CONCLUSIONS
Corpus cavernosography is an invasive vascular procedure used to study the competency of the penile venous system. It is

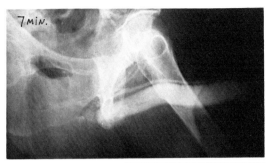

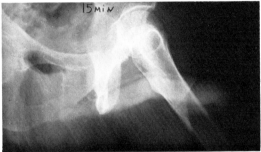

Figure 14-20. Cavernosograms (7- and 15-min) of 41-year-old patient known to have penile arterial obstruction producing impotence.

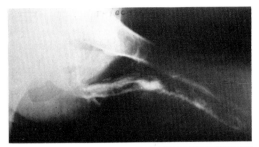

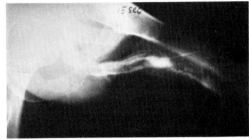

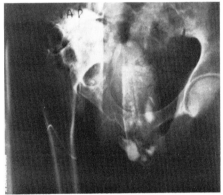

most pertinent when an impotent man complains of an unsustained erection, yet his clinical and noninvasive studies show no explanation for this complaint. It has been employed most successfully as an assessment of rapid drainage from the corpora cavernosa. It is also used for evaluation of the capacity, morphology and possible pathologies of the corpora. The invasive nature of this procedure requires strict adherence to the indications and is not to be used routinely.

Further studies in cavernosography may open new avenues of therapy for vascular erectile failure [6]. Cavernosogram, in conjunction with PA, offers evaluation of both phases of penile circulation.

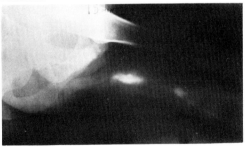

Figure 14-21. Cavernosogram after priapism. Impotent 31-year-old patient (same patient as in Fig. 14-11).

OTHER INVASIVE STUDIES
Radioisotope Penogram
Since 1970, Shirai and co-workers [34] have been developing the radioisotope penogram, to be used for differential diagnosis between functional and organic impotence.

Originally, they had difficulty in finding an isotope with the following characteristics: It had to remain in the blood for a certain period of time; it had to have a sufficient output of photons; it could not cause radiation side effects. Consequently their studies were delayed.

In 1975, however, Shirai started using $99^{m}T_{c}O4$. In a study of 11 cases, eight patients were classified as having possible organic impotence and three were designated as having nonorganic impotence.

Their study involved the IV injection of the radioisotope in doses of 150 to 700 mCi. Changes in penile blood flow were recorded as a penogram curve.

After identification of the penogram curve, a visual sexual stimulation was given to the patients studied. The patients who demonstrated a positive response to the stimulation through a rise in the penogram curve were classified as functionally impotent.

Since the radioisotope penogram reportedly produces only one curve, it might be that it offers only a total blood volume evaluation of the penis. However, the same authors believe the radioisotope penogram procedure is suitable for clinical routine. The method may have the same usefulness in evaluating impotence as the plethysmographic or PBP noninvasive methods used for study prior to invasive investigation.

Penile Scan

Casey [2] reported using penile scan by injecting technetium-99 postoperatively to verify the blood flow to the penis through the bypass artery. The method deserves further evaluation as a possible diagnostic tool for more precise penile blood flow determination.

CONCLUSIONS

Penile angiography has shown a high sensitivity in the detection of pathologic arterial lesions in impotent patients.

If the indications are observed, penile arteriography can yield as high as 93 to 97 percent abnormal findings in penile arteries. By using the standard percutaneous angiographic technique, the angiographer familiar with the use of gastrointestinal angiography should not encounter significant technical difficulties.

Corpus cavernosography visualizes the cavernosal bodies and the penile venous drainage system. The technique is familiar to urologists. It offers intriguing potential for better understanding of vasculogenic impotence, which in some patients may be produced by rapid drainage of the corpora cavernosa.

Radioactive studies of the penis have not been explored enough to assess their potential in vascular diagnosis of impotence. They could be significant if separate studies of functional penile blood flow become available.

Much progress has been made in understanding and evaluating the etiology of impotence in recent years. This is particularly true of vascular causes of impotence, even though the etiology was suggested almost a century ago. We are indeed grateful to those who have developed the noninvasive and invasive studies for the peripheral vascular system that are currently being applied to the investigation of impotence.

This rapid and aggressive development of noninvasive studies for vascular diseases finally has had an impact on our stereotypic, nonobjective past evaluation of impotence. Far-seeing investigators applying these methods in urology have made a great contribution in this field and are responsible for a giant step forward.

Although many of the cliches of impotence appear to have been explained, and the doors are opening for conservative and surgical correction of vasculogenic impotence, further research and progress in this field awaits new generations of clinicians and investigators. However, the concerned clinician has at his disposal methods already proved to be of diagnostic and therapeutic value. These methods, intelligently applied, can do much to help his patients enjoy a normal life.

REFERENCES

1. Canning, J. R., et al. Genital vascular insufficiency and impotence. *Surg. Forum* 14:298, 1963.
2. Casey, W. C. Revascularization of the corpus cavernosum for erectile failure. *Urology* 14:135, 1979.
3. Cohen, M. S., et al. Morphology of the corpus cavernosum arterial bed in impotence. *Proceedings of the First International Conference on Corpus Cavernosum Revascularization.* 13:103, 1980.
4. Conti, W. C. L'erection du penis humain et ses bases morpho-logico-vasculaire. *Acta Anat.* 14:217, 1952.
5. Datta, N. S. Corpus cavernography prior to insertion of penile prostheses. *Urology* 10:142, 1977.

6. Ebbehoj, J., and Wagner, G. Insufficient penile erection due to abnormal drainage of cavernous bodies. *Urology* 13:507, 1979.
7. Evans, I. L., and Young, A. E. Internal pudendal arteriography after priapism. *Br. J. Surg.* 60:329, 1973.
8. Fetter, T. R., Yenen, J. R., and Dodd, G. Application of cavernosography in the diagnosis of lesions of the penis. *Am. J. Roentgenol.* 90:169, 1963.
9. Fitzpatrick, T. J. Spongiosograms and cavernosograms: A study of their value in priapism. *J. Urol.* 109:843, 1973.
10. Fitzpatrick, T. J. Venography of the deep dorsal venous and valvular systems. *J. Urol.* 111:518, 1974.
11. Fitzpatrick, T. J. The corpus cavernosum intercommunicating venous drainage system. *J. Urol.* 113:494, 1975.
12. Fitzpatrick, T. J. The venous drainage of the corpus cavernosum and spongiosum. *Proceedings of the First International Conference on Corpus Cavernosum Revascularization.* 20:181, 1980.
13. Fitzpatrick, T. J., and Cooper, J. F. A cavernosogram study on the valvular competence of the human deep dorsal view. *J. Urol.* 113:497, 1975.
14. Ginestié, J. F., and Romieu, A. *L'exploration radiologique de l'impuissance.* Paris: Maloine, 1976.
15. Ginestié, J. F., and Romieu, A. *Radiologic Exploration of Impotence.* The Hague: Martinus Nijhoff, 1978.
16. Hamilton, R. E., and Swann, J. C. Corpus cavernosography in Peyronie's disease. *Br. J. Urol.* 39:409, 1967.
17. Jevtich, M. J. Importance of penile arterial pulse sound examination in impotence. *J. Urol.* 124:820, 1980.
18. Jevtich, M. J. Experience with penile arterial pulse sounds. *Proceedings of the First International Conference on Corpus Cavernosum Revascularization.* 4:31, 1980.
19. Lipsky, H. Über die pathogenese des idiopathischen priapismus. *Urol. Int.* 25:377, 1970.
20. Lowsley, O. S., and Bray, J. L. The surgical relief of impotence. *J. A. M. A.* 107:2029, 1936.
21. Lydston, G. F. The surgical treatment of impotence. *Am. J. Clin. Med.* 15:157, 1908.
22. May, F., and Hirtl, H. Das cavernosogramm. *Urol. Int.* 2:120, 1955.
23. Michal, V., et al. Direct arterial anastomosis to the cavernous body in the treatment of erectile impotence. *Rozhl. Chir.* 52:587, 1973.
24. Michal, V., et al. Vasculogenic impotence: Arteriography of the internal pudendal arteries and passive erection. *Proceedings of the First International Conference on Corpus Cavernosum Revascularization.* In press.
25. Michal, V., Kramar, R., and Pospichal, J. Femoropudendal bypass, internal iliac thromboendarectomy and direct arterial anastomosis to the cavernous body in the treatment of erectile impotence. *Bul. Soc. Internat. Chirurgie* 4:343, 1974.
26. Michal, V., and Pospichal, J. Phalloarteriography in the diagnosis of erectile impotence. *World J. Surg.* 2:239, 1978.
27. Millin, T. Impotence and its surgical treatment, with reference to a new operative procedure. *Proc. R. Soc. Med.* 29:817, 1936.
28. Newman, H. F., Northup, J. O., and Devlin, J. Mechanism of human penile erection. *Invest. Urol.* 1:350, 1964.
29. Ney, C., Miller, H. L., and Friedenburg, R. M. Various applications of corpus cavernosography. *Radiology* 119:69, 1976.
30. Padula, G. Problems of pudendal angiography. *Proceedings of the First International Conference on Corpus Cavernosum Revascularization.* 17:143, 1980.
31. Ružbarsky, V., and Michal, V. Morphologic changes in the arterial bed of the penis with aging. *Invest. Urol.* 15:194, 1977.
32. Scheer, A. Impotence as a symptom of arterial vascular disorders in the pelvic region. *Munch. Med. Wochenschr.* 102:1713, 1960.
33. Schelling, R. H., and Maxted, W. C. Major complication of silicone penile prosthesis. *Urology* 15:131, 1980.
34. Shirai, M., and Nakamura, M. Diagnostic discrimination between organic and functional impotence by radioisotope penogram with $^{99m}Tc_{O4}$. *Tohuku J. Exp. Med. (Jpn.)* 116:9, 1975.
35. Simpson, S. L. Impotence. *Br. Med. J.* 1:692, 1950.
36. Waltman, A. C., et al. Technique of left gastric catheterization. *Radiology* 109:732, 1973.
37. Wooten, J. S. Ligation of the dorsal vein of the penis as a cure for atonic impotence. *Texas Med. J.* 18:325, 1902–1903.
38. Zorgniotti, A. W., Padula, G., and Rossi, G. Impotence caused by pudendal arteriovenous fistula. *Urology* 14:161, 1979.

15

Evaluation of the Impotent Male: A Sex Therapist's View

STEVEN C. FISCHER
ALMA DELL SMITH

The purpose of this chapter is to acquaint the physician who is not a sex therapist with fundamental aspects of assessing erectile insufficiency, e.g., difficulty in attaining and/or maintaining erections. Sex therapists make a number of sequential assessments. First, an assessment of etiology is made. Second, the appropriateness of sex therapy is considered. Finally, an evaluation is made regarding the type and sequencing of experiences necessary for successful therapy outcome. In addition, psychologic evaluation of men with organic erectile insufficiency is necessary to identify motivation for surgery and unrealistic expectations regarding surgical outcome, to identify patients for whom surgery could precipitate emotional distress, and to prepare patient and partner for postsurgical adjustment [13]. The remainder of this chapter will be limited, however, to the first type of assessment—etiology from a sex therapist's perspective.

DETERMINING ETIOLOGY

Assessment of etiology is complex. Traditionally, there has been a tendency to view erectile insufficiency as *either* organic *or* psychogenic. This appears to be an oversimplification; there often may be an interaction between the two. There may, for example, be subtle but significant organic changes that result in relatively minor disturbances in a man's ability to attain or maintain an erection. His reaction or his partner's reaction to these changes, however, may have a major role in determining the future course of their sexual relationship. Their expectations and attitudes could result in a mutually satisfying sexual relationship or could result in a significant erosion of their sexual activities and satisfaction. Consequently, it is essential to assess the interaction between psychologic and organic factors. Erectile insufficiency can be psychogenic or biogenic or can result from an interaction between the two aspects.

Historically, estimates of psychologic etiology ranged from 80 to 95 percent. These estimates probably will decline as increasingly sophisticated medical examinations proliferate. Finding positive physical signs does not, in itself, rule out predominant or significant psychologic components. Similarly, finding psychologic aspects does not rule out predominant or significant organic factors. A thorough assessment should attempt to determine the multiplicity of factors leading to erectile problems and their relative importance, an ideal seldom achieved in clinical practice.

A reasonable working hypothesis is that organic and physical factors can set the limits of sexual functioning and that psychologic factors determine the variability within those limits. In a healthy male with no physical or organic impairment, erectile insufficiency may be assumed to be psychogenic. In a male quadriplegic it may be assumed to be organic. A third example, however, could be a male with vascular disease who attains 80 percent of penile blood volume. In the absence of anxiety this male could achieve erections sufficient for intercourse and be able to maintain a satisfying and fulfilling sexual relationship with his partner. Alternatively, this man could become anxious or despondent about his decrease in "arousal," or his partner's reaction to it, and could experience a further deterioration in their sexual relationship with increased erectile problems.

Attempting to determine the relative importance of physical and psychologic factors is of utmost importance because treatment choice is dependent on it. A couple who have sexual difficulties that are psychogenic are more likely to be offered and to accept sex therapy than a surgical implant. A couple whose sexual problems result from organic impairment are more likely to be offered and to accept a surgical implant. A man whose erectile problems result from a combination of organic and psychologic factors is in a more ambiguous situation, in which sex therapy and/or surgical implantation could be the most appropriate treatment(s). Optimal assessment and treatment requires coordinated effort from several specialties and disciplines.

METHODS OF ASSESSMENT
Psychologic Testing
Psychology historically has emphasized the importance of psychologic testing. In recent years, many psychologists have questioned the utility of all psychologic testing, whereas others argue that testing yields useful information about people globally but not specifically [12].

Before we review the research regarding the utility of psychologic testing in determining etiology, there are several basic issues of testing with which we should like to familiarize the reader. Before any psychologic test can be used to assess etiology, it must first be predictive. A study that takes two groups of men (one known to be organically impotent and one known to be psychogenically impotent), tests, and finds differences between the two groups is not predictive. This type of procedure may, however, be a necessary or desirable first step in determining what salient characteristics should be utilized or tested in a predictive study. A careful study may find ways in which two mutually exclusive groups differ. Whether these differences can now be used to predict into which group a new, previously untested person will fall remains an unanswered question. Moreover, there is a need for replication, repeating the experimental procedure on a similar sample. Thirdly, cross validation is required. This means a new sample is drawn from a different group and the same test and decision rules are used with the new group. If the test still predicts, confidence is increased regarding its utility.

Even if the above steps are taken, there is an additional problem: determining into which group a person belongs on the basis of an individual score without knowledge of the group distribution. Figure 15-1A depicts two hypothetical group distributions with significantly different means. An individual could easily be sorted into one of the groups, depending on his score. Figure 15-1B depicts two other hypothetical distributions also with significantly different means. However, these distributions grossly overlap. It would be impossible to know to which group a person belonged if he obtained a score in the shaded area.

One will appreciate the importance of this issue if the hypothetical distributions referred to males diagnosed as "organically" and

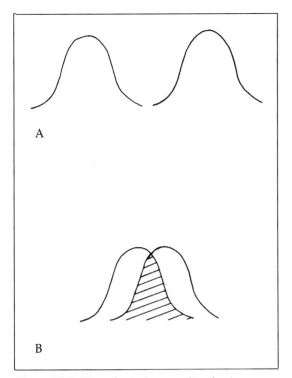

Figure 15-1. Hypothetical group distributions.

"psychogenically" impotent. The dependent measure could be a score on a physical or psychologic test. Anyone scoring in the shaded area would be impossible to accurately diagnose.

These are only some of the potential pitfalls of testing. Researchers and readers of research need to be aware of these issues to evaluate claims of others adequately.

The Male Impotence Test (MIT) was developed by Senoussi [14]. Ellis [5] raised several cogent methodologic problems with this test, and Beutler and co-workers [3] attempted to cross-validate the MIT using more clearly delineated groups. He found the MIT was unable to discriminate between biogenic and psychogenic impotence.

The Minnesota Multiphasic Personality Inventory (MMPI) is a widely used and extremely well researched psychologic inventory. The MMPI has 566 items to which respondents answer "true" or "false." It is an empiric test, meaning *every* item differentiates a psychopathologic group from a "normal" population. There are three validity scales that give an indication of the consis-

tency of the subject's response, his ability to understand the questions, his willingness to reveal psychologic difficulties. There are 10 clinical scales that yield information about the subject's general personality. Since the MMPI is an established instrument Beutler and co-workers [3] investigated whether personality variables assessed through the MMPI could distinguish biogenic from psychogenic impotence.

Beutler and co-workers took a sample of 32 impotent males and selected 10 subjects, six clearly psychogenic and four clearly biogenic, on the basis of nocturnal tumescence studies. The 10 subjects had their MMPI profiles studied and two decision rules were established that correctly placed those 10 into either a psychogenic or organic group. The decision rules were then applied to the remaining 22 subjects. Their classification based on decision rules was compared with their classification based on NPT (nocturnal penile tumescence) studies. This method correctly identified 90 percent of them (20 of 22).

An additional finding was that there was no clear personality type associated with either psychogenic or biogenic impotence. Biogenic impotence cuts across personality types, as does psychogenic impotence. The utility of the MMPI in predicting etiology was, however, only a tentative finding. The authors indicated the need to conduct further studies with different samples. Similarly, Beutler indicated that positive findings using the MMPI were preliminary [4].

Marshall, Surridge, and Delva [9] attempted to use the decision rules developed by Beutler in a cross-validation study. They found that a *complete reversal* of decision rules correctly identified 75 percent of their subjects. Stated differently, 75 percent were misidentified in using decision rules developed by Beutler.

To date, psychologic testing has not been able to yield information regarding etiology. It is clear there is no personality profile for either biogenic or psychogenic impotence. It is also clear that initially promising results of testing have not held up under additional studies. Any future claims must be considered tentative until the above considerations have been addressed adequately. Against this historical perspective caution is mandated.

Nocturnal Penile Tumescence

Nocturnal penile tumescence (NPT) studies are a promising advance in the behavioral assessment of erectile insufficiency. Masters and Johnson [10, 11] were among the first objectively to identify and describe physical changes humans experience when sexually aroused. They primarily relied on visual observation with relatively little physiologic measurement.

Penile tumescence studies use mechanical strain gauges [2] directly to measure changes in tumescence or detumescence in response to various stimuli. Originally developed to determine subjects' response to various sexual stimuli (e.g., homosexual versus heterosexual slides or videotapes) this technology has been extended to aid in the assessment of erectile insufficiency.

Zuckerman [15] and Barlow [1] have reviewed the use of physiologic measures to assess male sexual arousal to erotic stimuli and found them to be valid and widely accepted. Several cautions, however, need to be cited in the use of penile tumescence studies to assess erectile insufficiency. First, the assessment should occur at night during sleep. It is assumed that NPT studies obviate issues of anxiety that would likely occur if testing were done in a laboratory setting. In addition, it has been reported that men attain several erections during sleep, generally related to rapid eye movement (REM) sleep cycles [7, 8]. Consequently, lack of erections during sleep are presumed to result from something other than anxiety, even though anxiety-evoking dreams inhibit erections [6]. Second, the patient should be asked to use the equipment on several nights. Presently, most clinicians and researchers request two or three nights. This allows the subject to adapt to sleeping with a strain gauge around his penis and minimizes the possibility of erroneous data due to equipment error or failure. Third, we do not know how frequently men normally attain erections during sleep. Does attaining two erections during sleep mean the same

thing as attaining eight? Tumescence changes during sleep vary with age [7, 8]. Fourth, EEG should be monitored. If erections are correlated with REM cycle and a male fails to attain an erection, it would be impossible to know whether he is organically impotent or merely REM-sleep–deprived.

NPT studies are promising but should be considered experimental at this stage of development. Much additional research needs to be done before the NPT can be relied on as a primary assessment tool.

Interview

The interview remains the primary assessment device for the sex therapist. It provides a format by which the interviewer can establish the context in which the problem occurs, and its functional relationship to other events or situations. It is preferable to interview the partners together and separately. Often, one partner will perceive circumstances quite differently from the other or can provide information that the other partner cannot.

GENERAL ASSUMPTIONS. *Psychogenic erectile insufficiency results from anxiety.* Many patients, as well as professionals, believe psychologic etiology means the problem is "in the head." Many also believe that psychologically based treatment will require some form of long-term psychologic therapy. Neither of these assumptions is warranted. Anxiety is an autonomic response incompatible with sexual arousal. Given sufficient levels of anxiety, sexual arousal will be decreased or eliminated. Anxiety may result from beliefs and cognitions as well as conditioning. The most common form of anxiety has to do with performance, fears about being able to attain or maintain an erection. Finding anxiety does not in itself, however, rule out organic etiology. It is extremely important to distinguish between anxiety that *leads to* erectile insufficiency and that which *results from* erectile insufficiency. The latter can occur with organic etiologies.

What initiates a problem is frequently not what maintains it. For example, a man may be placed on antihypertensive medication and begin to have erectile problems. As a "test" several months later he may be asked to discontinue the medication in an attempt to determine whether the medication elicited these problems. If the medication is discontinued and erectile problems persist a potentially in-incorrect assumption may be made that medication did not affect erections. It is entirely possible medication initiated the problem but that an *autonomous* fear of failure presently maintains it. Similarly, a man may have too much to drink and be unable to attain or maintain an erection. On successive occasions, this person may continue to have erectile problems when abstaining from alcohol because he is afraid erectile insufficiency will recur.

In cases of anxiety (psychologic) etiology there should be a predictable response pattern and/or predictable history. If anxiety plays a role there would be an expectation of increased likelihood of sexual arousal when anxiety is minimal and of less sexual arousal when anxiety is heightened. In addition, it is likely that anxiety will be present early in the history of the problem. A man may have erectile insufficiency because he fears failure with women he knows well but can function reasonably well with novel women because there is less concern and risk about failing with them. Still another man may function sexually in close, emotionally supportive relationships, in which he knows his partner well, but he may have erectile insufficiency in novel relationships because he wants to make a good impression and fears failing more intensely. The above two examples are not merely theoretic possibilities but have been seen by the authors. Similarly, a man initially may have no difficulty attaining an erection with fellatio or when masturbating but may usually lose it at the point of penetration, a time when performance pressures are heightened. These patterns, however, should *not* be expected to remain stable over time. Anxiety may begin earlier or may generalize to other stimulus conditions as the problems persist.

Listed below are commonly seen patterns that can lead to erectile insufficiency. This list is not intended to be exhaustive or mutually exclusive.

1. *Drinking, fatigue, or physical illness.* Each of these can affect the ability to become sexually aroused and attain erections. It is not necessary for a man to be inebriated before sexual arousal is affected. Several drinks over a prolonged period may interfere without a subjective experience of intoxication.

2. *Premature ejaculation.* The authors have seen several men whose insufficiency was predated by a history of premature ejaculation. Concern and anxiety about delaying ejaculation as well as anxiety about the partner's reaction to premature ejaculation can lead to erectile problems. Other men begin to think distracting thoughts (e.g., the 1952 World Series) in an attempt to delay ejaculation. Unfortunately, thinking distracting thoughts can decrease sexual arousal and lead to loss of erection.

3. *Paucity of sexual repertoire.* Couples who have a limited sexual repertoire and whose primary means of sexual stimulation and expression is through intercourse place an inordinate amount of pressure on a man to maintain erections for long periods of time to satisfy his sexual partner. Helping a couple to increase their sexual repertoire can aid in decreasing these pressures.

4. *Concern over perceived changes in sexual arousal.* Masters and Johnson [10] report young men experiencing excitement-phase levels of sexual tension over an extended period of time will attain full erection, partially lose, and fully regain it several times during any sexual cycle. Older men, however, may have difficulty returning to full erectile performance when an erection is lost without ejaculation. Masters and Johnson [10, 11] report other changes in older men. Men in their sixties and older may require 2 to 3 times longer to achieve erection than the young man's 3 to 5 sec. Time required to ejaculate also increases in older men. In addition, older men frequently do not attain

full penile erection until just before the ejaculatory experience. Men over 50 expel the ejaculate 6 to 12 in. in contrast to the 12 to 24 in. reported for younger men. When erection has been maintained for long periods, there may be seminal fluid seepage rather than expulsion under pressure. Refractory periods increase for older men. Penile detumescence immediately after ejaculation is very rapid. These changes, which may be considered a normal part of the aging process, might cause anxiety and produce a fear that a man's sexually active years may soon be over. The resulting anxiety can lead to psychogenic impotence. Both anxiety and physical changes may be occurring, yet sex therapy may be the treatment of choice in some instances.

5. *Long periods of sexual abstinence.* The termination of a relationship, followed by a long period of abstinence, can lead to erectile dysfunction. This frequently is referred to as the widower's syndrome.

6. *Misinformation and unrealistic expectations.* Misinformation and unrealistic expectations lead to an unrealistic standard to strive for. When men fall short, anxiety levels increase, and erectile insufficiency can result.

7. *Medication effects interfering with sexual arousal.* Many psychotropic and antihypertensive medications militate against attaining erections.

8. *Relationship with partner.* If a couple is having marital problems or have conflict about certain aspects of their relationship (e.g., whether to have children) erectile problems can result.

9. *Psychopathology.* People may consult the physician about erectile difficulties but may, in fact, be experiencing a depressive reaction or other major psychiatric disorder.

10. *Traumatic event.* An anxiety-provoking traumatic event can lead to erectile difficulties. One male, recently seen, dated erectile problems to the time he tore his foreskin during intercourse.

11. *Partner's vaginismus.* It is not uncommon for a male to have erectile problems

related or secondary to his partner's vaginismus.

12. *Special times.* The authors have seen men whose erectile insufficiency began during a special time, when anxiety was heightened. Examples include first intercourse and attempting to sire a child.

CONCLUSIONS

Assessing erectile insufficiency is complex and requires the coordinated efforts of several disciplines. Searching for a single etiology is very often an oversimplification. Frequently, multiple causes may be found. In such cases the interaction between causes and their relative weighting should be investigated to ensure maximum understanding and appropriate treatment. To date, psychologic testing has not aided in determining etiology. Nocturnal penile tumescence studies appear promising but should be considered experimental until additional basic research is completed. The interview remains the primary assessment tool of the sex therapist. A detailed interview involving both partners with an experienced sex therapist is a necessary step in the complete assessment of erectile insufficiency.

REFERENCES

1. Barlow, D. H. Assessment of Sexual Behavior. In R. A. Ciminero, K. S. Calhoun, and H. E. Adams (eds.), *Handbook of Behavioral Assessment.* New York: Wiley, 1977.
2. Barlow, D. H., et al. A mechanical strain gauge for recording penile circumference change. *J. Appl. Behav. Anal.* 3:73, 1970.
3. Beutler, L. E., et al. MMPI and MIT discriminators of biogenic and psychogenic impotence. *J. Consult. Clin. Psychol.* 43:899, 1975.
4. Beutler, L. E., Scott, F. B., and Karacan, I. Psychological screening of impotent men. *J. Urol.* 116:193, 1976.
5. Ellis, A. The Male Impotence Test. In O. K. Buros (ed.), *The Seventh Mental Measurement Yearbook.* Highland Park, N.J.: Gryphon, 1972.
6. Karacan, I. Clinical value of nocturnal erection in the prognosis and diagnosis of impotence. *Med. Asp. Human Sex.* 4:27, 1970.
7. Karacan, I., Hursch, C. J., and Williams, R. L. Some characteristics of nocturnal penile

tumescence in elderly males. *J. Gerontol.* 27:39, 1972.

8. Karacan, I., et al. Some characteristics of nocturnal penile tumescence in young adults. *Arch. Gen. Psychiatry* 26:351, 1972.

9. Marshal, P., Surridge, D., and Delva, N. Differentiation of organic and psychogenic impotence on the basis of MMPI decision rules. *J. Consult. Clin. Psychol.* 48:407, 1980.

10. Masters, W. H., and Johnson, V. E. *Human Sexual Response.* Boston: Little, Brown, 1966.

11. Masters, W. H., and Johnson, V. E. *Human Sexual Inadequacy.* Boston: Little, Brown, 1970.

12. Mischel, W. *Personality and Assessment.* New York: Wiley, 1968.

13. Osborne, D. Psychologic evaluation of impotent men. *Mayo Clin. Proc.* 51:363, 1976.

14. Senoussi, A. E. *The Male Impotence Test.* Los Angeles: Western Psychological Services, 1964.

15. Zuckerman, M. Physiological measures of sexual arousal in the human. *Psychol. Bull.* 75:347, 1971.

16

Neurologic Impotence

IRWIN GOLDSTEIN

Neurologic impotence may be defined as the impaired ability of the patient to generate or sustain a penile erection because of abnormal neurologic factors. These factors may be related either to abnormal penile sensation [17, 26], abnormal vasomotor control of the penile circulation (to direct arterial blood into the trabecular spaces of the corporal bodies) [11], or abnormal cerebral initiation (modulation) of the sacral erection reflex [22]. Neurologic lesions causing impotence may be classified as infrasacral-sacral or suprasacral in location. Patients with peripheral neuropathies after radical pelvic surgery or patients with cauda equina or sacral cord injury may have abnormalities in infrasacral-sacral erectile pathways. Complete lesions in these pathways may result in total loss of erectile capability [4, 15]. Patients with multiple sclerosis, suprasacral spinal cord tumors, spinal cord trauma, transverse myelitis, cerebrovascular accidents, or Parkinson's disease may have lesions in suprasacral erectile pathways. Complete lesions involving these pathways may result in abnormal nocturnal penile tumescence with poorly sustained, less rigid erections.

The diagnosis of neurologic impotence should always be considered as an etiology of erectile dysfunction. If a neurologic etiology exists but is not recognized, unnecessary and prolonged psychotherapy or endocrinologic manipulation might result. Furthermore, microvascular surgical repair [23] might have a poor clinical outcome (despite a technically successful blood vessel anastomosis) if neurologic impotence coexists with vasculogenic impotence. Less commonly, a missed diagnosis of neurologic impotence might delay identification of a potentially treatable neurologic disease. An occult herniated vertebral disk is a prime example [28].

How is the diagnosis of neurologic impotence established? Usually, suspicion for neurologic involvement is made with the initial history and physical examination. Subsequent abnormal neurophysiologic evaluations help identify the presence and location of neurologic pathology. Neurologic impotence alone is then confirmed by abnormal nocturnal penile tumescence (NPT) studies, abnor-

I would like to thank Marcia M. Davidson for her excellent technical assistance in performing genitocerebral evoked response testing.

mal neurophysiologic evaulations, and the lack of other organic etiologies causing impotence. This chapter will review the considerations and techniques involved in diagnosing neurologic impotence.

The presence of an antecedent neurologic history should be considered important when discovered on the initial patient interview. Impotence in patients with a past history of head trauma, alcoholism, diabetes, transverse myelitis, or cervical spondylolisthesis should be considered as possibly having a neurologic etiology. In addition, neurologic causes should be suspect in patients without antecedent neurologic history but who complain of loss of erectile potency associated temporally with the appearance of classic neurologic symptoms such as headaches, impaired vision, change in mental status, paresthesias, back pain, and changes in bladder or bowel habits.

Whereas questions concerning neurologic history are important, questions concerning sexual performance or sexual activity are generally not useful in diagnosing a specific neurologic dysfunction. For example, information concerning the ability to attain a penile erection (either nocturnal or with sexual stimulation), the quality of the erection (rigid or not), and the circumstances in which erections are lost (with different partners or with different coital movements) are more helpful when used to differentiate between psychogenic and organic impotence. The partial, poorly sustained erection secondary to an incomplete sacral cord lesion or complete suprasacral cord lesion may be indistinguishable (by history alone) from one secondary to arterial vascular insufficiency.

Neurologic examination should include sensory testing of the perineum and lower extremities, motor testing of the upper and lower extremities and reflex testing of the quadriceps, Achilles tendon, and bulbocavernosus reflexes [25].

In particular, patients with peripheral neuropathies secondary to alcoholism or diabetes may have pain and touch sensory losses in a stocking-and-glove distribution. Patients with posterior column disease (tabes dorsalis)

may have associated pain and position sensory losses. Those with herniated disk may have loss of sensation in the lateral aspect of the leg (L4–L5 disks) or lateral aspect of the foot (S1–S2 disks).

Motor system examinations may help identify the location of a particular abnormality. Paraplegia involves cord lesions below the upper thoracic segments, whereas quadriplegia usually involves a cervical cord lesion. Parkinson's disease and multiple sclerosis are associated commonly with cerebellar motor dysfunction.

Examination of reflex activity provides information on segmental spinal cord function as well as suprasegmental neurologic control. Hypoactive or absent quadriceps reflex (L3, L4), Achilles tendon (L5, S1, S2), or bulbocavernosus reflex (S2, S3, S4) suggest segmental abnormalities. Hyperactive reflexes imply suprasegmental corticobulbar lesions. In particular, the bulbocavernosus reflex is useful in assessing the segmental function of the important S2–S4 segments [25]. This reflex can be found clinically in 70 percent of normal males [3] and by evoked response testing in almost 100 percent. Variants of the bulbocavernosus reflex include the trigonal reflex and the anal wink [28].

After the initial history and neurologic examination, the clinician should have an index of suspicion for the existence of neurologic impotence. Working in conjunction with a neurologist, the clinician subsequently could order skull x rays, brain scan, electroencephalography, carotid angiography, computerized tomography, and myelography to help define the location of a suspected neurologic lesion. Several neurourologic examinations have been developed recently that may provide objective information on specific neurologic pathways involved in erection.

The indications for these neurourologic evaluations include suspicion of neurologic impairment based on initial patient evaluation, history of bladder dysfunction suggestive of neurologic detrusor areflexia (abdominal straining, dribbling, retention), and abnormal nocturnal penile tumescence studies [2, 13, 18] in the presence of normal vascular and

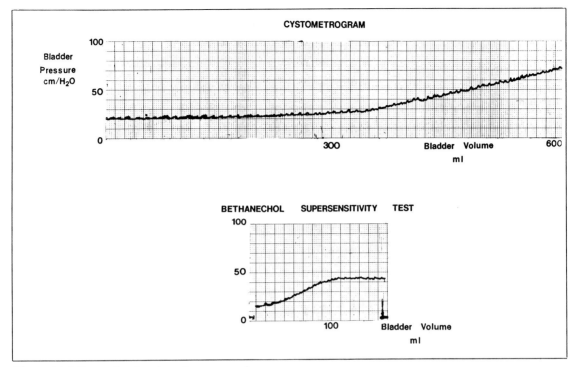

Figure 16-1. Example of cystometrogram and bethanechol testing in a patient with cauda equina syndrome and impotence. Intravesical pressure at 100 ml volume rises from 20 to 44 cm H_2O following bethanechol (5 mg) subcutaneous injection, indicating parasympathetic denervation.

endocrinologic erectile function tests. In our experience neurourologic testing on all impotent patients as a routine screening procedure has not been rewarding.

NEUROUROLOGIC TESTING

The peripheral nervous system as it pertains to the erection mechanism may be considered to involve only the pelvic nerves (parasympathetic) and pudendal nerves (somatic). There does not appear to be any role for the thoracolumbar sympathetics in the generation or maintenance of an erection [30].

Evaulation of the parasympathetic pelvic nerves is performed at the vesical parasympathetic plexus by cystometrography (CMG) and bethanechol supersensitivity testing [1, 21] (see Fig. 16-1). Patients who have had radical pelvic surgery or who have diabetes

and autonomic neuropathy [10, 11] are at risk for having lesions in the pelvic nerves. In our experience, however, CMGs and bethanechol testing for impotence evaluation generally have been useful only if suspected patients had concomitant voiding dysfunction. It is hoped that in the future parasympathetic evaluation for impotence will be done directly at the level of the corporal parasympathetic plexus. In this manner, patients who have abnormal corporal parasympathetic function with normal proximal vesical parasympathetic pathways may become identifiable.

The pudendal nerves (S2–S4) supply sensation from the penile skin and provide motor innervation to the bulbocavernosus, ischiocavernosus, and external urethral sphincter muscles. The integrity of the sensory aspect of the pudendal nerve is important in the development of a normal erection [17, 26]. In contrast, the motor aspect of the pudendal nerve may play a greater role in ejaculation [27]. Examination of the somatic pudendal nerve is best performed by perineal electromyography (EMG) and sacral latency testing (SLT) (see Fig. 16-2).

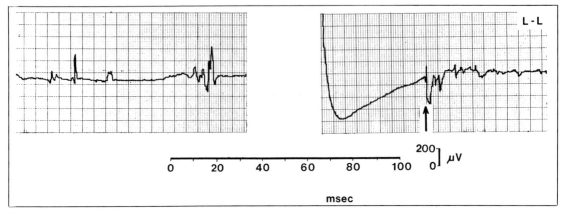

A

Figure 16-2. A. Perineal EMG (left) and sacral
evoked response (right) in a patient with lumbar
disk disease and impotence is presented. Perineal
EMG demonstrates abnormal polyphasic
potential. Sacral latency time is 45.8 msec.
B. Myelogram with L5–S1 defect.

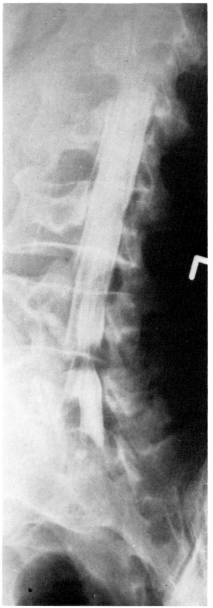

B

Perineal electromyography is a recording of the motor unit potentials from the perineal striated muscles. It has been used to identify denervation states and to recognize occult subclinical disturbances in the motor pudendal pathway. This test is especially useful in toxic and metabolic disorders that result in peripheral neuropathy (e.g., alcoholism, diabetes) or postpelvic trauma in which the peripheral pudendal nerve may have been injured [28]. The sacral latency test is an electrophysiologic representation of the bulbocavernosus reflex. The presumed pathway of this crossed polysynaptic somatic-somatic reflex [19] involves pudendal afferents, sacral cord segments S2–S4, pudendal efferents, and the perineal striated bulbocavernosus muscle [6, 9, 12, 30]. Documentation of suspected sacral cord injury (multiple sclerosis, spinal cord trauma, spinal cord tumors, herniated intervertebral disk) is the major use of this procedure. In situations involving somatic sacral cord injury, conclusions can be drawn concerning the function of autonomic nerves. Parasympathetic sacral neurons are anatomically located close to the central pudendal somatic pathway [28, 29].

Examination of the suprasacral afferent pathways recently has become possible by the pudendal (genitocerebral) evoked response (GCER) [14, 16]. In this evaluation, objective information is obtained by electrically stimulating the peripheral pudendal nerve at the penis and observing the evoked potential or waveform at various sites proximally within the central nervous system. The presumed pathway of this evaluation includes somesthetic receptors in the skin of the penis, pudendal sensory axons to sacral dorsal root ganglia, ascending second-order fibers, presumably to the region of the thalamus, and finally to third-order fibers in the contralateral primary sensory area deep in the interhemispheric fissure [8]. The evaulation can be divided conveniently into peripheral conduction time (penis to sacral cord) and central conduction time [8, 16] (sacral cord to cerebral cortex) to help localize neurologic lesions. "Upper motor neuron" impotence may thus be objectively assessed using this technique.

Technical Considerations

Cystometrography and bethanechol testing have been well described previously [1].

Perineal electromyography and sacral latency testing are performed with the patient supine on the examining table, without sedation or medication. A neurologic examination documenting perineal and lower extremity sensation, deep tendon reflexes (ankle and knee), flexor plantar responses (Babinski's sign) and bulbocavernosus reflex is obtained. The patient is then placed in the lithotomy position, and the bulbocavernosus muscle is defined by placing the index finger over the perineum during a Valsalva or cough maneuver. A fine No. 25 electromyographic concentric needle electrode is placed into the muscle on one side of the midline. Proper placement is assured by audio and oscilloscopic control.

Electromyographic assessment is performed by observing (1) individual motor unit action potential configuration [5]; (2) presence of neuropathic potentials (positive sharp waves, polyphasic potentials, or fibrillation potentials); (3) ability to contract voluntarily the bulbocavernosus muscle; and (4) degree of motor unit action potential recruitment (interference pattern) during a bulbocavernosus reflex or cough.

Sacral latency testing is performed by taping a block skin-stimulating electrode on the ipsilateral side of the penile shaft. Square-wave stimuli are delivered at a frequency of 1/second, with a duration of 1 millisecond. Stimulation begins at 0 V and is increased slowly to determine sensory threshold (first sensation), reflex threshold (first consistent bulbocavernosus muscle contraction); and minimum latency. Usually, 8 to 32 stimulations are averaged on the final response. In a lateralization study, the contralateral penile shaft is stimulated, and the previous EMG recording electrode placement is maintained. Subsequently, the contralateral bulbocavernosus muscle is used, and the study is repeated with ipsilateral and contralateral penile shaft stimulation. A complete lateralization evaluation therefore results in four latency values [19] (see Fig. 16-3).

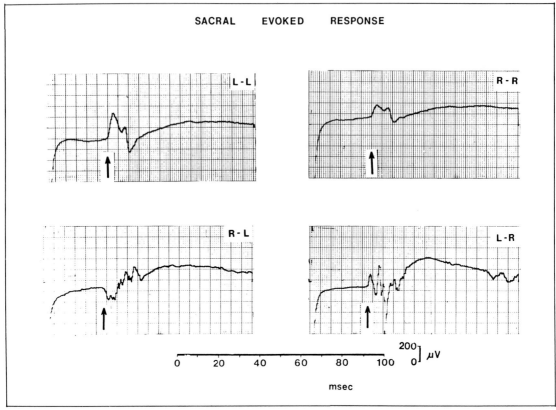

Figure 16-3. A typical sacral evoked potential lateralizing study is presented. Note the four values that can be derived by this technique.

Figure 16-4. Genitocerebral evoked response study from a patient suspected of having neurogenic impotence. Note that the N2 peak is at 42.0 msec, and the P2 peak is at 38.4 msec, representing a normal study.

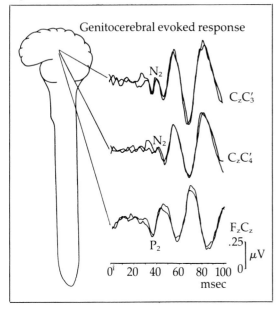

Genitocerebral evoked response testing is performed with a cooperative, unmedicated patient in the supine position, relaxed on a comfortable recliner. The room is temperature controlled and the lights are dimmed throughout the study.

Recording electrodes (silver-silver chloride cup electrodes with felt pads) are attached by collodion and filled with conductive paste. Electrode impedances are kept below 3000 ohm. Active electrodes for peripheral pathways can be chosen over vertebral L1 for the sacral cord, and vertebral L3, L5 for the cauda equina. Reference electrodes have been used over the suprasacral cord at verebral T4. Cortical recording electrodes have been chosen over the sites C3′, C4′ (approximately 2 cm back and 7 cm lateral to C_z according to the International Coding System), and F_z. Reference electrodes for the cerebrum have been used over C_z (based on noncephalic field potential studies) (see Fig. 16-4).

Block skin-stimulating electrodes are taped over the left and right sides of the penile shaft. Adequate preparation of the penile skin with a pumice scrub helps keep stimulation impedances below 5000 ohm. A ground electrode is placed between the stimulus site (penis) and the recording sites (the lowest is generally vetebral L1). A flexible metal strip, covered with a warm, saline-soaked cloth and wrapped around the lower abdomen, has been satisfactory, with ground impedances usually kept less than 5000 ohm.

Square-wave stimuli are delivered at a frequency of 1 per second, with a duration of 0.2 millisecond, and at a constant current of 6 to 15 ma. Generally, the latter level is chosen, based on appreciation of sensation and reflex contractions of the bulbocavernosus muscle. A photoelectric stimulus isolation unit is used to reduce stimulus artifact to a minimum and to provide an extra margin of patient safety.

During each study four bipolar recordings are obtained. These are usually, but not exclusively, chosen as T4–L1, F_z–C_z, C_z–C3′, and C_z–C4′ for bilateral penile stimulation and T4–L1, F_z–C_z, C_z–C3′, and C4′–C3′ for unilateral stimulation (left-sided in this example). Each recording is amplified approximately 500,000 times through the use of filters with bandpass of 30 Hz (low cutoff) and 3000 Hz (high cutoff). An automatic artificial reject with an adjustable reject amplitude has been found extremely helpful.

The digital averager used has 1024 total memory points; separated into four channels, it utilizes 256 memory points per channel. The intersample interval or time between each memory point is 400 microseconds. The total sweep duration is 102.4 milliseconds. A 2.56-msec delay is introduced, to assist in diminishing stimulus artifact [7, 8].

A typical study with a cooperative patient generally takes approximately 2 hours, including the time for electrode placement. In general, 256 samples per study suffice. A complete study includes runs with right and left penile stimulation and bilateral penile stimulation.

Neuroclinical Results

For the evauation of impotence, 159 SLT tests have been performed. The average values for the four responses in the overall population was L–L, 37.6 milliseconds; R–L, 40.1 milliseconds; R–R, 39.8 milliseconds; and L–R, 40.2 milliseconds. Of those patients who had at least one abnormal latency value, the average abnormal values were L–L, 49.1 milliseconds; R–L, 54.1 milliseconds; R–R, 54.8 milliseconds; and L–R, 53.2 milliseconds (see Table 16-1).

For the evaluation of impotence, 24 GCER tests have been performed. The average value for normal *total* latencies (penis to cerebral cortex) was 40.66 ± 1.33 milliseconds. This was distributed as peripheral conduction time 12.39 ± 1.33 milliseconds and central conduction time 28.45 ± 1.68 milliseconds.

Abnormal results were recorded in three distinct groups: (1) patients with infrasacral-sacral impotence and abnormal peripheral conduction times with normal central conduction times, (2) patients with suprasacral impotence and abnormal central conduction times with normal peripheral conduction times, and (3) patients with both infrasacral-

Table 16-1. Sacral latency testing

	Left to left (msec)	Left to right (msec)	Right to right (msec)	Right to left (msec)
Average sacral latency values (129 tests)	37.6	40.0	39.9	40.1
Average abnormal sacral latency values (25 tests)	49.1	53.2	54.8	54.0

Source: New England Male Reproductive Center, University Hospital, Boston.

Table 16-2. Genitocerebral evoked response

	Peripheral conduction time (msec)	Central conduction time (msec)	Total latency (msec)
Average normal values (14 patients)	12.39 ± 1.33	28.45 ± 1.68	40.66 ± 1.33
Average abnormal values (13 patients)	19.81 ± 0.71	38.15 ± 6.72	52.71 ± 6.91

Source: New England Male Reproductive Center, University Hospital, Boston.

sacral and suprasacral impotence and abnormal peripheral and central conduction times. Average latencies in the three groups are recorded in Table 16-2.

CONCLUSIONS

Neurologic factors may cause impotence by interference with penile sensation, interference with corporal vasomotor control, or interference with cerebral initiation or modulation. Neurologic involvement is usually first suspected with the initial patient evaluation. It is then confirmed by objective neurophysiologic testing, such as, perineal electromyography, sacral latency, and genitocerebral evoked response testing. These procedures attempt to identify abnormalities in the somatic pudendal pathway. Motor parasympathetic pathways to the corporal helicine blood vessels are presently not evaluated by direct objective testing. Inference of parasympathetic nerve function is made on cystometrography and bethanechol supersensitivity testing. Recognition and diagnosis of abnormal neurologic factors causing organic impotence is essential in the proper management of patients with erectile dysfunction.

REFERENCES

1. Blaivas, J. G. A Critical Appraisal of Specific Diagnostic Techniques. In R. J. Krane and M. B. Siroky (eds.), Clinical Neuro-Urology. Boston: Little, Brown, 1979. Pp. 69–109.
2. Bohlen, J. G. Sleep erection monitoring in the evaluation of male erectile failure. Urol. Clin. North Am. 8:119, 1981.
3. Bors, E., and Blinn, K. A. Bulbocavernosus reflex. J. Urol. 82:128, 1959.
4. Bors, E., and Comarr, E. A. Neurologic disturbances of sexual function with special reference to 529 patients with spinal cord injury. Urol. Surv. 10:191, 1960.
5. Bradley, W. E. Urinary bladder dysfunction in multiple sclerosis. Neurology 28:52, 1978.
6. Chantraine, A., de Laval, J., and Onkelinx, A. Motor Conduction Velocity in the Internal Pudendal Nerves. In J. E. Desmedt (ed.), New Developments in Electromyography and Clinical Neurophysiology. Basel:Karger, 2:433, 1973.
7. Chippa, K. H., and Ropper, A. H. Evoked potentials in clinical medicine (part 1). N. Engl. J. Med. 306:1140, 1982.
8. Chippa, K. H., and Ropper, A. H. Evoked potentials in clinical medicine (part 2). N. Engl. J. Med. 306:(20) 1205, 1982.
9. Dick, H. C., et al. Pudendal sexual reflexes: Electrophysiologic investigations. Urology 3:376, 1974.
10. Duchen, L. W., et al. Pathology of autonomic neuropathy in diabetes mellitus. Ann. Intern. Med. 92:301, 1980.
11. Ellenberg, M. Impotence in diabetes: The neurologic factors. Ann. Intern. Med. 75:213, 1971.
12. Ertekin, C., and Reel, F. Bulbocavernosus reflex in normal men and in patients with neurogenic bladder and/or impotence. J. Neurol. Sci. 28:1, 1976.
13. Fisher, C., et al. The assessment of nocturnal REM erection in the differential diagnosis of sexual impotence. J. Sex Marital Ther. 1:277, 1975.
14. Goldstein, I. Tests for organic impotence. Fam. Pract. Recert. 4:67, 1982.
15. Goldstein, I., et al. Neurourologic abnormalities in multiple sclerosis. J. Urol. 128:541, 1982.
16. Haldeman, S., et al. Pudendal evoked responses. Arch. Neurol. 39:280, 1982.
17. Herbert, J. The role of the dorsal nerves of the penis in the sexual behavior of the male rhesus monkey. Physiol. Behav. 10:293, 1973.
18. Karacan, I., et al. Nocturnal penile tumescence and diagnosis in diabetic impotence. Am. J. Psychiatry 135:191, 1978.
19. Krane, R. J., and Siroky, M. B. Studies on sacral-evoked potentials. J. Urol. 124:872, 1980.
20. Krane, R. J., and Siroky, M. B. Neurophysiology of erection. Urol. Clin. North Am. 8:91, 1981.
21. Lapides, J., et al. Denervation supersensitivity as a test for neurogenic bladder. Surg. Gynecol. Obstet. 114:241, 1962.
22. MacLean, P. D., Denniston, R. H., and Dua, S.

Further studies on cerebral representation of penile erection: Cauda thalamus, midbrain, and pons. *J. Neurophysiol.* 26:273, 1963.

23. Michal, V., Kramer, R., and Pospichal, J. Femora-pudendal by-pass, internal iliac thromboendarterectomy, and direct arterial anastomosis to the cavernosus body in the treatment of erectile impotence. *Bull. Soc. Int. Chirc.* 4:343, 1974.

24. Osborne, D. Psychological aspects of male sexual dysfunction. *Urol. Clin. North Am.* 8:135, 1981.

25. Sax, D. S. The History and Examination in Neuro-Urology. In R. J. Krane and M. B. Siroky (eds.), *Clinical Neuro-Urology,* Boston:Little, Brown, 1979.

26. Semans, J. H., and Langworthy, O. R. Observations on the neurophysiology of sexual function in the male cat. *J. Urol.* 40:836, 1938.

27. Siroky, M. B., and Krane, R. J. Physiology of Male Sexual Function. In *Clinical Neuro-Urology.* R. J. Krane and M. B. Siroky (eds.), Boston:Little, Brown, 1979. Pp 45–62.

28. Siroky, M. B., Sax, D. S., and Krane, R. J. Sacral signal tracing: The electrophysiology of the bulbocavernosus reflex. *J. Urol.* 122:661, 1979.

29. Truex, R. C., and Carpenter, M. B. *Human Neuroanatomy* (5th ed.) Baltimore: Williams & Wilkins, 1964. P. 244.

30. Vacek, J., and Lachman, M. Bulbocavernosus reflex in diabetes with erective disorders. Clinical and electromyographic study. *Cas. Lek. Cesk.* 116:1015, 1977.

31. Weidman, C. L., and Northcutt, R. C. Endocrine aspects of impotence. *Urol. Clin. North Am.* 8:143, 1981.

17

Nocturnal Penile Tumescence

ALAN J. WEIN
KEITH VAN ARSDALEN
TERRENCE R. MALLOY

Nocturnal penile tumescence (NPT) was described first by Halverson in 1940 as a sleep phenomenon in infants [7], and was subsequently reported in adults by Ohlmeyer in 1944 in the German literature [21]. A major discovery of the 1950s was the description of rapid eye movement (REM) sleep by Aserinsky and Kleitman [1]. Further extensive observations on NPT as a naturally occurring phenomenon, monitoring techniques, and normal measurable parameters were more or less simultaneously published in the mid-1960s by two groups, Fisher and co-workers [4] and Karacan and co-workers [8–14], which have continued to make very significant contributions in this area. Karacan first suggested the use of NPT monitoring as a clinical tool for the diagnosis and prognosis of impotence in 1970 [11]. Since that time, much discussion has been engendered regarding the efficacy of NPT monitoring as a definitive diagnostic tool in the evaluation of erectile failure [3, 5, 15, 17, 19, 20, 25].

Penile erection for the purpose of sexual gratification is a complex, cerebrally initiated, neurovascular phenomenon that occurs within a certain hormonal milieu. The exact psychologic, neurologic, vascular, and hormonal mechanisms involved are unknown, as are their interrelationships in the cascade of events that culminate in tumescence and rigidity of the penis, which continues during a sexual act. Failure of any one, or a combination, of these factors can result in erectile dysfunction. Categorization of the etiology of such dysfunction is often difficult, even into the relatively broad categories of psychogenic or organic. There is no technique in common clinical use that reproducibly will stimulate a nonsexual erection. Such a phenomenon would indicate the organic factors involved in the erectile process were functioning sufficiently for at least the initiation of erection and thereby would permit categorization of the cause of repeated failure to achieve an erection (although not necessarily to maintain one during intercourse) as psychogenic in origin. Simply, *nocturnal penile tumescence* is the phenomenon of naturally occurring, nonsexual, sleep-related erections. As such, its occurrence in an individual with erectile failure would logically suggest a psychogenic origin for the sexual dysfunction.

As will become obvious, some facts and many opinions concerning NPT unfortunately, are not entirely clear-cut or consistent, and its role as a diagnostic tool in the evaluation of erectile failure is not yet agreed on by all workers in the field. This chapter will describe the basic characteristics of NPT in normal males and in various categories of patients, the place of NPT monitoring in the diagnostic evaluation of erectile failure, and the controversies that presently surround its use.

SLEEP CHARACTERISTICS AND NPT

REM sleep is characterized by rapid, jerky and binocularly symmetric eye movement associated with a stage-1 EEG pattern, dreaming, and increased dream recall [1]. Also noted is a diffuse activation of the autonomic nervous system and body activity, with increases in the respiratory and heart rates, overt body movements, bruxism, and changes in the galvanic skin response [9]. Such periods generally occur 4 or 5 times each night, with each episode lasting 20 to 25 minutes. There is a periodicity of approximately 90 minutes, such that total REM time accounts for 20 to 25 percent of the total sleep time [4]. The REM stage of sleep is considered distinct from the calmer nonREM (NREM) aspect of sleep, as well as the waking state, and it is found from birth to old age. It involves cortical as well as phylogenetically older centers of the brain. Its physiologic or psychologic role is not known, but its universality and regularity suggest that it must be of biologic importance. It seems probable that the physiologic alterations described antedate the psychologic process of dreaming [4].

The rhythmic nature of NPT was described before the REM sleep cycle, and the concurrence of these two events was subsequently documented. Fisher and co-workers [4] showed that erections were associated with 95 percent of 86 REM episodes monitored in 17 interns, residents, or hospital employees at their insitution [4]. They also noted the strik-

ing temporal relationship of the beginning and end of the erectile periods to the REM periods. Karacan, in his initial work, noted that 80 percent of REM sleep periods were accompanied by erection. Erections were noted also during NREM sleep in his study [9]. The characteristics of NPT are now well described. Four or five erections occur nightly, and the great majority of episodes have a significant portion occurring within REM sleep, although this is not exactly correlated. In fact, in patients deprived of REM sleep, the erectile episodes continue to occur and do so in the NREM periods, indicating some independence of these two phenomena [5]. Additional evidence of at least some degree of independence is that, while erections begin and end at approximately the same time as the REM periods, it is not unusual to find an erection to begin several minutes before the onset of a REM period. Less commonly, the onset of erection occurs several minutes after a REM period has begun. Full erection usually occurs for some time within a given REM period, but tumescence is never maximal all during a given episode. Detumescence usually begins before the end of REM and is generally not complete until after the end of REM. The NPT episode is therefore usually slightly longer than the REM period, lasting 25 to 35 minutes and accounting for approximately 20 to 40 percent of sleep time, depending on age [8, 12–14]. Total sleep time and total REM time decrease during the teen years and then stabilize. Total tumescence time is maximal during the teen years, and the total tumescence time as a percentage of total REM time is also maximal during this period. Each tends to decline gradually until the age of 70 to 80. The duration of each tumescence episode also is shortened gradually. Although this age-related decline is noted, it also should be noted that normal elderly males still have three or four erections per night, accounting for approximately 20 percent of sleep time [14].

As with REM sleep, the ubiquity of NPT would suggest some vital functional significance for the organism. The ontogenic trends in Karacan's data [14], with the highest amount of tumescence during the prepubertal and pubertal years and the decline thereafter, may indicate a possible relationship to psychosexual development. Fisher feels that NPT is a primary physiologic phenomenon that secondarily becomes associated with dreaming [5].

Of particular note are other lesser known characteristics of NPT, namely that recent sexual gratification does not affect the cycle of sleep-related erection, and that the dream content of REM-related erectile episodes is usually not erotic in nature [5]. "Morning erections" are simply erectile episodes similar to the nocturnal tumescence states, but are noted because awakening occurs while they are present. They therefore represent the last NPT episode of sleep. Karacan disproved the still commonly held belief that these erections are secondary to a distended bladder [11]. Subjects were awakened to void 2 hours before their usual awakening time. They then returned to sleep until their usual arising time. There was no difference in the occurrence of morning erections in this group than in controls. It should be emphasized that such erections are noted only if one awakens during their occurrence and has adequate awareness at that time. A person who awakens slowly may not notice such erections. Moreover, clinical correlation between history taking and NPT monitoring suggests that one's psyche may choose to ignore their presence.

In summary, NPT is a highly stable and prominent sleep phenomenon that has been described in normal males from birth to old age. A gradual decline in the quantity of tumescence episodes is noted over this period, but the phenomenon does not normally disappear. NPT occurs most commonly in association with REM sleep, and the normal frequency and duration of both generally have been well defined.

NPT IN THE DIAGNOSTIC
EVALUATION OF ERECTILE FAILURE

The problem of impotence always has been a difficult one for the patient and clinician. It is one of the few medical problems in which the diagnosis is made by the patient before seeing the physician. However, there is no practical direct way to evaluate erectile capacity in the situation in which the patient is symptomatic, and there are no direct tests available to identify all possible deficits in the erectile cascade. Medical and surgical diseases may be identified by the history, physical examination, and laboratory studies, but whether they are truly etiologic or simply coexist with erectile failure often is not known. Likewise, significant psychopathology may be identified, but it is difficult directly to prove a cause-and-effect relationship. The traditional approach to the differential diagnosis of impotence as organic or psychogenic has been based on such associations. A patient with no demonstrable neurologic, vascular, hormonal, or end-organ abnormality is felt to have psychogenic impotence. Psychogenicity often is diagnosed in this fashion, even in the absence of positive psychogenic factors in the history. This approach undoubtedly accounts for the overestimate, found predominantly in the older literature, that as many as 90 percent of cases of secondary impotence are psychogenic in origin. Conversely, if an organic abnormality that has been associated with impotence is identified, then the diagnosis of organic impotence on this basis often has been made without thoroughly excluding other potential organic factors and etiologic or associated psychologic factors as well.

Proper classification of the etiology of erectile failure is necessary for very practical reasons. It is important to try to prevent unnecessary reconstructive or prosthetic surgery if a psychologic remedy is possible, and to prevent unproductive and expensive psychotherapy and delay in proper treatment for the organic group. In our initial evaluation, the chief complaint is clarified to allow us to be sure we are dealing with a purely erectile problem. The history and physical examination are completed and laboratory tests obtained, including urinalysis, complete blood count, SMA-12 (serum electrolytes, liver enzymes, creatinine, BUN), testosterone and prolactin levels. A Minnesota Multiphasic Personality Inventory (MMPI) is then given and, prior to leaving, the patient is given educational material to review before his return appointment. In the interim, the MMPI is scored, and the results of other tests obtained. A tentative classification is formulated. The unquestionably psychogenic patient (i.e., classic history of nondisease- or trauma-related sudden onset and/or selective occurrence and/or normal nonsexual erections with a normal examination and laboratory values) is referred to a sexual therapist for further evaulation. The therapist may then make a decision as to the possible therapeutic value of NPT monitoring. Patients with actual or suspected endocrine disease or deficiency are evaluated further for this and treated without further other evaluation. In all other patients, however, we consider NPT monitoring to be the single most valuable additional diagnostic adjunct available, with an approximately 80 to 85 percent efficiency. The basic assumption is that NPT monitoring provides a valid and reliable index of the potential awake erectile capacity of the individual, because the physiology of erection does not change in proportion to the level of consciousness. The sleep state is thought to bypass psychic conflict, so patients with psychogenic impotence and intact physiology have normal nocturnal erections, whereas patients with organic impotence have persistently impaired physiologic mechanisms and therefore absent or abnormal NPT [5]. Karacan first discussed the use of NPT monitoring for categorization therapy and prognosis in impotent diabetic patients [11]. He subsequently recommended that NPT evaluation precede any extensive or expensive treatment for impotence whether or not a medical, surgical, or psychologic etiology was initially suspected. Fisher and co-workers, with detailed case presentations, came essentially to the same conclusions and noted that a most important distinction was the discrepancy between NPT status and performance in a sexual situation in patients with psychogenic impotence and the close correspondence of the characteristics of sleep erections with those in the awake state in patients with organic impotence [5].

A major problem in the use of NPT monitoring in the differential diagnosis of im-

potence was recognized by Schiavi [22], who noted that, although much work had been done in defining NPT values for normal individuals, remarkably little information was available on the patterns of nocturnal erection in men with either psychogenic or various types of organic impotence. The problem, as previously noted, is that the precise etiologic mechanisms of both psychogenic and organic impotence are not known. Therefore, the value of NPT monitoring cannot be tested exactly against a known standard. Rather, the proof of the validity of NPT monitoring is indirect and consists of the correlation of NPT characteristics in groups defined as normal or in groups having either a very high probability of organic etiology or a very high probability of psychogenic etiology. Wasserman and co-workers state that the basic assumption that NPT monitoring can distinguish the two categories of impotence has never been validated in a large group of patients shown to be psychogenically or organically impotent independent of the NPT measurements themselves [25]. Marshall and co-workers also challenged this basic assumption on the same grounds and further noted, as others have recognized, that it is theoretically possible that nocturnal and sexual erections do *not* occur by the same mechanism and are not under the same controls [19, 20]. It therefore would be possible for the NPT mechanism to be intact while the sexual mechanism is impaired, and if that were so, a normal NPT would not necessarily indicate psychogenic pathology.

Moreover, the basic question of whether (and, if so, how much) purely psychologic factors can inhibit NPT has never been answered completely. Karacan originally investigated the relationship of dream anxiety to the erection cycle and found a significant difference between the number of full as compared to partial or no erections and the dream content as analyzed by Gottschalk's anxiety score [9]. REM periods having dreams with a high anxiety content showed poor or absent erectile activity. Fisher mentioned a similar phenomenon in his original work [4]. Abnormal findings due to the new and unfamiliar conditions of the first night of testing in the sleep laboratory were first noted by Jovanovich (cited by Wasserman [25]) and are now well recognized. This is further evidence of a potential psychologic inhibitory effect on nocturnal penile tumescence, because normal recordings are usually found on subsequent nights after a patient without significant organic disease adjusts to these surroundings. One can speculate that this first-night effect may not be limited to the first night in some individuals. Jovanovich (cited by Fisher [6]) also has reported abnormal NPT data in patients judged to have psychogenic impotence.

Although the extent of the psychologic influences on NPT has not been completely resolved, two points made by Kaya and co-workers [17] are important. First, in their extensive experience in over 15 years, they have yet to observe a normal subject without a sexual dysfunction or a sleep disturbance who did not show a normal NPT. Second, although negative psychologic factors may cause NPT fluctuation, they do not appear to inhibit erections, if still a physiologic possibility, over an entire night or a series of nights. Nevertheless, Karacan [15] recognizes, as does Fisher [6], a group of important patients, comprising 15 to 20 percent of all those tested, who have abnormal NPT but no recognizable organic pathology. Karacan's group seems to feel it most likely that there are patients with undetected organic pathology, while Fisher and co-workers feel that some of these do in fact represent patients with psychogenic impotence. Recently, Schmidt and Wise [23] supported the possibility of at least one type of heretofore unrecognized pathology with their description of some impotent patients of what may be a central nervous system syndrome consisting of impaired penile tumescence with other sleep abnormalities, including frequent apnea and hyperventilation with decreased oxygen saturation, myoclonic jerks, and bradycardia.

In summary, the measurement of NPT for the evaulation of impotence is based on several clinically relevant and sound assumptions, which are intellectually logical but which have not really been proved by a truly scientific method. Exceptions to the "rules" do exist, and, in fact, in 15 to 20 percent of patients, abnormal NPT is noted without an identifiable organic etiology. NPT monitoring, however, provides objective evidence for accurate presumptive categorization in the remaining 80 to 85 percent of patients. Impotent patients with NPT characteristics within the range of normal have a very high probability of a psychogenic etiology. Impotent patients with no NPT activity or markedly diminished activity have a very high probability of an organic etiology.

TECHNIQUES OF NPT MONITORING

Complete sleep monitoring obviously is performed best in a formal sleep laboratory, but any controlled environment can suffice simply for the detection of the NPT phenomenon. At-home monitoring with a portable device also has been advocated. In any case, alcoholic beverages, unnecessary drugs, and distractions must be avoided. Many parameters may be monitored simultaneously with penile circumference. These include the electroencephalogram (EEG), the electrooculogram (EOG), and electromyogram (EMG) from the bulbocavernosus, ischiocavernosus, or the external anal sphincter muscle, respiratory rate, systemic and penile blood pressure, penile blood flow, and oxygen saturation [16]. For the most thorough clinical evaluation, we have found simultaneous monitoring of the EEG and EOG (both eyes) to be helpful. Although these are not necessary in the vast majority of cases, their measurement ensures that NPT occurs or is absent in a setting of normal sleep, and that sleep as a whole is not disturbed. The rate of change of the penile parameters during the development and disappearance of any erectile activity would intuitively seem to be important, but accepted guidelines and specific abnormal patterns associated with particular pathologic conditions have yet to be defined.

Changes in penile circumference are measured by two loop strain gauges that are positioned around the penis — one just behind the corona and one at the base. Each must be com-

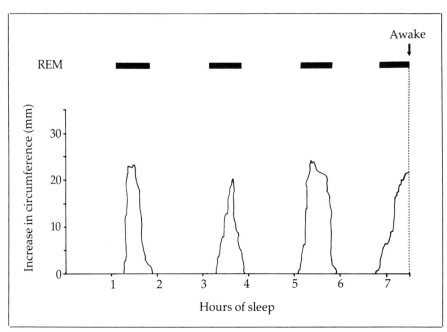

Figure 17-1. Condensed NPT tracing showing concurrent REM sleep periods. Patient is a 46-year-old man with psychogenic impotence. Note that "morning erection" is REM-associated and represents the last NPT episode before arising.

fortable enough so as not to inhibit sleep or erection, and each must remain in place all night to provide continuous monitoring. Many devices have been described for measuring changes in penile circumference, but the thin, mercury-filled silicone tubing loop, as perfected by Karacan [10], has been used most extensively. The loop forms one limb of a Wheatstone bridge, in such a way that stretching causes the mercury column inside to be narrowed and the electrical resistance thereby increased. Very small variations can be amplified and recorded. It is important to tape the leads securely to the patient to prevent movement artifacts once the guages are in place. Initially, Karacan [10] monitored only the change behind the penile glans and Fisher [4] monitored this only at the base. Each now uses the two-gauge technique, but their "normal" data are derived from comparisons made according to their original study locations.

Monitoring takes place for one to three nights. The first night serves as a period of adjustment. The first-night effect has been mentioned previously and various sleep and NPT patterns may be atypical. Obviously, if all parameters are normal on the first night, it is not necessary to go beyond this. The basic NPT data generally are collected for a given

patient on the second night. Episodes are characterized as "full" or "partial" erections, and the maximum circumference change for the patient is determined. A normal study shows 3 to 5 erectile episodes per night; the duration of each episode is 10 to 25 minutes; and expansion varies from 15 to 30 mm (Fig. 17-1). "Normal" represents a tip increase of 16 to 20 mm for Karacan [16] and for Fisher, a base increase of 24 mm [6]. During the third night, data from the previous night are used to define the best time for direct observation and for awakening the patient, that is, during a maximal episode of expansion. At that time, the erection may be photographed, an estimate of the degree of the erection is made and compared to an idealized full erection, and an estimate of the rigidity as sufficient or not for vaginal penetration is made by the patient and an observer. The observer, an essential part of the entire procedure, checks for sources of error and artifact within the system, takes part in the estimation of the erections as noted above, and compares his estimation with that of the patient. Characteristically, patients with organic impotence will estimate accurately the degree of erection that occurs (compared to an idealized 100%) and report that this degree is similar to what they experience in a sexual situation. Patients with psychogenic impotence who achieve normal erections during sleep will characteristically state that these erections, although they may approach an idealized normal, are greatly in excess of those achieved in a sexual situation. They may also report that, even though they themselves have noted some nonsexual erectile activity in the past, the erections experienced during the testing sequence are superior to the nonsexual erections noted outside of the testing situation.

One significant potential source of error that makes the presence of an observer desirable is the phenomenon of significant expansion without rigidity sufficient to effect vaginal penetration. Although this phenomenon was mentioned early by both the Fisher [5] and Karacan groups [17], it received surprisingly little attention in the urology literature until recently. Karacan noted that in 90 percent of his patients a penile circumference increase of 16 to 20 mm produced rigidity sufficient for penetration, but that in 10 percent these values may not indicate sufficient penile rigidity for vaginal penetration [16]. We found that 17 percent of a consecutively studied group of 134 impotent patients exhibited episodes of penile expansion within the range of normal that proved, on examination, to be insufficient for penetration [26]. Base expansion in this group varied from 15 to 30 mm, whereas coronal expansion varied from 10 to 28 mm. Although the number of episodes of expansion per night was generally less than in the normal group, the number of episodes varied from 1 to 5, and the duration of many of these was well within the range of normal. Karacan has developed a device to measure buckling pressure and has found that at less than 60 mm Hg buckling pressure the penis is not adequate for penetration. Between 60 to 100 mm Hg, penetration ability is questionable, and at greater than 100 mm buckling pressure the penis is definitely of sufficient

Table 17-1. Comparative value of NPT monitoring in different settings

Setting	1	2	3	4	5
Sleep laboratory	+	+	+	+	+
Observer and controlled environment	+	+	+	−	−
Home	+	−	±	−	−

Key: 1 = accurate and reproducible recording, assuming equipment intact and properly fitted and no patient malingering; 2 = estimate of rigidity; 3 = estimate of maximum episode to preimpotence erection and idealized normal; 4 = data to evaluate sleep characteristics; 5 = data to further research NPT characteristics.

rigidity [16]. Wabrak also advises the use of a "rigidometer" and suggests that the future role of NPT monitoring may be in deciding when to check rigidity measurements [24]. Because no standard device is accepted or available at this time, direct observation and palpation by an examiner during a maximal episode of expansion is essential. It is interesting to speculate on possible etiologies of this phenomenon of expansion without rigidity. In our series of 23 such patients, although there were etiologic or situational organic associations implied for 16, four patients had absolutely no detectable psychologic, organic, or sleep abnormality, whereas three had only disturbed REM sleep and/or significant anxiety.

Although the advantages and disadvantages of each setting for NPT monitoring are obvious (Table 17-1), each clinician must decide which of the available parameters he is most interested in and which method is most appropriate and practical for his practice situation. The use of a portable home unit without an independent observer may be very useful and cost-efficient in some situations [18], especially if the NPT pattern is perfectly normal or totally absent and the resultant inference from the study is perfectly compatible with the extra-NPT impression of the patient's erectile failure. The use of a device that measures breaking strength alone (the "postage stamp" technique [2] or a variant thereof) would seem still simpler and perhaps useful in some situations, but has obvious potential drawbacks.

CONCLUSIONS

The characteristics of REM sleep and NPT are now well recognized. The duration and characteristics of each phenomenon varies somewhat with age, but their occurrence seems to span the life of the normal individual, implying a basic physiologic or psychologic significance that is not presently understood. The proper assessment of a patient into a category of psychogenic or organic impotence is essential. The use of observer-related NPT monitoring in the evaluation and prognosis of erectile failure has proved to be a useful clinical tool for categorization of patients, but only when reviewed in the context of and correlated with the entire history, physical examination, and laboratory findings. In this fashion, the great majority of patients may be assessed as having a high probability of one form of impotence or the other. The assumptions on which NPT monitoring are based have been challenged, as the proof of these is largely indirect and a still significant number of patients (15–20%) cannot be adequately classified by this means. This probably represents our own limitations in totally understanding the psychophysiologic mechanisms of erection.

The techniques of monitoring have been described. Direct observer and patient observation are essential to fully evaluate rigidity and adequacy for vaginal penetration, regardless of the absolute normal values. In addition to its use as a diagnostic tool, other potential benefits of NPT monitoring include (1) showing the psychogenically impotent patient that he can in fact get an erection and thereby improve body image, (2) reassuring the organically impotent patient that his impotence is not in fact psychogenic, and (3) reassuring the physician of the patient's motivation to follow recommendations and continue a logical search for an etiology and proper treatment. As yet unresolved and important questions include (1) the effects of various types of psychopathology on NPT and the mechanism(s) by which these occur, (2) the effects of various medications on NPT, and (3) the effects, if any, of disuse and their reversibility.

REFERENCES

1. Aserinsky, E., and Kleitman, N. Regularly occurring periods of eye motility and concomitant phenomena during sleep. *Science* 188:273, 1953.
2. Barry, J. M., Blank, B., and Boileau, M. Nocturnal penile tumescence monitoring with stamps. *Urology* 15:171, 1980.
3. Casey, W. C. Phallography: Techniques and results of nocturnal tumescence monitoring. *J. Urol.* 122:752, 1979.
4. Fisher, C., Gross, J., and Zuch, J. Cycle of penile erection synchronous with dreaming (REM) sleep. *Arch. Gen. Psychiatry* 12:29, 1965.
5. Fisher, C., et al. The assessment of nocturnal REM erection in the differential diagnosis of sexual impotence. *J. Sex Marital Ther.* 1:277, 1975.
6. Fisher, C., et al. Evaluation of nocturnal penile tumescence in the differential diagnosis of sexual impotence. *Arch. Gen. Psychiatry* 36:431, 1979.
7. Halverson, H. M. Genital and sphincter behavior of the male infant. *J. Genet. Psychol.* 56:95, 1940.
8. Kahn, E., and Fisher, C. REM sleep and sexuality in the aged. *J. Geriatr. Psychiatry* 2:181, 1969.
9. Karacan, I., et al. Erection cycle during sleep in relation to dream anxiety. *Arch. Gen. Psychiatry* 15:183, 1966.
10. Karacan, I. A simple and inexpensive transducer for quantitative measurements of penile erection during sleep. *Behav. Res. Meth. Instru.* 1:251, 1969.
11. Karacan, I. Clinical value of nocturnal erections in the prognosis and diagnosis of impotence. *Med. Asp. Human Sex.* 4:27, 1970.
12. Karacan, I., Hursch, C. J., and Williams, R. L. Some characteristics of nocturnal penile tumescence in elderly males. *J. Gerontol.* 27:39, 1972.
13. Karacan, I., et al. Some characteristics of nocturnal penile tumescence in young adults. *Arch. Gen. Psychiatry* 26:351, 1972.
14. Karacan, I., et al. Sleep-related penile tumescence as a function of age. *Am. J. Psychiatry* 132:931, 1975.
15. Karacan, I. Impotence: psyche vs. soma. *Medical World News* 17:28, 1976.
16. Karacan, I., Salis, P. J., and Williams, R. L. The Role of the Sleep Laboratory in the Diagnosis and Treatment of Impotence. In *Sleep Disorders: Diagnosis and Treatment*. R. L. Williams, I. Karacan, and S. H. Frazier (eds.), New York: Wiley, 1978.

17. Kaya, N., Moore, C., and Karacan, I. Nocturnal penile tumescence and its role in impotence. *Psychiatr. Ann.* 9:426, 1979.

18. Kenepp, D., and Gonick, P. Home monitoring of penile tumescence for erectile dysfunction. *Urology* 14:261, 1979.

19. Marshall, P., Morales, A., and Surridge, D. Unreliability of nocturnal penile tumescence recording and MMPI profiles in assessment of impotence. *Urology* 17:163, 1981.

20. Marshall, P., Morales, A., and Surridge, D. Diagnostic insignificance of penile erections during sleep. *Urology* 20:1, 1982.

21. Ohlmeyer, P., Brilmayer, H., and Hullstrung, H. Periodische Vorgäuge in Schlaf. *Pfluegers Arch.* 248:559, 1944.

22. Schiavi, R. L. Sex therapy and psychophysiological research. *Am. J. Psychiatry* 133:562, 1976.

23. Schmidt, H. S., and Wise, H. A. Significance of impaired penile tumescence and associated polysomnographic abnormalities in the impotent patient. *J. Urol.* 126:348, 1981.

24. Wabrak, A. J. Penile Rigidity: Concepts and Correlations. Presented at Fifth World Congress of Sexology, June 23, 1981.

25. Wasserman, M. D., et al. Theoretical and technical problems in the measurement of nocturnal penile tumescence for the differential diagnosis of impotence. *Psychosom. Med.* 42:575, 1980.

26. Wein, A. J., et al. Expansion without significant rigidity during nocturnal penile tumescence testing: A potential source of misinterpretation. *J. Urol.* 126:343, 1981.

18

Diagnostic Approach to the Impotent Patient

ROBERT J. KRANE
MIKE B. SIROKY

The number of effective therapeutic modalities for erectile dysfunction has continued to increase in recent years. This has changed the diagnostic approach to the impotent patient, which previously was often of the nihilistic or the "shotgun" variety. The availability of more sophisticated diagnostic techniques (sacral latency, penile blood pressure, angiography) as well as therapies (behavior modification, penile prostheses, and penile revascularization) has mandated a well-planned diagnostic approach that is intended (1) to provide a probable diagnosis, (2) to enable one to select the appropriate therapeutic options, and (3) to provide a factual basis for counseling the patient.

Before we describe specific diagnostic techniques, it seems reasonable to discuss the varied reasons that cause patients to seek medical attention for erectile dysfunction, as well as some of the preconceptions and prejudices that they bring to the initial office visit. During the past 3 years, we have seen approximately 450 patients with erectile dysfunction at our clinic. Most come with varying amounts of information as well as misinformation concerning impotence and its treatment.

These preconceived ideas usually are associated with (1) a type of therapy (e.g., "I'm sure a shot of male hormone will take care of the problem," or "I have come to see you about implanting one of these new penile devices."); or (2) an etiologic diagnosis (e.g., "I'm sure I don't have any psychologic problems causing this."). Many patients come with very little knowledge of the diagnostic and therapeutic capabilities now available in evaluating and treating impotence. Thus, it is important to view the initial visit as a diagnostic, as well as a teaching, situation. The physician should explain fully to the patient the diagnostic approaches that are available and, probably more important, the therapeutic options that exist.

This type of approach may impact strongly on the ultimate diagnostic and therapeutic regimen. As an example, after a discussion of surgical, hormonal, and psychologic therapy, the patient may realize that one or more of these options is not suitable for him. The subsequent diagnostic plan should take this decision into account.

It is important to remember that some patients come not for therapy but merely for information regarding the etiology of the problem. For instance, patients receiving psychologic therapy without much response may wish to rule out organic disease. Similarly, other patients are interested in identifying an organic etiology for psychosocial reasons. The latter type of patient is often past middle age and has had a long and stable marriage. His wife may have interpreted his loss of erectile function as a loss of affection toward her, and this may have led to marital problems. Identifying an underlying organic problem often suffices because the sexual dysfunction itself was not particularly disturbing to such a couple.

It cannot be overemphasized that an open discussion of the diagnostic and therapeutic options should be undertaken during the initial interview, rather than at a later date. Patients who feel negative about surgery or who would not consider psychologic therapy can have a diagnostic approach tailored for their situation.

We shall now turn to a brief description of our diagnostic approach to the patient with erectile dysfunction. This begins with history taking and physical examination, as outlined in Chapter 12. Clues relating to hormonal, neurologic, vascular, or psychologic disease are sought, and the evaluation proceeds in accordance with those findings.

Screening Tests

As initial screening for organic impotence, all of our patients undergo a hormone profile and nocturnal penile tumescence (NPT) monitoring. The purpose of hormone screening is to detect hypogonadism and hyperprolactinemia. Although these conditions are uncommon in our experience, we feel that hormone screening is worthwhile because hormonal imbalance, when present, is often occult, and, when diagnosed, is easily treated. For these reasons, we recommend serum testosterone (T), luteinizing hormone (LH), and prolactin determinations (PRL) as adequate

screening for hormone imbalance. Most patients with decreased T levels in the initial sample will be found to have normal T levels when repeat samples are drawn in the morning (or on tripooled samples). If these latter tests are abnormal, a full endocrine evaluation is warranted. In our experience, only about 15 percent of patients with initially decreased serum T are found to require full endocrinologic evaluation by this approach. On the other hand, we feel it is important to document androgen deficiency completely before instituting replacement therapy, because one is embarking on a long-term course of therapy that is not without risk.

The NPT examination is an excellent means of differentiating organic from psychogenic impotence, although it is not without false-positives and false-negatives. Its accuracy is increased if monitoring is carried out for two or three nights. This need not be performed in a sleep laboratory and is quite effectively accomplished with a portable unit used in the patient's home. A false-positive tracing (normal-appearing erections in the presence of organic impotence) may occur if the patient's penis increases in circumference but does not attain sufficient rigidity for intercourse. A false-negative tracing (absent or poor erections in the presence of psychogenic impotence) may occur if the patient does not fall asleep, if there is an equipment failure, or if, as in some cases, there is severe psychologic disturbance.

Nevertheless, the NPT examination remains an excellent source of corroborating information. For example, a patient with a history of partial erections may show low-amplitude, poorly sustained circumferential change on NPT, and thus the diagnosis of vasculogenic impotence is corroborated. Conversely, the same patient may show excellent, well-sustained erectile activity, leading one to suspect psychogenic impotence. In any case, the NPT examination should not be considered an absolute discriminant between psychogenic and organic impotence in and of itself, but it is probably the best means of corroborating the findings of other examinations.

Specific Tests

In our experience, sophisticated neurologic testing such as the evoked potential studies described in Chapter 16 have not been of particular value in diagnosing occult neurologic lesions causing impotence. Every patient with an abnormal evoked potential study (genitocerebral or sacral) was suspected on other grounds to have a neurologic lesion. Evoked potential studies are useful, however, even in the presence of known neurologic disease as a specific assessment of the pudendal sensory and motor pathways. For example, the patient with multiple sclerosis, minimal neurologic disability, and erectile dysfunction would be an excellent candidate for an evoked potential study.

In contrast, testing for penile vascular insufficiency has proved to be extremely useful both in corroborating suspected disease and in detecting occult disease. In our experience, approximately 45 percent of patients thought to have organic impotence have been found to have abnormally low penile blood pressure indices. This proportion can be increased to almost 60 percent by performing pelvic and lower extremity exercise to bring out cases of marginally decreased blood flow. Measurement of penile temperature may be used to corroborate Doppler findings.

There is little question that abnormal vascular findings are quite common in patients thought to have organic impotence (e.g., flat NPT tracing). The problem remains, however, of demonstrating a cause-and-effect relationship between the vascular findings and the erectile dysfunction. In our view, such a relationship may be presumed to exist if one or both of the following obtain: (1) the history contains features typical of a vasculogenic etiology (e.g., slow onset, loss of erection during intercourse, preservation of ejaculation) or (2) therapeutic maneuvers that increase penile blood flow (e.g., vasodilator drugs, angiodilatation, penile revascularization) result in restoration or improvement in erectile function.

Finally, we need to address the question of arteriography and its role in the evaluation of the impotent patient. Certainly, patients with impotence who are undergoing femoral arteriograms should have a simultaneous selective study of the hypogastric and pudendal vasculature. This will add little to the morbidity of the procedure and will yield useful information to the vascular surgeon in planning any necessary surgery. The indications for arteriography are not clear in the patient with abnormal penile Doppler studies but no lower extremity symptoms. It is our feeling that properly performed Doppler studies and NPT examinations are sufficient to permit diagnosis of vasculogenic impotence. Pudendal arteriography therefore should be reserved for patients in whom penile revascularization is being considered.

Almost all of our patients obtain an evaluation interview by a sex therapist-psychologist. In many cases, considerable amounts of data are generated by these interviews and impact significantly on subsequent therapy. Even in cases of organic impotence, it is useful to explore a couple's attitude toward penile prosthesis. Finally, one must remember that, in our present state of knowledge, a considerable number of patients cannot be neatly categorized as either organic or psychogenic. Indeed, in many cases, both etiologies are pertinent to the patient's erectile dysfunction. In such a situation, it is our feeling and practice to recommend a course of behavior therapy prior to considering more irreversible modes of treatment. This may be considered a therapeutic trial, because a positive response to sex therapy is characteristic of psychogenic impotence. In cases that do not respond, one feels much less reluctant to consider surgical intervention.

In summary, our diagnostic approach is heavily influenced by our therapeutic options. The various methods of treatment are discussed quite early in the evaluation process. Most patients obtain NPT and hormone profiles for screening, as well as penile Doppler studies and psychologic interviews for the reasons outlined above. Evoked potential studies and arteriography are reserved for specific cases, as was previously discussed. As therapy is refined in the future (e.g., penile revascularization), a concomitant adjustment in diagnostic approach will be necessitated.

19

Behavioral Treatments of Erectile Insufficiency

ALMA DELL SMITH
STEVEN C. FISCHER

Prior to the work of Masters and Johnson, the usual treatment of sexual dysfunction was some form of psychoanalytically oriented psychotherapy. The prevailing view was that treatment of the sexual dysfunction itself was not appropriate. Consequently, patients would be involved in psychotherapy that would not address directly problems of sexual functioning. The behavioral revolution in psychotherapy that began in the early 1960s, however, amply demonstrated that more direct therapies centered primarily in the here-and-now were extremely effective. Wolpe [10] and Masters and Johnson [7] have shown that direct symptomatic treatment could be used to ameliorate sexual dysfunctions. It has been further demonstrated that symptom substitution has not occurred when behavior therapy has been utilized [11]. This chapter will describe behavioral treatment for erectile insufficiency and problems of premature ejaculation. The latter is included because it can be a precursor to erectile insufficiency.

In planning psychologic treatment for the sexually dissatisfied individual, it is essential to assess all aspects that contribute to, and are functionally related to, the problem. These may be seen as problems of information, of anxiety, of skill or technique, and of marital relationship. All of these problems are interrelated and often must be addressed simultaneously. Occasionally, but probably infrequently, providing information is sufficient to reduce or eliminate sexual dysfunction. Unfortunately, information is often poor or insufficient because of the patient's or physician's anxiety. For example, telling people to "relax" or "go slower" is unlikely to help patients and may increase their frustration because they try and fail. Often, persons with sexual problems feel that because the initial advice was not helpful, nothing further can be done. It would be far more helpful to *teach* patients how to relax and how to go slower. It would be even more helpful to structure treatment in a manner that forestalls "failure" by prescribing specific exercises to enhance technique, and that provides assistance for problems in treatment as they arise. The therapist should be prepared to use a combination of psychotherapeutic techniques; the usual goals of the sex therapy include:

1. Correcting myths and misinformation by providing information
2. Ensuring that the patient receives a high level of physical and psychologic stimulation by increasing a couple's sexual repertoire and communication about sexual matters
3. Eliminating anxiety and performance demands that may interfere with erection.

Addressing hostility, resentments, and conflicts in the marital relationship, or treatment of other nonsexual problems may have to precede effective use of sex therapy techniques, but such methods are beyond the scope of this chapter.

ESTABLISHING MUTUAL RESPONSIBILITY

A preliminary stage of all sex therapy treatments is the establishment of the understanding by both parties that sexual dysfunctions are shared problems and that the couple has a mutual responsibility for future change. In most cases, one member of the couple is identified as dysfunctional, and expectations are that treatment will be directed to that person. Yet sexual dissatisfaction or dysfunction affects both partners. For instance, the woman's fear of having painful intercourse due to insufficient lubrication may inhibit her responsiveness to the man, who then perceives her as rejecting, which increases his anxiety and leads to increasing difficulty with erections. What may have started as one partner's problem, soon becomes a mutual problem, the solution to which rests with both partners. Circumventing the issue of blame is more likely to foster a spirit of cooperation. Both must realize that each has something to gain from therapy. In general, and with sex in particular, one receives what one gives. Sex therapists view the couple's sexual relationship as the identified problem. Consequently, both sexual partners usually are seen together in sex therapy. In-

deed, treatment-outcome studies [1] have shown that involvement of a cooperative spouse in treatment has been associated with a more positive outcome. However, some treatment successes have been reported for persons without partners or whose partners refuse to participate in treatment [8].

TREATING PROBLEMS OF INFORMATION

When the onset of the sexual problem has been acute, one of the earliest and easiest interventions that can be made by the sex therapist, urologist, or primary physician is providing the client with basic information about human sexual anatomy and functioning, the possible causes of his particular problem, and correcting misinformation and myths about sex. Such information impacts on anxiety levels as well as on sexual skills and affects the client's cognitive set regarding sexuality. An example of misinformation creating unrealistic expectations and anxiety is the belief held by some men that any male should be able to have an erection under any circumstances with any woman. A most common misconception is that size of erection determines female satisfaction. Another example is the belief that simultaneous orgasm is essential to one's being considered a good lover. Not meeting his own criteria of adequacy, the male may begin to perceive himself as a failure. This perception then begins the cycle of evaluation, anxiety, and further decreases in arousal.

Misinformation and lack of information accrue from folklore, cultural stereotypes, sexual role stereotypes, religious prohibitions, pornographic reading material, and a myriad of other sources. Through discussions, provision of alternative material, and most important, through individualized, structured experiences, such misinformation can be corrected, and the individual male can discover what is true for him, and deemphasize comparisons.

Informing the male about the four stages of male sexual arousal identified by Masters and Johnson [6] (excitement, plateau, orgasm, and resolution), and what occurs in each phase may also reduce unrealistic expectations he may have about performance. For instance, the excitement phase depends on one's receiving an adequate amount of appropriate stimulation with no inhibiting factors present. For some men, "adequate stimulation" may be simply the thought of their partner's body. For others, or for the same man at a different time, adequate stimulation may necessitate manual or oral direct stimulation plus fantasy. The plateau stage of arousal also differs from one person to another, or from one time to another, and differs for men and women. Average time of thrusting to orgasm is about 2 minutes for men. Most women require much longer to reach orgasm with thrusting, or may not have orgasms with intercourse at all [6]. Information about differences in the resolution phase has also proved important in some instances. Some woman have little or no resolution phase and can have repeated orgasms. Depending on his age, state of health, level of fatigue, and the sexual situation, the male's resolution time varies widely, from 30 minutes to several hours.

Basic information about sexual functioning seems especially important for the young, inexperienced man and for the aging man. The former have had less experience with which to correct myths learned "on the street," whereas the latter may be judging their current sexual functioning by comparing it to their functioning while in their youth. Information about changes in physiologic function due to age are especially appropriate for older men, who may interpret normal changes as pathologic. It has been shown that older men require increased amounts of stimulation during the excitement phase to become aroused. Moreover, the amount of erection may be reduced, even though it may still be adequate for intercourse. Frequently, older males may lose the erection during foreplay, yet regain it if stimulated again sufficiently. Finally, the older male may need a longer resolution phase before again attempting intercourse [3]. One can note that the common purpose of providing information is to provide more realistic expectations for the man who is con-

cerned about his performance.

The male may also need extensive information about female sexual functioning, so that he may have a more accurate understanding of his partner's needs and be better able to please her. Anatomy books and pictures currently available for this purpose may be one, nonthreatening way to convey such information. Many males do not know the exact location of the clitoris and do not know the most effective type of stimulation to the clitoris. Techniques of foreplay are often learned through trial and error, with little specific feedback from an equally naive partner. Such learning may be quite inhibited by anxiety in early years, or effectiveness of technique may differ from woman to woman. If the male is comfortable with looking at pictures, visual and tactile exploration of his partner's body, and feedback from her will facilitate learning her specific needs better. As with basic anatomy, information about sexual technique may be given by the therapist through books, films, or discussion. Although such information may be necessary initially, however, it usually is not sufficient for complete treatment and should be followed up with the exercises described later in this chapter.

Another source of concern of many men complaining of sexual dysfunction is the "cause" of their problem. They wonder repeatedly if they are not organically impaired or wonder who is at fault. Information on the role of performance anxiety, spectatoring (mentally watching oneself), frequent evaluation thoughts, the role of anxiety about partner satisfaction, birth control, or other anxieties, and on the role of miscommunication may be needed to allow him to focus on psychologic factors. Information regarding statistics, of psychogenic, organic, and combined factors, or why the therapist has concluded that the etiology is largely psychologic enlists the cooperation of the male in the treatment. In this vein, it is also helpful to inform the couple of the nature of the treatment, and what is to be expected of them (e.g., home practice, reading).

In addition to altering expectations, information is intended to alter the couple's cognitive set regarding the goals of sexuality. Information is given for the purpose of reducing anxiety and for enhancing enjoyment, not to reinforce the patient's notion that performance is what counts. This theme of enjoyment, not performance, should be present throughout all discussions and home practice.

TREATING PROBLEMS OF ANXIETY

The second major area of therapy intervention is treating problems of anxiety and distraction. Sexual arousal occurs naturally, assuming that a person is receiving adequate physical and psychologic sexual stimulation and it is not blocked in some fashion, either anatomically or by inhibiting thoughts and anxiety. Although all factors contributing to sexual arousability are unknown, in general, sexual arousal depends on discharges of the autonomic nervous system. Erection in the male and vaginal engorgement in the female are primarily parasympathetic functions [5]. Discharges of the sympathetic division of the autonomic nervous system caused by anxiety, irritation, conflict, or hostility tend to inhibit arousal. Similarly, much of sexual stimulation is psychologic, i.e., the perception of sexual events, fantasies, or attention to particularly arousing touch; and attentional focus directed toward guilt, tension, or ultimate performance goals, rather than to immediate pleasurable sensations, will block positive psychologic stimuli. Treatment of these two inhibitions, anxiety and distraction, involves devising specific instructions and exercises for the couple to allow them increasing experiences of relaxation and pleasure associated with sexuality.

Treatment development depends on the specific anxieties of a given couple. Anxiety may be provoked by early parental or social prohibitions against certain activities such as masturbation or oral sex, by residuals of previous traumatic experiences related to sex, or by negative attitudes such as aversion to genital odors and textures. More commonly, though, anxiety is evoked by concerns regarding performance and the partner's reactions. Although somewhat similar, treatments for anxiety will be divided between

treatment of performance anxiety and treatment for other anxieties based on negative attitudes or previous trauma.

Some anxieties based on social prohibitions can be counteracted by simple permission giving from an authoritative person. For young or inexperienced persons with a strict background that has prohibited sexual expression, and whose sexual problem is related to thoughts that what they are doing is wrong, permission from the physician to engage in a variety of sexual activities such as masturbation, extended foreplay, or oral sex may be helpful. Reassurance that the activities are normal and healthy further reduces anxiety. For others, more extensive discussions of the origins of their anxieties may be required, with the addition of training in relaxation and provision of experiential exercises.

The purpose of experiential exercises is to associate the sexual experience with relaxation and pleasure, rather than anxiety and tension. These experiences are generally graduated (step by step). Clients can participate in the sequence of experiences either (1) vicariously, by reading or viewing films; (2) by imagination; or (3) directly, by home practice (alone or with the partner). The vicarious experience of reading books or viewing fims of sexual activity may be the least anxiety provoking, especially if the client can select and regulate the amount of stimulation he is receiving and can have the experience alone. Similarly, being able to imagine a particular anxiety-provoking situation in the safety of the therapist's office contributes to a reduction in anxiety. This kind of imaginary practice also occurs during discussions of the activity with the therapist or partner and can be further encouraged with discussions with the partner at home. In some cases, a structured, systematic desensitization program [10] may be devised, whereby the individual is first trained in deep muscle relaxation and in the creation of clear images. The images are then presented to the client in vivid detail as he remains in a state of deep relaxation. The situations that were first imagined are then practiced at home.

An example of graduated, direct experiences would be those suggested to a man who had a distaste for vaginal texture and odor, which engendered anxieties about manual foreplay and penile insertion. He was first instructed simply to look at his wife's genitalia, next to massage her back and legs with a lotion (simulating the texture of vaginal lubricant), next to touch her labia briefly, and so forth, until he gradually became comfortable with all aspects of manual or penile vaginal containment. Progression from one step to another depends solely on the level of comfort at the previous step. Another example of direct, graduated experiences is masturbation practice given to a young man who had previously experienced pain on intercourse due to organic disease and who was reluctant to allow his penis to be touched except in very restricted ways. He was told to refamiliarize himself with pleasurable sensations by extending his own masturbation patterns and then gradually instructing his partner in how to touch him without bringing on his fear of the previous pain. Masturbation practice is also useful in treating men without partners, or men for whom the initial steps of sensate focus are too anxiety-provoking in the presence of a partner.

"PLEASURE NOT PROWESS": TREATING PERFORMANCE FEARS

Performance fears parallel other anxieties, in that they are distracting and inhibiting. A man preoccupied with judging his performance, speculating on his ability to achieve erection, and wondering what his partner's reactions will be is an anxious observer, not a relaxed participant. The source of the performance fear may arise from imaginary concerns or from previous experience with a partner who was critical of his ability to satisfy her due to awkward technique, premature ejaculation, or inability to achieve an erection sufficient for intercourse. Educating the partner about her contribution to his problem may help to elicit a more supportive attitude. The therapist should not reinforce the notion that erection is the ultimate goal, but rather should foster the idea that sexuality is for pleasure and enjoyment, not performance. Home practice in sensate focus is directed toward achieving this goal.

Before initiating the sensate-focus practice, a clear understanding is reached that no attempts will be made to have intercourse or to achieve orgasm. The couple is then encouraged to provide sensuous pleasure for each other, alternating the giving and receiving roles. If other thoughts intrude they are encouraged to pause briefly in their play in order to refocus attention on the pleasuring session. In the first exercises, breast and genital touching is prohibited. If arousal occurs, it is to be ignored. In subsequent pleasuring sessions, teasing stroking of genitals is permitted but with the continued prohibition of intercourse or orgasm. This permits the couple to learn that erections will occur during relaxed play, that if the erection subsides, another may occur, and that intercourse is not necessary each time arousal occurs.

As the couple grows more confident, vaginal containment with the female astride is encouraged, initially with no movement, then gradually increasing stimulation with slow, followed by vigorous, thrusting. As problems frequently arise with the home practice, it is important in follow-up to address difficulties that the couple experiences. Failure to schedule a practice session or not following instructions and thus reexperiencing difficulty are common problems.

TREATING PROBLEMS OF SKILL

Problems of skill or technique are wide ranging. They include rarely spending time on precoital activities, having a limited sexual repertoire, and engaging in sexual activities virtually the same way every time. Analysis of a couple's problems often reveals sexual patterns that are limited and repetitive and that are no longer stimulating. Couples in treatment also reveal, often for the first time, that they dislike a particular activity or that certain of their partner's behaviors turn them off. Such dissatisfactions are readily conveyed, often nonverbally, and if unresolved, add to the tensions between the couple. In the case of inadequate skills, the couple needs training in how to set up an atmosphere conducive to sexual interest, how to initiate and refuse sexual activity gracefully, how to communicate effectively about sexual likes and dislikes, and how best to arouse their partner and to be aroused.

If sex is a low-priority activity as compared with work, child care, household tasks, or social responsibilities, sex may be relegated to a hurried, late-night activity, engaged in when both partners are tired or have had little opportunity to relax together. Similarly, if the couple has rigid sex role separation, the problem may lie in an inability to alter household tasks in such a way as to provide a more relaxed setting. Arranging dates with each other or rearranging schedules to provide more time for intimacy tends to make the sexual experiences more positive. Arranging a romantic setting free of interruptions from children or telephones, with time to talk about mutual interests or concerns, enables the couple to work out any tensions that block intimacy and to be free to enjoy each other.

Most distressed couples report that sexual initiation takes place in a tentative, indirect way that minimizes risk or that is so direct as to preclude a warm-up or transition phase. In the former approach, a misunderstanding regarding the partner's interest can be interpreted as yet another refusal. In the latter case, the partner may be turned off or may refuse because of anticipation of an unsatisfactory, hurried intercourse. Couples can avoid such misunderstandings by describing to each other how they might effectively approach each other. Rehearsing ways to refuse an approach by expressing one's feelings rather than criticizing the partner can be practiced with the therapist present to offer suggestions. Saying, "I'd like to make love tonight, honey, but I feel too upset about work just now to relax" gives the partner much more insight into the refusal than "Not now." Information about feelings also may lead to a resolution of the problem that is contributing to the refusal.

Communicating about sexual likes and dis-

likes during foreplay and intercourse enhances reciprocal pleasuring. This can be done by sharing fantasies of what they would like to have done to them, or by reading or viewing sexual material and sharing their reactions with each other. The couple may be encouraged to demonstrate their own masturbatory technique to their partner, or to describe what kind of pressure or touch is most pleasurable. Because preferences may change depending on mood or stage of intercourse, nonverbal guiding of the partner's hands or speed of movement helps communicate a change of response. Care should be taken as to how feedback is given, in that positive suggestions such as, "a light touch feels better" is preferred to punishing, critical feedback such as "Don't! That doesn't do a thing for me." Sexual technique is also enhanced through the sensate-focus exercises already described, during which couples are encouraged to explore other body areas of sexual sensitivity and different ways to arousal.

TREATMENT OF PREMATURE EJACULATION

The relatively common problem of a rapid ejaculatory reflex or premature ejaculation may result in secondary impotence in the male. If the partner is not usually satisfied, due to too brief intercourse, the sexual relationship may become increasingly tense and further problems may ensue. In the past, treatments for premature ejaculation were aimed at minimizing erotic or tactile stimuli in order to prolong the erection. Recommendations to do mental computations, wear condoms, or apply anesthetics to the penis may briefly delay ejaculation but also may contribute to the problem.

The most effective treatment, devised by Semans in 1956, involves teaching the male to focus more, rather than less, on his penile sensations. He or his partner are instructed to stimulate the penis manually until he feels the sensations of ejaculatory inevitability, at which time the stimulation is discontinued. This procedure is followed until he can tolerate increasing stimulation for longer periods of time. They then gradually learn intra-vaginal control, usually beginning with a female-superior position.

This treatment has been found to be quite effective for couples in the intensive Masters and Johnson sex therapy program. Howe and Mikulas found that 9 of 10 couples who received written instructions were able to achieve satisfactory ejaculatory control. Similarly, Kaplan and her colleagues simultaneously instructed four couples in six group sessions with Howe practice. All four couples reported attaining voluntary ejaculatory control by the 2-month follow-up. It is apparent from these studies that the Semans approach is preferred in cases in which erectile dysfunction is secondary to problems of ejaculatory control. Again, identification of etiology is of primary importance in devising treatment.

CONCLUSIONS

Sex therapy is a complex process. Typically, a couple is seen together because it is their sexual relationship that is seen as needing therapy. A number of assessments are made regarding the causes of the dysfunction. Generally they include problems of information, anxiety, or skill. Treatment is directed at all problem areas and usually includes some form of experiential exercises that are structured to enhance relaxation and enjoyment, enabling sexual arousal to emerge. Specific techniques to augment these exercises may include relaxation training, systematic desensitization, communication skills training, and bibliotherapy.

REFERENCES

1. Cooper, A. J. Disorder of sexual potency in the male: A clinical and statistical study of some factors related to short-term prognosis. *Br. J. Psychiatry* 52:709, 1966.
2. Howe, J. C., and Mikulas, W. L. Use of written material in learning self-control of premature ejaculation. *Psychol. Rep.* 37:295, 1975.
3. Kaplan, H. S. *The New Sex Therapy.* New York: Brunnel/Mazel, 1974.
4. Kaplan, H. S., et al. Group treatment of premature ejaculation. *Arch. Sex. Behav.* 3:443, 1974.
5. Lazarus, A. A. Overcoming Sexual Inadequacy. In A. A. Lazarus (ed.), *Behavior Therapy and Beyond.* New York: McGraw-Hill, 1971. Pp. 141–162.
6. Masters, W. H., and Johnson, V. E. *Human Sexual Response.* Boston: Little, Brown, 1966.
7. Masters, W. H., and Johnson, V. E. *Human Sexual Inadequacy.* Boston: Little, Brown, 1970.
8. Reckless, J., and Geiger, N. Impotence as a Practical Problem. In J. LoPiccolo and J. LoPiccolo (eds.), *Handbook of Sex Therapy.* New York: Plenum, 1978.
9. Semans, J. Premature ejaculation: A new approach. *South. Med. J.* 49:353, 1956.
10. Wolpe, J. *Psychotherapy by Reciprocal Inhibition.* Stanford, Calif.: Stanford University Press, 1958.
11. Wolpe, J. *The Practice of Behavior Therapy.* New York: Pergamon, 1969.

Surgical Treatment of Peyronie's Disease

PAT O'DONNELL
GARY LEACH
SHLOMO RAZ

François de la Peyronie was a French surgeon who was summoned to Paris by Louis XIV and eventually became court surgeon to Louis XV [68]. He was founder of the Royal Academy of Surgery of Paris. In a paper entitled "Some Observations Opposing the Normal Ejaculation of Semen," he described a condition of fibrous thickening of the shaft of the penis with pain and curvature on erection [68]. For over 200 years attempts to elucidate the pathophysiology of the disease have proved fruitless.

The therapy Peyronie recommended was that his patients bathe in the Spa of Bareges. He found excellent initial responses [68]. However, responses reported by others were less favorable, and the treatment fell into disuse. Over the past 200 years, this has been the course of events with almost every therapeutic agent that has ever been used for treatment of Peyronie's disease.

The lack of information on pathophysiology, the confusion regarding therapy, and the unpredictability of the disease makes the approach to its management a difficult problem. The clinical experiences of a number of investigators are reviewed, and a management approach is presented for this perplexing illness.

CLINICAL PRESENTATION

The common presenting symptoms of Peyronie's disease are pain on erection, curvature on erection, and a mass in the penis. When the penis is flaccid, the patient is usually asymptomatic. The salient symptom in 95 percent of patients is curvature of the penis during erection [47]. A less common complaint is that of painful erections, which usually occur earlier in the course of the disease. The presence of a lump in the penis is the third most common complaint, although a palpable plaque is present in 97 percent of patients. Often, patients are concerned that the mass is malignant; however, malignant degeneration has never been reported [33]. Patients are usually relieved to learn that the lesion is benign [51, 58].

Table 20-1. Incidence of Peyronie's disease by age

Decade	Number of cases	Percentage (%)
20–29	5	3
30–39	12	7
40–49	35	19–90
50–59	76	41–71
60–69	52	27–30
70–79	4	2–3
80–89	2	1
Total	186	100

Patients with Peyronie's disease present most often in middle age [59]. The average age of presentation is 53 years [4]. Table 20-1 gives the distribution of Peyronie's disease by age.

As can be seen from Table 20-1, 30 percent of patients are above age 60, 71 percent are above age 50, and 90 percent are above age 40. Thus, Peyronie's disease is primarily a disease of aging men.

Peyronie's disease has been thought by some to be more prevalent in the white population than the black [47]. However, most authors have noted no particular racial prevalence [26, 88].

The average duration of symptoms at the time of presentation is 6 months [4]. Fifty-four percent are seen by a urologist within 6 months from the onset of symptoms, and 91 percent are seen by the end of 1 year. The lesion is usually solitary, although multiple lesions are present in approximately 20 percent of patients [59]. The direction of curvature is toward the location of the plaque [31]. The most frequent location is on the dorsum of the penis (in 72% of patients) [4, 47]. The location is on the lateral surface in 21 percent, and it is ventrally located in only 7 percent [47]. The lesion is located in midshaft in 51 percent, the distal shaft in 26 percent, and the proximal shaft in 23 percent [4]. The direction of curvature is upward in 58 percent, downward in 10 percent, to the left in 16 percent, and to the right in 12 percent [59]. The size of the plaque may vary from 0.5 × 1.5 cm to as large as 2 × 8 cm; however, the average plaque size is 2 × 3 cm. Sixty-eight percent of patients have difficulty with intercourse, although it is the chief complaint in only 18 percent [40].

The average patient presenting with Peyronie's disease is a 53-year-old black or white male complaining of dorsal curvature of the penis of over 6-month's duration that produces sexual dysfunction. A solitary 2 × 3 cm plaque may be palpable on the dorsal midshaft of the penis.

DIAGNOSIS OF PEYRONIE'S DISEASE

The diagnosis of Peyronie's disease usually can be made by history and physical examination. A mass almost always can be felt on palpation. It is often difficult to determine precisely the size and the outline of the plaque. The size of the lesion found at time of surgery is consistently larger than that estimated preoperatively by examination [49]. Multiple areas of plaque formation or intraseptal extension may be difficult to delineate on physical examination [16].

Because of the limitations of physical examination in determining the extent of disease, corpus cavernosography has been advocated to better outline the plaque [16, 46, 95]. This procedure has been helpful especially in evaluating intraseptal extension of Peyronie's plaque.

Cavernosography is performed by applying a rubber tourniquet to the base of the penis and injecting approximately 20 ml of 60% Urografin into either one of the corpora cavernosa. Patients who have had previous surgery for Peyronie's disease, or who have received radiation therapy are at increased risk of complications from cavernosography and should be excluded from the study [16].

An alternative to cavernosography is the use of diagnostic ultrasound [66]. Through use of this technique, the lesion can be outlined accurately and the location of multiple lesions can be determined. Diagnostic ultrasound can be helpful in planning a surgical approach in patients who have extensive involvement with plaque. Moreover, the study is useful in evaluating the response of Peyronie's plaque to nonsurgical management.

Plain x-ray films and xeroradiography can be helpful in determining the presence of calcification as well as estimating the extent of the lesion [34], but these studies usually offer no advantage over diagnostic ultrasound in determining size of the lesion, presence of multiple lesions, or calcification of lesions.

NATURAL HISTORY OF PEYRONIE'S DISEASE

Many clinical reviews of patients having Peyronie's disease have been studies of consecutive patients treated with a single therapeutic modality. Therefore, the influence of the natural history of the disease on the clinical results has been uncertain. The information presently available on the outcome in patients receiving no treatment is helpful in decisions for both surgical and nonsurgical management of Peyronie's disease. Burford reported that of 19 patients receiving no treatment, only 1 improved and 18 remained unchanged [10]. However, this rather poor outcome in untreated patients has not been confirmed by others. Ashworth [2] studied 32 patients, eight of whom were followed without treatment. In follow-up at 5 years, two patients showed disappearance of the lesion and two others had decrease in the size of the plaque. Thus, 50 percent of the patients had improvement in the lesion without treatment, but none of the patients had normal sexual function. Two patients were impotent and six others had decrease in potency. Therefore, the apparent improvement in the pain and curvature may have been a result of a decrease in sexual function.

Williams reviewed 21 patients, 12 of whom were untreated and were followed for as long as 8 years [105, 106]. There was complete resolution in 4 (33%), improvement in 5 (42%), and only 3 (25%) were unchanged. In patients having complete resolution of the plaque, the average time for resolution was 4 years. Pain was the first symptom to disappear. Plaque resolution usually occurred somewhat later. Therefore, it has been suggested that Peyronie's disease may be fully manifest when first seen, and the natural history is one of gradual resolution [105].

Bystrom studied seven untreated patients with follow-up of 1 to 7 years [15]. In three patients having pain on erection, disappearance of symptoms occurred in all three. Disappearance of plaque occurred in five (71%), and resolution of curvature occurred in two of five (40%) patients. The natural history seems to favor lessening of pain, and this most frequently is followed by plaque resolution, and finally, resolution of curvature.

Furlow reviewed 26 patients who had no treatment for Peyronie's disease [40]. The follow-up results for symptoms of pain, plaque, and curvature are shown in Table 20-2.

These results indicate that the symptoms of Peyronie's disease, if untreated, tend to improve. Pain on erection completely resolved in 82 percent of patients and improved in the remaining 18 percent. Fifty-eight percent had resolution or improvement of the plaque, and over one-half had improvement or resolution of curvature. Therefore, in clinical studies the influence of the natural history can lead to erroneous conclusions when one is evaluating the results of a therapeutic modality without untreated controls. In untreated pa-

Table 20-2. Natural history of untreated Peyronie's disease [40]

Symptoms	Number of patients	Symptom gone	Symptom improved	Symptom unchanged	Symptom worse
Plaque on penis	26	10 (39%)	5 (19%)	7 (27%)	1 (4%)
Curvature of penis	23	3 (13%)	9 (39%)	6 (26%)	3 (13%)
Painful erection	11	9 (82%)	2 (18%)	None	None

Source: W. Furlow, H. Swenson, and R. Lee, Peyronie's disease: A study of its natural history and treatment with orthovoltage radiotherapy. *J. Urol.* 114:69, 1975.

tients, over a period of time, one can expect resolution of pain in over 80 percent, decrease in plaque size in over 50 percent, and improvement in curvature in about one-half of the patients.

PATHOLOGY OF PEYRONIE'S DISEASE

The symptoms of Peyronie's disease are produced by a localized abnormal deposition of collagen in the tunica albuginea. There is inelasticity of the tunica albuginea at the point of abnormal collagen deposition that produces curvature of the penis on erection.

The lesion originates as an inflammatory cellular infiltrate of the loose areolar connective tissue that separates the corpus cavernosum from the tunica albuginea [89]. The lesion may extend through the tunica albuginea to involve Buck's fascia and occasionally extends around the neurovascular bundle, producing anesthesia of the glans. The lesion also may extend deep into the corpus cavernosum.

The early lesions histologically show lymphocytic and plasmacytic infiltration of the areolar connective tissue layer, with the inflammatory cells primarily located perivascularly [89]. As the lesion progresses, there is a decrease in cellularity and an increase in fibrosis [69, 89].

In a study of 100 routine autopsies, 23 patients had some form of involvement of the areolar connective tissue sleeve as seen in early Peyronie's disease [90]. The median age for this group was 43 years. This compares with 53 years as the average age for the clinical presentation of Peyronie's disease [4]. Seven of the 23 patients with early Peyronie's had evidence of urethritis. This finding again raises the question of the role of urethritis in the etiology of the disease.

The etiology of this abnormal collagen deposition in the loose areolar connective tissue layer remains unknown. The plaques contain virtually no smooth muscle. In vitro digestion of plaque tissue with highly specific collagenase has shown this tissue to be well over 80 percent collagen on a weight basis [41, 43]. Infrequently, mineralization with cancellous

bone formation occurs on an organic bone matrix that is 90 percent collagen by weight. The noncollagen fibrous component of tunica albuginea is largely elastin. These fibers have been observed to be fragmented focally in cases of Peyronie's disease, with a complete absence of elastic fibers in the plaques [41].

On histologic examination of the normal tunica albuginea, the elastic fibers are seen to be oriented in a circular pattern. The collagen fibers are oriented longitudinally. Fluid-filled cylinders such as the corporal bodies will have the greatest wall tension at the area of the greatest diameter. Therefore, the wall tension producing elongation is much greater than that producing increase in diameter and requires the longitudinal orientation of the collagen fibers, which have the greater tensile strength. The arrangement of the collagen fibers allows for elongation. An abnormal arrangement of the collagen deposition of Peyronie's disease prevents the normal longitudinal expansion of the collagen fibers and produces the curvature of the penile shaft [42].

A protein-polysaccharide ground substance consisting of hyaluronidase and other proteoglycans embeds the collagen fibers in the tunica albuginea. This material is also present in Peyronie's plaques, although diluted by the increased collagen density. Intralesional injections of hyaluronidase have been used to dissolve ground substance and reduce the deformity. However, clinical trials of this agent have failed to demonstrate any beneficial effect. Hyaluronic acid in connective tissue affects the viscosity of the gel-like ground substance, but it apparently does not contribute to the mechanical properties of the tissue. Experimentally measuring tissue stiffness has shown that there is no increase in the rate of linear extension under constant load in rat skin and cervix treated with hyaluronidase. It is interesting that there is a marked decrease in tissue stiffness after treatment with trypsin. Trypsin itself does not digest collagen. This indicates that other, unidentified proteins are present that affect the mechanical properties of the tissue [41, 42].

Since collagenase is a highly specific enzyme, it has been proposed as a possible treatment for the contracture caused by Peyronie's disease [41]. The enzyme does not have the ability to digest the noncollagenous ground substance, and this tends to keep the enzyme localized, adding to the safety of local injection of the enzyme.

Dupuytren's contracture, another local disorder of abnormal collagen deposition, is present in 10 percent of patients with Peyronie's disease [47]. Other local collagen abnormalities are fibrosis of the auricular cartilage and plantar fibromatosis, both of which have been associated with Peyronie's disease [22]. It has been speculated that these are local manifestations of a generalized systemic collagen disorder. However, there is an absence of systemic symptoms in Peyronie's disease, and the purely localized character of non-involvement of neighboring areas of the same tissue is not characteristic of a systemic disease.

There have been isolated associations of Peyronie's disease with other diseases such as sclerosing cholangitis [97], α-1-antitrypsin deficiency [73], propranolol therapy [72, 98], and carcinoid syndrome [5, 50]. Seven of eight patients with Peyronie's disease had an antigen for the B7-cross-reacting group [107]. This perhaps raises the possibility that there exists an identifiable causative agent that produces disease selectively in the genetically predisposed patient.

NONSURGICAL MANAGEMENT OF PEYRONIE'S DISEASE

Since the original description of Peyronie's disease in 1743, a variety of therapeutic regimens have been used for treatment, but the efficacy of each is very limited. However, medical management continues to be the initial approach to therapy of Peyronie's disease, because the combined effect of the natural history and medical management results in improvement in most patients [103]. Tocopherols have become the most widely used initial treatment [27, 49, 51, 103]. Their use was first described by Scott and Scardino in 1948 [87]. In 23 patients treated with a daily dose of 300 mg of mixed tocopherols or 200 mg of synthetic α-tocopherol, they found an excellent response in 11 patients (48%), improvement in 10 (43%), and no change in two (9%). Devine advocated 6 months of medical therapy using vitamin E before considering a surgical approach [27]. In 30 patients, he noted a disappearance of the lesion in six patients (20%), improvement in 14 (46%), and no change in six (20%). Burford combined oral tocopherols 50 mg daily with radium plaque treatment in 31 patients, and, on follow-up of 2 years or more, 84 percent of patients showed improvement or cure from the treatment [13].

Steroids in the treatment of Peyronie's disease represent a widely used form of non-surgical therapy. It was first described by Teasley [94] in 1954. He used a solution of 25 mg of cortisone (Cortone) injected directly into the plaque. His initial report showed favorable results in 24 patients.

Table 20-3 shows the results of intralesional injection of steroids.

Bystrom [15] studied different types of treatment of Peyronie's disease with the results shown in Table 20-4. The period of observation varied between 1 and 16 years, with a mean of 5.5 years.

In a review of 250 patients, Chesney [22] compared the various methods of medical therapy. Some of these results are shown in Table 20-5. He felt that the use of steroids had improved both the immediate and late results of Peyronie's disease. Improvement was especially marked in younger patients having a short history of disease.

The rationale for use of steroids in the treatment of Peyronie's disease is that Peyronie's plaque is composed primarily of collagen. Steroid injection into the laboratory-produced granulomas decreases the collagen formation. Steroids are known to depress fibroblastic activity and collagen formation. The inhibitory effect is not specifically directed against collagen synthesis alone but may represent generalized depression of connective tissue–forming cells. It appears that the primary action of steroid therapy in Peyronie's disease is depression of basic cellular meta-

Table 20-3. Results of intralesional injection of steroids

Author	Drugs	Number of patients	Improved (%)
Bodner [6]	Steroids & hyaluronidase	17	88
Furey [40]	Hydrocortisone, meticortelone	13	61
Ekstrom [30]	Prednisolone	18	94
Descantis [29]	Dexamethosone	14	85
Toksu [96]	Dermojet, triamcinolone	5	100
Winter [108]	Dermojet, dexamethosone	21	86
Taranger [93]	Dermojet, triamcinolone, hydrocortisone	7	29

Table 20-4. Results after various forms of treatment for Peyronie's disease

Type of treatment	Number of patients	Good	Moderate	No improvement
Local steroid	30	3	6	21
Vitamin E	17	0	1	16
Radiotherapy plus vitamin E	19	0	4	15
Local steroid plus vitamin E	11	1	2	8

Table 20-5. Results of medical therapy of Peyronie's disease

Method of therapy	Number of patients	Good results	Partial improvement	Not improved	Not known
Local corticosteroid injection	23	15 (65%)	4 (17%)	2 (7%)	2
Local corticosteroid injection and vitamin E	47	26 (55%)	11 (23%)	5 (11%)	5
Local corticosteroid injection, oral prednisone, and vitamin E	16	9 (56%)	6 (38%)	1 (6%)	
Prednisolone tablets and vitamin E	28	9 (32%)	10 (36%)	3 (11%)	6
Vitamin E tablets	79	19 (24%)	29 (37%)	10 (13%)	21
vitamin E in methyltestosterone	7	1 (14%)	6 (86%)		

bolic processes that result in collagen synthesis [70]. Dimethyl sulfoxide (DMSO) has been used with some success in the treatment of Peyronie's disease. The drug was used by Scheinman in treatment of four patients [85]. He noted improvement in three patients; Persky used DMSO for treatment of 13 patients and found improvement in six (46%) [76].

DMSO has been used in the past as an in-dustrial solvent and was found useful in preserving cells against freezing. DMSO also has a local analgesic effect and anti-inflammatory properties. The drug is absorbed rapidly through the skin and is said to produce a smell of garlic or oysters on the patient's breath. The drug is now considered experimental, because of laboratory evidence of association with cataracts [4].

Local injections of parathyroid hormone into the plaque also have shown favorable results [67]. In a study of 12 patients receiving weekly injections for 8 weeks, eight patients (67%) had improvement in the lesion and a decrease in curvature. The rationale for this treatment was that excess parathyroid hormone depresses collagen synthesis and promotes collagen degradation.

Zarfonetis [109] described the use of potassium p-aminobenzoate (Potaba) for treatment of Peyronie's disease. p-Aminobenzoate was given orally in a dosage of 12 gm/day divided into four or six equal doses. The medication can be given in the form of a chilled 10% aqueous solution or in 0.5-gm capsules. The reason for the large dose requirement is that potassium p-aminobenzoate is rapidly excreted in the urine. A total of 21 patients were treated. Of 16 patients having pain on erection, 16 (100%) showed complete resolution of symptoms. In 17 patients having penile deformity, there was improvement in 14 (82%), and no change in three (18%). In 21 patients having plaque formation, there was improvement in 16 (76%), and no change in five (24%). Side effects of p-aminobenzoate include anorexia and nausea. Hypoglycemia may result if the patient has a poor dietary intake. Sulfonamide compounds are metabolic antagonists of p-aminobenzoate and should not be administered concomitantly.

Helsop described the use of ultrasonic therapy in nine patients and found early relief of pain in all patients so treated [48]. Approximately two-thirds were able to resume intercourse. Frank studied 25 patients treated with ultrasound and found subjective improvement in 23 (95%) [35]; there was a decrease in the plaque size in 19 (76%). A course of ultrasonic therapy consisted of 12 treatments for 5 minutes each on consecutive days, except weekends. Iontophoresis [83, 101], and diathermy [23, 100] have been used with some success, although neither is used commonly today.

Procarbazine was introduced for treatment of Peyronie's disease in 1970 and was thought to have promise as a therapeutic agent [18, 22]. However, in a study [68] of 22 patients who completed a full 12-week course of treatment, 9.1 percent improved, and 90.9 percent either remained the same or became worse. Thus, the cytostatic side effects of therapy outweighed the benefits [71]. The response to the different therapeutic agents is quite variable and the treatment of this disease is far from satisfactory.

Although Peyronie's disease has been known for over 200 years, little progress has been made in understanding the disease process. Many factors contribute to this poor understanding. First, the disease is relatively uncommon. The clinical experience of most investigators is fairly limited. The onset and resolution of symptoms are gradual so that results are not readily appreciated. The natural history is unpredictable but favors improvement of symptoms, which can be interpreted as response to therapy.

Randomized control studies with untreated patients are lacking. There are no current means for objective measurement of response to therapy. Varying subjective responses to each symptom often are reported. Of the major symptoms of Peyronie's disease, curvature is the least affected by the natural history and is the most common limitation to function. The degree of curvature, together with plaque size, may be amenable to objective measurement. Valid clinical evaluation of response to medical therapy will require randomized studies with placebo-treated controls, followed by objective measurement of changes in symptoms. If curvature and plaque can be measured objectively, it would seem the standard by which response to medical therapy should be judged.

RADIOTHERAPY

In 1912, Bernasconi described a case of Peyronie's disease that was cured by roentgen therapy. Compared with other modes of therapy in use at that time [77], radium therapy was an attractive alternative. Radium therapy and later, orthovoltage radiation therapy, became the most frequently used treatments for Peyronie's disease. Regulating the dose of radium was sometimes difficult, and the treatment

Table 20-6. Results of radiotherapy for Peyronie's disease

Author	Radiation source	Number of patients	Marked or moderate improvement	Mild improvement	No improvement
Griff [45]	Radium	15	5 (33%)	8 (53%)	2 (13%)
Soiland [92]	Orthovoltage	10	9 (90%)		1 (10%)
Schourup [86]	Orthovoltage	10	3 (30%)	3 (30%)	4 (40%)
Aquino [1]	Cobalt	32	21 (66%)		10 (31%)
Dahl [24]	Radium	96	19 (20%)	34 (35%)	43 (45%)
Fricke [36]	Radium	112	42 (38%)	20 (18%)	50 (45%)
Dunlap [28]	Orthovoltage	23	21 (91%)		2 (9%)
Duggan [27]	Orthovoltage	87	30 (35%)	42 (48%)	15 (17%)
Helvic [47]	Orthovoltage	40	29 (72%)		11 (28%)
Feder [32]	Orthovoltage	36	20 (56%)	9 (25%)	7 (19%)

Table 20-7. Comparison of radiotherapy and no treatment

	Gone (%)	Improved (%)
No treatment (26 patients)		
Plaque	39	19
Curvature	13	39
Radiotherapy group I (22 patients)		
Plaque	39	23
Curvature	18	32
Radiotherapy group II (19 patients)		
Plaque	33	11
Curvature	6	33

occasionally burned the skin. Orthovoltage was associated with fewer skin problems. Results of some of the clinical studies using roentgen therapy are presented in Table 20-6.

Furlow compared three groups of patients, one having no treatment, a second group receiving one treatment of radiotherapy of 250 to 600 roentgen, and a third group receiving two treatments of orthovoltage radiotherapy [59]. The results are given in Table 20-7, which surveys only the common symptoms of curvature of the penis and plaque of the penis. These results indicate that the symptoms of radiation-treated patients are not improved in comparison to those of untreated patients. However, the symptom of painful erection showed improvement in 9 months with treatment compared to 16 months without.

Whether radiation therapy in Peyronie's disease is effective is difficult to state with certainty, but it most likely is of very limited value. Moreover, radiation therapy is not an innocuous treatment [58, 103].

SURGICAL THERAPY

A surgical approach to the treatment of Peyronie's disease usually is reserved for patients who have had a trial of medical therapy for 6 months to 1 year [27, 51]. This allows enough time to detect any improvement due to medication. It also allows time for improvement due to the natural history of the disease to occur. During this period, however, the patient may experience varying degrees of anxiety. Even when seen initially by the physician, he is usually somewhat anxious. The anxiety that is associated with this poorly understood disease has been well recognized for many years [3, 33, 58, 102]. The problem may become severer during the initial period of medical therapy, in which there is no symptomatic response. Often, severer psychic disturbances are seen, and an occasional patient may become suicidal [7, 58]. Burford stated: "Sexual disability occasionally gives rise to neuropathic conditions, even to grave melancholia. The younger the victim is, usually the more nervous, morose, hypochondriacal or even suicidal he becomes [10]." In younger, sexually active patients, marital problems related to sexual dysfunction can greatly exacerbate the anxiety. At such times, a great deal of supportive therapy may be required for the patient to accept conservative management. It often may be difficult for the physician to delay surgical intervention in these patients.

After an adequate period of medical therapy, patients with persisting symptoms that prevent successful penetration, such as continued pain on erection, worsening of curvature, or significant decrease in potency may be considered for a surgical approach to therapy. Since the etiology of Peyronie's disease is unknown, the goal of surgery can not be curative; it is rather alleviation of symptoms and preservation of function. The persistence of pain on erection after medical therapy occasionally will require surgical intervention for relief; but pain usually will resolve with medical therapy alone and is not often an indication for surgery.

Historically, the first successful operative procedure in Peyronie's disease was done in 1728 by McClellan [34]. In the late 1800s, there were a number of cases having excision of Peyronie's plaque, often for pathologic examination to rule out neoplasm [52, 104]. Occasionally, those patients had good function after surgical excision of the plaque, but fibrosis and recurrence of curvature was often the outcome. As a result, surgery for treatment of Peyronie's disease did not become widely accepted. The introduction of radiotherapy as a method of treating Peyronie's disease offered an alternative to surgery that became widely used.

It was not until Lowsley introduced the graft inlay technique in 1946 that an interest in the surgical approach was renewed [59]. He treated 27 patients who had plaque excision and closure of Buck's fascia over the defect. Seventeen patients (58%) either were cured or markedly improved. In 10 patients, he used a fat graft from the abdomen to repair the defect in the tunica albuginea. Seven of these patients (70%) either were cured or markedly improved.

In 1949, he reported the results of surgical treatment of 50 consecutive cases [58]. Of 17 patients having simple plaque excision, nine (53%) were cured, and four (24%) were markedly improved. Of 33 patients operated on with the use of a fat graft, 20 (61%) were cured and six (18%) showed marked improvement. In 1957, Fogh-Andersen treated eight patients with the fat-inlay graft technique, with results similar to those of Lowsley [34]. This procedure was a significant improvement over previous surgical approaches. It also offered a method for treatment of patients in whom conservative therapy had failed.

From these early experiences with the graft inlay technique, the following observations were made [34, 59]:

1. The best results are obtained in younger men.
2. Poorest results occur in patients who have plaque extension to the lateral or ventral surface of the corpus cavernosum.
3. Better results are obtained if operation is done early in the course of the disease.
4. Patients having previous ionizing radiation have a much greater number of wound complications postoperatively.

These important observations have proved to be true also with the other graft inlay procedures.

Poutasse [79] felt that although curvature often persisted after simple plaque excision, the procedure alone usually would decrease curvature from a disabling 75 to 90 degrees to a functional 0 to 20 degrees. Without the use of a graft inlay material, however, fibrosis at the site of plaque excision has been a frequent occurrence, and it produces recurrent curvature [102].

In the laboratory, Horton [51] examined different autogenous grafting materials in dogs. He compared autogenous dermal graft, arterial wall graft, vein graft, and fascia lata. All grafts except dermis had scarring and contraction that resulted in curvature of the penis. Only the dermal grafts survived without significant contraction. The adnexal glands and hair follicles underwent atrophy and did not form inclusion cysts. A similar technique was used clinically in the treatment of

Peyronie's disease. In eight patients, the plaque was excised, and a dermal graft inlay was placed to cover the defect in the tunica albuginea. One patient was impotent after surgery, and seven (88%) were able to sustain an erection for intercourse. There was no recurrence or extension of disease in the group. Hicks and co-workers [49] operated on 15 patients using the dermal graft procedure and found that 12 (80%) were cured, one was improved (6.7%), and only two (13%) were failures.

In a follow-up series of 50 patients treated with the dermal graft inlay technique [103], more than 70 percent of the patients were satisfied postoperatively with their sexual performance. There was a reduction of curvature in 84 percent and a reduction of pain on erection in 83 percent of patients. In patients who were unable to perform coitus preoperatively, however, only 53 percent were able to have intercourse postoperatively. Results in 30 percent of patients operated on were considered unsatisfactory, due to persistent pain, curvature, and impotence [103].

The combined experiences of many investigators have more clearly defined the results and specific problems with the dermal graft procedure. The following factors often are associated with postoperative problems: (1) previous treatment with ionizing radiation, (2) decrease in sexual potency of the patient, (3) previous steroid injection therapy, (4) extensive plaque formation, and (5) lateral and ventral plaque extension. Previous radiotherapy and previous steroid injection are associated with an increase in local wound complications [103]. Of poor surgical results, 75 percent have been in patients having previous radiotherapy [58]. Occasionally, plaque formation may be quite extensive. When the erectile tissue is extensively involved with plaque formation, there is little chance of potency after excision of the fibrous plaque [74]. Therefore, management of these patients with a graft inlay technique is unlikely to result in preservation of potency. Also, in patients with lateral extension of the plaque, surgical correction is more difficult, and this accounted for six of seven patients requiring reoperation in Lowsley's series [59].

Other autogenous grafting materials have been used for the graft inlay technique. Rectus muscle aponeurosis has been used in four patients who had no operative complications and showed encouraging early results [8]. Corpus spongiosum taken from the bulbous urethra has been used in four patients, with surgical failures in two of them (50%) [63]. A greater-saphenous-vein graft was used in one patient, who was able to have normal sexual intercourse postoperatively [84]. Certainly, a much greater clinical experience with these tissues is required before their efficacy can be determined.

Lyophilized human dura has been studied in dogs and found to be satisfactory in replacing the tunica albuginea for the graft inlay procedure [54]. After the laboratory studies, seven patients underwent excision of plaques and replacement of tunica albuginea with lyophilized human dura. On follow-up from 2 months to 4.5 years, no complications occurred, and all patients had a straight penis and effective sexual function. The lyophilized human dura appears to be a satisfactory alternative to dermal graft and obviates the need for the graft excision [54, 55].

In a laboratory study, a comparison of fat graft, dermal fat graft, and dermal graft was done in dogs [17]. The dermal fat graft, which used a very thin fat layer, appeared more suitable because it was more easily manipulated during surgery than was the fat graft. Moreover, there was an improvement in hemostasis over the dermis graft. The layer of fat on the dermis graft should be kept very thin. All grafts were shown to be replaced gradually by fibrous tissue, and a certain amount of scarring and contraction resulted. Therefore, the graft should be slightly larger than the defect, to allow for subsequent fibrosis [17].

Surgical Procedure
The operative technique currently used for the dermal graft inlay procedure begins with an initial circumcising incision proximal to the corona. The foreskin is mobilized and retracted to the base of the penis [51]. Buck's fascia is opened longitudinally, lateral to the dorsal nerves and vessels, and the plaque is exposed. A tourniquet is applied to the base

of the penis and saline is injected into the corporeal body, producing an erection that demonstrates the extent and location of the lesion. The neurovascular bundle is dissected from the corpora and retracted. The plaque is then removed from the underlying erectile tissue, and a dermal graft is placed. The dermal graft is taken from the lower abdomen or thigh by excising a split-thickness graft of $^{12}/_{1000}$ in. of epidermis and removing the underlying dermal graft. It is partially defatted, to a thickness of about 1 mm, and excised approximately one-third larger than the excised plaque. It is placed into the defect with the fat side down and secured in place with interrupted 5-0 Prolene sutures [103]. Running sutures of the same material are used to suture the graft in place, and a second erection is produced, to check for leaks and to determine whether the curvature has been corrected. After skin closure, a pressure dressing is applied to decrease bleeding and edema. A small drain is left for 24 hours; a catheter is usually not necessary. Postoperative erections are controlled with diazepam and inhaled amyl nitrite [103].

Even in the hands of the most experienced surgeons, this technique yields unsatisfactory results in almost one-third of patients [103]. Others have had even less encouraging results. In treating seven patients by means of the dermal graft, Melman [65] found that despite a technically good surgical result, all seven were impotent on postoperative follow-up of 1 year or longer. Palomar and co-workers [74] treated 10 patients by using the dermal graft procedure and found that seven (70%) became impotent postoperatively. Pryor treated eight patients with a dermal graft procedure, and all were impotent on follow-up [80].

Some of the problems experienced in the graft inlay technique that contributed to failures include the following: (1) formation of additional plaque in other areas along the shaft of the penis, which results in recurrence of curvature; (2) postoperative impotence; (3) fibrosis of the graft, resulting in recurrent curvature; (4) persistent curvature despite an apparently successful operative procedure.

Surgery itself does not alter the basic disease process. Therefore, plaque may recur at other sites in the tunica albuginea at any later time, resulting in a surgical failure.

The problem of impotence in patients having Peyronie's disease has long been recognized as occurring as well with any therapy as with no therapy at all [2, 32, 59]. The occasional occurrence of a flaccid penis distal to the plaque has led to the speculation that there are vascular abnormalities associated with the plaque that decrease the erectile function. Ashworth [2] stated that although the process may be self-limiting and capable of spontaneous regression, "the onset of Peyronie's disease heralds the end of effective sexual life." Wesson [100], in 1943, stated, "Frequently following surgery there is complete loss of erectile power; hence, it is wise never to operate while the patient still has any sexual function." The reason for loss of erectile power is as uncertain now as it was then. Whether it is related to damage of the vascular supply of the corpora or simply a manifestation of the natural history of Peyronie's disease is not known. Nonetheless, impotence after either medical or surgical treatment for Peyronie's disease has been a frequent cause for failure of therapy [2].

The frequent loss of sexual function after use of current surgical techniques led to the use of the Small-Carrion prosthesis as an initial surgical procedure for the management of Peyronie's disease [81]. This approach is relatively simple and achieves the objectives of surgical therapy — relief of symptoms and maintenance of sexual function.

The most common symptom requiring surgery is persistent curvature. Placement of the prosthesis alone without plaque incision will correct curvature in most patients [54, 75, 82], but sometimes incision of the plaque is required to make the penis completely straight [81, 88] (Figs. 20-1 through 20-5). After insertion of the prosthesis, the penis should be examined, and if residual curvature is present, plaque incision should be done. After placement of the prosthesis, the penis will remain straight even if the plaque becomes larger or if new plaque formation oc-

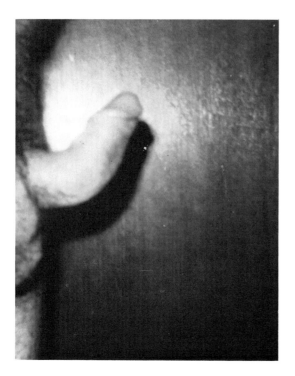

Figure 20-1. Typical "home" photograph taken to illustrate upward curvature of penis secondary to plaque is shown.

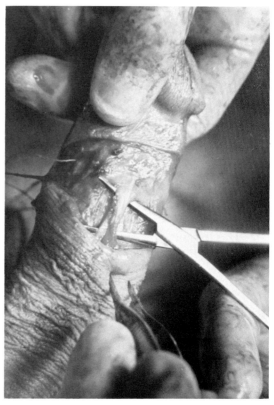

Figure 20-2. The dorsal neurovascular bundle is shown after being isolated from underlying plaque.

curs [54] (see Fig. 20-6).

In the initial clinical study, plaque incision and stenting with a Small-Carrion prosthesis was done in 12 patients [81]. Eleven patients (91%) had good surgical results and had excellent postoperative sexual functioning. One failure occurred due to infection of the prosthesis. Seven additional patients were treated and good results were obtained in six. In a total of 19 patients treated with the incision and stenting procedure, 17 patients (89%) had an excellent functional result [9].

Palomar and co-workers [74] compared patients having the dermal graft procedure with those having the penile prosthesis implant. Of 10 patients having the dermal graft, it was considered to have failed in seven, due to postoperative impotence. Of six patients treated with a prosthesis stenting procedure, five were sexually functional postoperatively.

The operative technique for prosthesis stenting is described by Raz and co-workers [81]. The patient is placed in the supine position with knees flexed and abducted to allow palpation of the corpora during insertion of the prosthesis. A circumcising incision is made in the skin just proximal to the glans. A tourniquet is applied at the base of the penis, and an erection is produced by injection of saline. Stay sutures are placed in the distal end of each corpus, and a longitudinal incision is made into each corpus cavernosum. The Small-Carrion prosthesis is introduced via the penile route. Introduction of the prosthesis places the nonelastic tissue of the plaque under stretch. The penis should then be examined for curvature, and if curvature is minimal at this point, no further treatment is necessary. If deformity is still present, however, the dorsal neurovascular bundle is isolated and protected. Single transverse incisions are made in each fibrotic plaque. As the penis straightens, the transverse incisions are transformed into diamond-shaped defects,

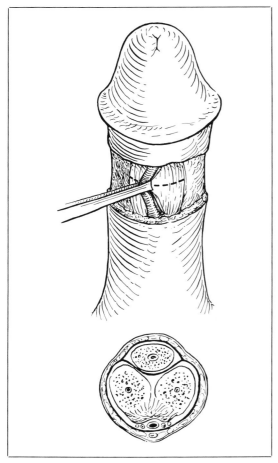

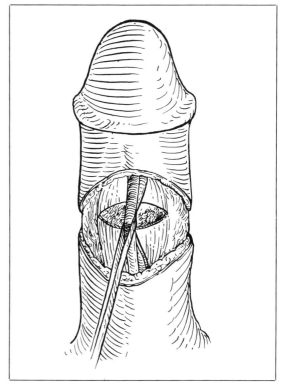

Figure 20-4. A transverse incision has been made through plaque and tunica albuginea.

Figure 20-3. The neurovascular bundle is being retracted to expose the underlying plaque. Dotted line shows where transverse incision in plaque is made.

which are covered with Buck's fascia. Broad-spectrum antibiotics are used preoperatively and continued for 6 days postoperatively. A Foley catheter is inserted and left in place for 24 hours. This procedure is easily performed and is well tolerated in most patients, with minimal postoperative problems.

Most patients requiring surgical correction of Peyronie's disease will be in the older age group. As is shown in Table 20-1, 71 percent of patients are above 50 years of age when seen initially. Patients below 40 years of age represent only 10 percent of those coming for treatment of Peyronie's disease. In this age group, the presence of normal preoperative potency makes the risk of impotence after a graft inlay procedure much lower than in the older patient [34, 58]. Moreover, younger patients prefer the possibility of normal non-prosthetic erections [54]. In a study of 22 patients, seven patients aged 25 to 46 underwent excision of Peyronie's plaque with a graft inlay procedure using lyophilized human dura. The remaining 15 patients (ages 45–78) had Small-Carrion prostheses placed. All patients had excellent postoperative results [54].

Patients who require surgery for treatment of Peyronie's disease may be selected for either a graft inlay procedure or a prosthetic stenting procedure. In patients over 45 years of age, the prosthetic stenting procedure will give excellent results in over 85 percent of cases. In patients below 45 years of age, one can expect similar results with the graft inlay procedure.

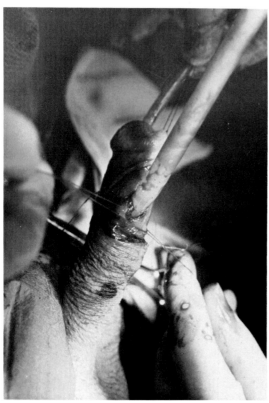

Figure 20-5. An incision into the corpus has been made to allow for implantation of a noninflatable penile implant.

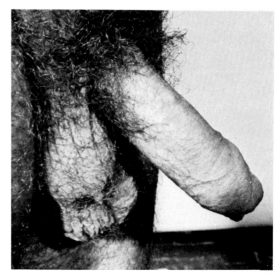

Figure 20-6. A result of surgical therapy is presented. Note the lack of dorsal curvature.

CONCLUSIONS

Although Peyronie's disease was described over 200 years ago, the etiology remains unknown and the pathogenesis is poorly understood. Patients with this disease present with curvature of the penis, pain on erection, and a palpable plaque. Pain is an earlier symptom followed by plaque formation and curvature. Pain has a tendency to resolve with all forms of therapy as well as with no therapy. Pathologically, the early lesion is a vasculitis of the loose areolar connective tissue layer between the tunica albuginea and the corpora cavernosum. Early lesions show infiltration with plasma cells and lymphocytes while advanced lesions show loss of cellularity and progressive fibrosis. It is likely that pain is associated with the early inflammatory lesion and disappears as the lesion becomes more fibrotic. The progressive fibrosis with abnormal deposition of collagen produces curvature, which responds poorly to medical therapy. Therefore, it is the most common indication for surgical therapy. The choice of the surgical procedure may be difficult since none is ideal. The graft inlay procedure results in a high incidence of impotence in older men. The prosthetic stenting procedure provides symptomatic relief and restores sexual function to this age group. However, the stenting procedure is less appealing to the younger age group. Since the graft inlay procedure is uniformly more successful in this group, it is the preferred surgical procedure for younger patients.

Surgery is considered when symptoms persist that prevent coitus after at least 6 months of medical therapy. Vitamin E is the preferred medical treatment. Potaba and intralesional steroids also appear efficacious. The role of the natural history of the disease in the clinical improvement with these drugs is unknown. Radiotherapy may also be of benefit; however, failures of radiotherapy are clearly greater surgical risks.

An arbitrary plan of management would consist of initial therapy with vitamin E, 300 mg daily for 1 year. Sexually motivated patients unable to achieve penetration following medical therapy would be considered for surgery.

Stenting with a penile prosthesis is recommended in patients over 45 years of age or in younger patients with decreased potency or extensive plaque formation. Patients below 45 years of age without extensive lesions are recommended for a dermis or lyophilized human dura inlay graft procedure.

An improved approach to treatment awaits a better understanding of this disease. Peyronie himself recommended to his patients that they bathe in the Spa of Bareges, which seemed to result in significant improvement One may seriously question whether anything of importance has been added since that time.

REFERENCES

1. Aquino, J. A., Cunningham, R. M., and Filbee, J. F. Peyronie's disease. *J. Urol.* 97:492, 1967.
2. Ashworth, A. Peyronie's disease. *Proc. R. Soc. Lond. [Biol.].* 53:20, 1960.
3. Beach, E. W. Peyronie's disease or fibrous cavernositis: Some observations. *Calif. West. Med.* 55:7, 1941.
4. Billig, R., et al. Peyronie's disease. *Urology* 6:409, 1975.
5. Bivens, C. H., Marecek, R. L., and Feldman, J. M. Peyronie's disease: A presenting complaint of the carcinoid syndrome. *N. Engl. J. Med.* 289:844, 1973.
6. Bodner, H., Howard, A., and Kaplan, J. Peyronie's disease: Cortisone-hyaluronidase-hydrocortisone therapy. *J. Urol.* 72:400, 1954.
7. Bromberg, P. Fibrous cavernositis: Induration of the corpora cavernosa. *South. Med. J.* 14:480, 1921.
8. Bruschini, H., and Mitre, A. Peyronie's disease: Surgical treatment with muscular aponeurosis. *Urology* 13:505, 1979.
9. Bruskewitz, R., and Raz, S. Surgical considerations in treatment of Peyronie's disease. *Urology* 15:134, 1980.
10. Burford, E. H. Fibrous cavernositis. *J. Urol.* 43:208, 1940.
11. Burford, C. E., Glenn, J. E., and Burford, E. H. Fibrous cavernositis: Further observations with report of 31 additional cases. *J. Urol.* 56:118, 1946.
12. Burford, E. H., Glenn, J. E., and Burford, C. E. Therapy of Peyronie's disease. *Urol. Cutan. Rev.* 55:337, 1951.
13. Burford, E. H., and Burford, C. E. Combined therapy for Peyronie's disease. *J. Urol.* 78:265, 1957.
14. Burns, A. B., and Persellin, R. H. Experi-mental penile corporal (auto-immune?) vasculitis in the rat. *Invest. Urol.* 9:241, 1971.
15. Bystrom, J., et al. Induratio penis plastica (Peyronie's disease): The results of the various forms of treatment. *Scand. J. Urol. Nephrol.* 6:1, 1972.
16. Bystrom, J., et al. Induratio penis plastica (Peyronie's disease): Cavernosography in assessment of the disease process. *Scand. J. Urol. Nephrol.* 8:155, 1974.
17. Bystrom, J., and Norberg, K. Free autogenous grafts into the penile cavernous tissue: An experimental study in dogs. *Urol. Res.* 3:145, 1975.
18. Bystrom, J. Induratio penis plastica: Experience of treatment with procarbazine (Napulan). *Scand. J. Urol. Nephrol.* 10:21, 1976.
19. Bystrom, J., and Rubio, C. Induratio penis plastica (Peyronie's disease): Clinical features and etiology. *Scand. J. Urol. Nephrol.* 10:12, 1976.
20. Callomon, F. Induratio penis plastica: The problem of its etiology and pathogenesis. *Urol. Cutan. Rev.* 49:742, 1945.
21. Cameron, H. Examples of some surgical diseases and accidents of rare occurrence. *Lancet* 1:841–885, 1884.
22. Chesney, J. Peyronie's disease. *Br. J. Urol.* 47:209, 1975.
23. Corbus, B. C. Chronic cavernositis cured by diathermy. *J. Urol.* 12:313, 1926.
24. D'Abreu, A. Peyronie's disease. *Br. J. Urol.* 15:90, 1943.
25. Dahl, O. The treatment of plastic induration of the penis (Peyronie's disease). *Acta Radiol.* 41:290, 1954.
26. Desanctis, P., and Furey, C. Steroid injection therapy for Peyronie's disease: A 10-year summary in review of 38 cases. *J. Urol.* 97:114, 1967.
27. Devine, C., and Horton, C. Surgical treatment of Peyronie's disease with dermal graft. *J. Urol.* 111:44, 1974.
28. Duggan, H. Effect of x-ray therapy on patients with Peyronie's disease. *J. Urol.* 91:572, 1964.
29. Dunlap, J., and Lathem, J. X-ray therapy in Peyronie's disease. *South. Med. J.* 62:485, 1969.
30. Ekstrom, T., and Hultengren, N. Peyronie's disease (plastic induration of the penis): Treatment by local injections of prednisone. *Acta Chir. Scand.* 124:163, 1962.
31. Etter, E. Plastic induration of the penis (Peyronie's disease). *Urol. Cutan. Rev.* 40:808, 1936.
32. Feder, B. Peyronie's disease. *J. Am. Geriatr. Soc.* 19:947, 1971.
33. Fister, G. Plastic induration of the penis. *Urol. Cutan. Rev.* 36:588, 1932.

34. Fogh-Andersen, P. Surgical treatment of plastic induration of the penis (Peyronie's disease). *Acta Chir. Scand.* 113:45, 1957.
35. Frank, I., and Scott, W. Ultrasonic treatment of Peyronie's disease. *J. Urol.* 106:883, 1971.
36. Fricke, R., and Olds, J. The radium treatment of Peyronie's disease. *Am. J. Roentgenol.* 42:545, 1939.
37. Fricke, R., and Varney, J. Peyronie's disease and its treatment with radium. *J. Urol.* 59:627, 1948.
38. Furey, C. Peyronie's disease: Treatment by the local injection of meticortelone and hydrocortisone. *J. Urol.* 77:251, 1957.
39. Furlow, W. Peyronie's disease and penile implantation. *J. Urol.* 120:647, 1978.
40. Furlow, W., Swenson, H., and Lee, R. Peyronie's disease: A study of its natural history and treatment with orthovoltage radiotherapy. *J. Urol.* 114:69, 1975.
41. Gelbard, M. Collagenase and Peyronie's disease: Experimental studies. Read before the Los Angeles Urological Society, June 3, 1980.
42. Gelbard, M. Personal communication, 1980.
43. Gelbard, M., Walsh, R., and Kaufman, J. Collagenase for Peyronie's disease. *Urology* 15:536, 1980.
44. Giles, R. Peyronie's disease or plastic induration of the penis. *Urol. Cutan. Rev.* 51:399, 1947.
45. Griff, L. Peyronie's disease: The role of radiation therapy and a general review. *J. Radium Ther. Nucl. Med.* 100:916, 1967.
46. Hamilton, R., and Swann, J. Corpus cavernosography in Peyronie's disease. *Br. J. Urol.* 39:409, 1967.
47. Helvie, W., and Ochsner, S. Radiation therapy in Peyronie's disease. *South. Med. J.* 65:1192, 1972.
48. Heslop, R., Oakland, D., and Maddox, B. Ultrasonic therapy in Peyronie's disease. *Br. J. Urol.* 39:415, 1967.
49. Hicks, C., et al. Experience with the Horton-Devine dermal graft in the treatment of Peyronie's disease. *J. Urol.* 119:504, 1978.
50. Highton, T., and Garrett, M. Some effects of serotonin and related compounds on human collagen. *Lancet* 1:1234, 1963.
51. Horton, C., and Devine, C. Peyronie's disease. *Plast. Reconstr. Surg.* 52:503, 1973.
52. Jones, S. Localized thickening in the corpus cavernosum. *Trans. Pathol. Soc. Lond.* 44:102, 1893.
53. Kaplan, I. Peyronie's disease. *Urol. Cutan. Rev.* 46:350, 1942.
54. Kelami, K. A. Peyronie's disease and surgical treatment. *Urology* 15:559, 1980.
55. Kelami, A. Replacement of tunica albuginea of corpus cavernosum penis using human dura. *Urology* 6:464, 1975.
56. Kretschmer, H. L., and Fister, G. M. Plastic induration of the penis: A report of 16 cases. *J. Urol.* 16:497, 1926.
57. Loeffler, R., and Sayegh, E. Perforated acrylic implants in management of organic impotence. *J. Urol.* 84:559, 1960.
58. Lowsley, O., and Boyce, W. Further experiences with an operation for the cure of Peyronie's disease. *J. Urol.* 63:888, 1950.
59. Lowsley, O., and Gentile, A. An operation for the cure of certain cases of plastic induration (Peyronie's disease) of the penis. *J. Urol.* 57:552, 1947.
60. Martin, C. Long-time study of patients with Peyronie's disease treated with irradiation. *Am. J. Roentgenol. Radium Ther. Nucl. Med.* 114:492, 1972.
61. McKenzie, D. Peyronie's disease. *J. Med. Assoc. Ga.* 67:426, 1978.
62. McRoberts, W. Peyronie's disease. *Surg. Gynecol. Obstet.* 129:1291, 1969.
63. Medgyesi, S. Surgical treatment of induratio penis plastica (Peyronie's disease) with a corpus cavernosum graft. *Br. J. Plast. Surg.* 32:129, 1979.
64. Melman, A. Experience with implantation of the Small-Carrion penile implant for organic impotence. *J. Urol.* 116:49, 1976.
65. Melman, A., and Holland, T. Evaluation of the dermal graft inlay technique for the surgical treatment of Peyronie's disease. *J. Urol.* 20:421, 1978.
66. Mohar, N., Rukavina, B., and Uremovic, V. Ultrasound diagnosis as a method of investigation of plastic induration of the penis. *Dermatologica* 159:115, 1979.
67. Morales, A., and Bruce, A. The treatment of Peyronie's disease with parathyroid hormone. *J. Urol.* 114:901, 1975.
68. Morgan, R., and Pryor, J. Procarbazine (Natulan) in the treatment of Peyronie's disease. *Br. J. Urol.* 50:111, 1978.
69. Mukherjee, A., et al. Plastic induration of the penis: Peyronie's disease — A histopathological study. *Indian J. Pathol. Microbiol.* 21:197, 1978.
70. Nocenti, M., et al. Collagen synthesis and C-14–labeled proline uptake and conversion to hydroxyproline in steroid-treated granulomas. *Proc. Soc. Exp. Biol. Med.* 117:215, 1964.
71. Oosterlinck, W., and Renders, G. Treatment of peyronie's disease with procarbazine. *Br. J. Urol.* 47:219, 1975.
72. Osborne, D. R. Propranolol and Peyronie's disease. *Lancet* 1:1111, 1977.
73. Palmer, P. E., Woolf, H. J., and Kostas, C. I. Multisystem fibrosis in alpha-1-antitrypsin deficiency. *Lancet* 1:221, 1978.
74. Palomar, J., Halikiopoulos, H., and Thomas, R. Evaluation of the surgical management of

Peyronie's disease. *J. Urol.* 123:680, 1980.

75. Pearman, R. Insertion of a Silastic penile prosthesis for the treatment of organic sexual impotence. *J. Urol.* 107:802, 1972.

76. Persky, L., and Stewart, B. The use of dimethyl sulfoxide in the treatment of genitourinary disorders. *Ann. N.Y. Acad. Sci.* 141:551, 1967.

77. Polky, H. Induratio penis plastica. *Urol. Cutan. Rev.* 32:287, 1928.

78. Poutasse, E. Peyronie's disease. *Trans. Am. Assoc. Genitourin. Surg.* 63:97, 1971.

79. Poutasse, E. Peyronie's disease. *J. Urol.* 107:419, 1972.

80. Pryor, J., and Fitzpatrick, J. A new approach to the correction of the penile deformity in Peyronie's disease. *J. Urol.* 122:622, 1979.

81. Raz, S., deKernion, J., and Kaufman, J. Surgical treatment of Peyronie's disease: A new approach *J. Urol.* 117:598, 1977.

82. Roen, P. Peyronie's disease and penile implantation. *J. Urol.* 118:1074, 1977.

83. Rothfield, S., and Murray, W. The treatment of Peyronie's disease by iontophoresis of C-21–esterified glucocorticoids. *J. Urol.* 97:874, 1967.

84. Sachse, H. Venous wall graft in Peyronie's disease. *Urologe [A]* 15:131, 1976.

85. Scheinman, L., and Miller, E. Use of dimethyl sulfoxide (DMSO) in Peyronie's disease. *Pacific Med. Surg.* 75:61, 1967.

86. Schourup, K. Plastic induration of the penis. *Acta Radiol.* (Stockh.) 26:313, 1945.

87. Scott, W., and Scardino, P. A new concept in the treatment of Peyronie's disease. *South. Med. J.* 41:173, 1948.

88. Small, M. Peyronie's disease and penile implantation. *J. Urol.* 119:579, 1978.

89. Smith, B. Peyronie's disease. *Am. J. Clin. Pathol.* 45:670, 1966.

90. Smith, B. Subclinical Peyronie's disease. *Am. J. Clin. Pathol.* 52:385, 1969.

91. Soiland, A. Peyronie's disease or plastic induration of the penis. *Radiology* 42:183, 1944.

92. Soiland, A., and Lindberg, L. Plastic induration of the penis. *Am. J. Cancer* 21:372, 1934.

93. Taranger, L., Robson, C., and Barkin, M. The surgical approach to Peyronie's disease. *J. Urol.* 114:404, 1975.

94. Teasley, G. Peyronie's disease: A new approach. *J. Urol.* 71:611, 1954.

95. Thomas, M., and Rose, D. Peyronie's disease demonstrated by cavernosography. *Acta Radiol.* (Stockh.) 12:221, 1972.

96. Toksu, E. Peyronie's disease: A method of treatment. *J. Urol.* 105:523, 1971.

97. Viteri, A., Hardin, W., and Dyck, W. Peyronie's disease and sclerosing cholangitis in a patient with ulcerative colitis. *Digestive Dis. Sci.* 24:490, 1979.

98. Wallis, A. A., Bell, R., and Sutherland, P. W. Propranolol and Peyronie's disease. *Lancet* 2:980, 1977.

99. Waters, C., and Colston, J. A report of three cases of fibrosclerosis of the penis treated by roentgenization without improvement. *Surg. Gynecol. Obstet.* 20:41, 1915.

100. Wesson, M. Peyronie's disease (plastic induration), cause and treatment. *J. Urol.* 49:350, 1943.

101. Whalen, W. A new concept in the treatment of Peyronie's disease. *J. Urol.* 83:851, 1960.

102. Whitacre, H. J. Plastic induration of the corpus cavernosum. *N.Y. State Med. J.* 91:586, 1910.

103. Wild, R., Devine, C., and Horton, C. Dermal graft repair of Peyronie's disease: Survey of 50 patients. *J. Urol.* 121:47, 1979.

104. Willett, E. Calcareous plate removed from the dorsum of the penis. *Trans. Path. Soc. Lond.* 44:102, 1893.

105. Williams, J., and Thomas, G. The natural history of Peyronie's disease. *Proc. R. Soc. Med.* 61:876, 1877.

106. Williams, J., and Thomas, G. The natural history of Peyronie's disease. *J. Urol.* 103:75, 1970.

107. Willscher, M., Cwazka, W., and Novicki, D. The association of histocompatibility antigens of the B-7 cross-reacting group with Peyronie's disease. *J. Urol.* 122:34, 1979.

108. Winter, C., and Khanna, R. Peyronie's disease: Results with Dermal-Jet injection of dexamethasone. *J. Urol.* 114:898, 1975.

109. Zarafonetis, C., and Horrax, T. Treatment of Peyronie's disease with potassium para-aminobenzoate (Potaba). *J. Urol.* 81:770, 1959.

21

Finney Flexirod Penile Prosthesis

ROY P. FINNEY

The Finney Flexirod penile implant has been designed to incorporate various features thought to be desirable in any semirigid implant. First and foremost, the implant should impart enough rigidity to the penile shaft and enough support at its proximal end to permit satisfactory coitus. The implant should have sufficient bulk to increase penile diameter over that of the normal flaccid penis. In addition, the implant should provide stability to the glans, because a lack of stability can make intromission quite difficult. The implant should be designed so that it can pass beneath the glans as far as possible since even ½ cm can make a considerable difference in patient satisfaction. Another important consideration is the patient's ability to conceal the permanently erect penis underneath his clothing. A significant bulge in the trousers, even in today's society, can produce embarrassment. All of these factors have to do with patient satisfaction, but, in addition to this, there is the surgeon to consider. An implant, the size of which can be determined prior to surgery, is also a highly desirable feature. This eliminates the need to have available a full set of penile implants of a different length for each case. This is not only cost-effective since a lower inventory may be kept, but it also decreases the initial investment necessary to begin this type of surgery in a given hospital.

DESIGN OF THE PROSTHESIS

With the above considerations in mind, the Finney Flexirod penile implant was designed. After the experience with single-rod silicone elastomer penile implants [5, 7], which have an excellent hinge action at their proximal end, a hinge was incorporated into the Flexirod. This hinge allows the implanted penis to hang in a more normal, dependent position inside the trousers and facilitates concealment to a considerable degree. Various designs were tried using a mechanical hinge, a ball-and-socket hinge, and even a hinge that could be locked into the erect position. The locking hinge did not seem to add any particular benefit since intromission is usually accomplished manually. After various tests, the simplest type of hinge with the lowest possibility of failure was chosen (Fig. 21-1). This hinge consists of a special soft, silicone elastomer and is designed to be positioned at the base of the penis beneath the pubis. Distal to the soft hinge segment is attached a firm, semirigid rod, and both are covered by a soft elastomer shell. This distal rod is designed to provide sufficient rigidity for normal coitus while still allowing enough flexibility to prevent undue penile trauma (Fig. 21-2).

The tip of the Flexirod implant, unlike that of other designs, incorporates a parabolic shape that more nearly conforms to actual penile anatomy. This shape accomplishes two highly desirable objectives. First, as is not true of blunt-tipped implants, there is little ball-and-socket action of the glans over the end of the implant. This is most important, because the unstable glans makes coitus much more difficult. Secondly, the parabolic tip is able to reach further under the glans to the extreme distal end of the corpus, without excessive dilation, which may contribute to extrusion. Each millimeter gained in this area improves stability to a considerable degree.

Since all men are not created equal, at least with regard to penile length, it was seen that in order to have the hinge positioned in the proper location, the distal rigid shaft would have to be supplied in different lengths. It was further found that the length of this rigid distal portion of the implant necessary to achieve proper hinge action in a given patient could be determined by penile measurement well in advance of surgery. On the other hand, the *total* length of the corpus cavernosum from the ischial tuberosity to the distal tapered end under the glans cannot be determined accurately by measurement before surgery. For this reason, the Finney Flexirod implant has a proximal, or tail, end that is divided into 0.5-cm segments. The tail end is designed to be longer than will be required, with the intention that it can be trimmed to fit the individual patient's *total* corporal length at the time of surgery.

SIZING THE IMPLANT

The Flexirod is available in 9-mm and 12-mm diameters. In the vast majority of patients, the larger diameter is used. Patients who have scarring of the erectile tissue after priapism, who have had infection of a previous implant that has necessitated removal, and possibly in rare cases of patients who have Peyronie's disease in whom the corpora cannot be dilated sufficiently, may require the 9-mm diameter implant. Every effort should be made to use the larger diameter.

The size (length) of implant required for a given patient may be determined well in advance of surgery by simple measurement with a metric ruler as confirmed by Barry [1]. Experience has revealed that many surgeons do not understand the basis for this measurement. In contrast to other semirigid penile implants, the length listed on the package is *not* the total length of the implant. It is important that everyone using the Flexirod penile implant understand this. The listed measurement is the length of the distal, more rigid, portion of the implant only, and it does not include the 5-cm hinge or the 8-cm tail portion (Fig. 21-3). This is purposely done because it is the more rigid shaft of the implant that is the key factor in sizing.

The object in sizing the patient for the Flexirod implant is to have 2 or 3 cm of the soft hinge extend beyond the pubic bone (Fig. 21-4). To accomplish this, one proceeds as follows. With the patient in the standing position, the penis is placed on firm horizontal stretch, and a metric rule is placed firmly against the pubis. It may be necessary to have certain men lie down and have an assistant retract the thick fat pad superiorly so that the ruler can be placed firmly against the pubis. With the penis on firm stretch a measurement is taken from the pubis to the mid-glans. The mid-glans is the approximate location of the distal ends of the corpora. This measurement, which in the average man is 12 cm, gives one the length of the corpora beyond the pubis or, to put it another way, the length of the pendulous portion of the corpora. Since, for

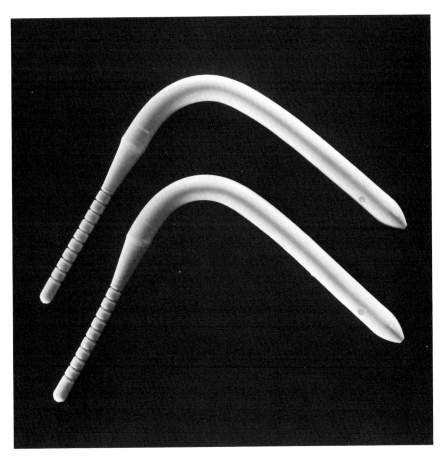

Figure 21-1. The completed prosthesis, bent to show the function of the hinged segment.

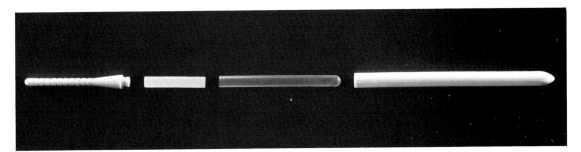

Figure 21-2. The various components before final bonding. From left to right: trimmable segmented proximal tail; soft, hinged rod; rigid distal rod; and soft outer covering and parabolic tip.

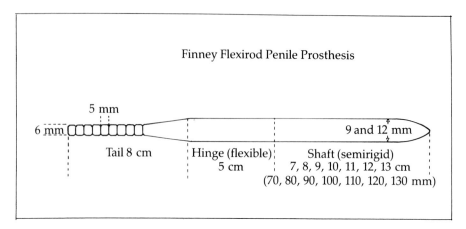

Figure 21-3. Diagram of the prosthesis components with dimensions. Implants are listed in sizes 70–130 mm. This is the length of the rigid shaft only.

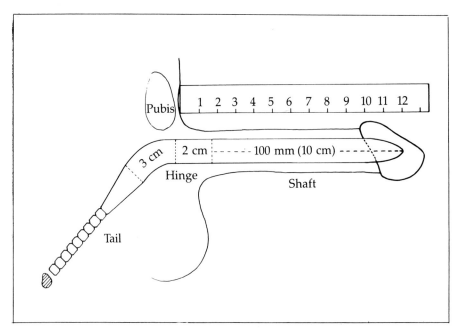

Figure 21-4. Placement of the hinge with 2 cm extending beyond the pubis. Pubis to midglans measurement in centimeters minus 2 cm = size of implant needed. This allows 2 cm of the flexible hinge to extend beyond the pubic bone.

proper hinge action, 2 or 3 cm of the soft, hinged section of the implant should extend beyond the pubis into the pendulous corpora, one subtracts 2 or 3 cm from the measured length. For example, if the measured pubis–

to–mid-glans length is 12 cm and one were to implant a 12-cm (120 mm) Flexirod implant, there would be no hinge beyond the pubis, and thus the hinge action of the penis would be poor. With a measurement of 12 cm, one subtracts 2 cm from this to allow 2 cm of the hinge to extend beyond the pubis and implants a 10-cm implant (Fig. 21-4). The 10-cm more rigid distal segment plus the 2-cm hinge segment equal the measured pendulous penile corporal length.

Originally, all patients were implanted with 2 cm of hinge extending beyond the pubis. It was found that although this worked quite well for men having a penis of average or longer length, the hinge action was less than optimal for men having a short penis. The mechanical leverage and extra weight of the longer penis causes it to hang quite well in a dependent position with a 2-cm hinge. Men having a penile measurement of less than 12 cm should have a 3-cm hinge to make up for this lack of leverage. This is accomplished by subtracting 3 cm from the penile measurement, rather than 2 cm. The number of centimeters subtracted from the measurement is the length of the hinge that will extend beyond the pubis, and the longer the hinge, the better the hinge action.

SURGICAL TECHNIQUES

The Flexirod prosthesis may be implanted by a number of techniques. Small, Carrion, and Gordon [8] have had extensive experience with the perineal route and have discussed this elsewhere. The Flexirod implant may be implanted quite easily through the perineum [3]. Since the length of the implant for proper hinge action has been determined preoperatively by measurement, one need only trim the tail end of the implant to the proper total length during surgery. This tail end may then be tucked in through the crus incision. In the vast majority of cases, the two implants should be cut to the same total length. This is accomplished by saving the trimmed portion of the first tail and removing the same amount from the second prosthesis. A word of caution: *This trimming process should be stepwise and gradual because another half centimeter can be removed; but if too much is cut, it cannot be replaced.* Some surgeons do not prefer the perineal approach, because it is adjacent to the anus, which must be very carefully excluded from the operative field.

The preferred method of implantation is through the penile base dorsally or [4, 6], if one is trying to avoid any penile scar, through the penile scrotal junction ventrally. For several days before surgery, patients wash the genitalia with povidone-iodine (Betadine) scrub. A 15-minute preoperative povidone-iodine scrub and careful draping including only the penis are used. Three ml of 3:1 dilute povidone-iodine solution is injected into the urethra, which is held by the assistant while the skin incision is made. The distal urethra often contains bacteria, and it is thought that this instillation helps to prevent infection. A 3- to 4-cm midline skin incision is made on the dorsum of the penis near its base, and this is extended downward until the superficial dorsal penile vein is visualized. An identification suture of 3-0 Dexon is placed just beside this vein for later identification of the midline neurovascular bundle. After one side is implanted, the corpora become distorted and the neurovascular bundle in the midline is displaced toward the contralateral side. This identification suture helps one to be certain that he is far enough laterally to make the incision for the second implant.

The skin is then retracted laterally and by using sharp dissection is deepened through the Buck's fascia to expose the tunica albuginea. The encircling vessels stand out quite clearly, and the surface of the tunica glistens once the Buck's fascia has been elevated laterally. It may be necessary to coagulate one set of encircling vessels, but an attempt should be made to avoid these. Stay sutures are placed above and below the intended site of the tunica incision, and the tunica is opened by sharp dissection for approximately 3 cm. The crus is dilated proximally with a No. 10 Hegar dilator, care being taken that it does not pass through the septum into the opposite crus. The No. 10 dilator is then passed distally under the glans. Following this, the No. 12 dilator is passed distally under the glans, but with no great force, and this is followed by passing the actual implant through the incision and out to the tip end of the distal corpus. The tapered tip of the implant accomplishes the final dilation and more accurately indicates the distal end of the

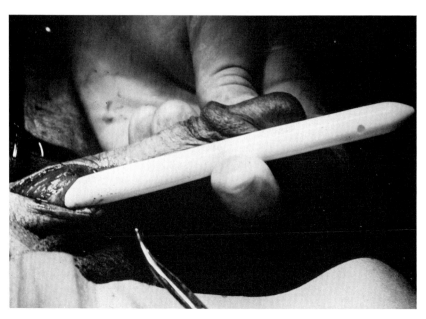

Figure 21-5. Technique of finding total implant length during surgery (*see text*).

corpus. The implant is then withdrawn from the distal penile shaft, and the implant's tail is inserted into the crus with a rotary tamping motion. One must be certain that the tail reaches the proximal end of the crus. One way to accomplish this is to use a No. 6 Hegar dilator as a depth gauge and transfer this length to the Flexirod implant. The penis is then placed on traction and the distal end of the implant is held beside it (Fig. 21-5). The distance between the mid-glans and the tip of the implant is taken. Commonly, the implant may be 5 cm or more too long. This indicates that approximately 5 cm of the tail of the implant needs to be trimmed for proper fit. The implant is removed from the crus and half this amount is trimmed from the implant tail. The implant is reinserted and then additional segments are trimmed until the implant appears to be the proper length. The implant may then be bent double and snapped into place. A suture or heavy skin hook at the distal end of the tunica incision aids in this maneuver. If difficulty is encountered in passing the entire implant into the penile shaft, the tunica incision should be lengthened. If there is any tendency for the implant to buckle or bend after insertion, it is too long, and additional tail segments should be removed.

With the implant in place, the tunica is closed with continuous 3-0 Dexon suture, and the identical procedure is performed on the contralateral side. It is at this stage that particular care must be exercised to avoid the displaced midline neurovascular bundle. After both implants are in place, the Buck's and Colles' fascia are closed together with continuous 4-0 Dexon, and the skin is closed with a similar subcuticular suture. Povidone-iodine ointment is applied to the incision, and a light gauze dressing with minimal pressure. Elastic tape is not used because cases of penile necrosis have been reported with excessive pressure. A No. 14F Foley catheter is left in overnight. This primarily serves to keep the dressing from becoming wet with urine as the patient tries to void into a urinal while in bed.

This same technique may be used through the penoscrotal junction [2]. Just as one must avoid the midline neurovascular bundle with the dorsal approach, one must carefully avoid the urethra with the penoscrotal approach. This is not difficult and may be facilitated by inserting a small Foley catheter at the start of surgery. We prefer to coat this Foley with povidone-iodine ointment to help prevent urethral contamination.

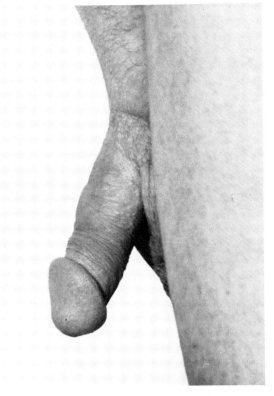
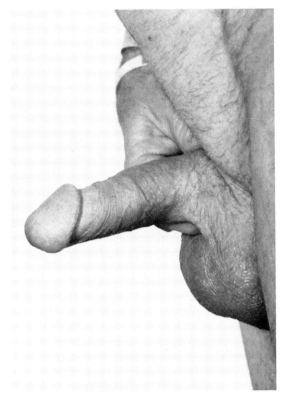

Figure 21-6. Patient with Finney Flexirod
prosthesis several weeks after surgery.

POSTOPERATIVE MANAGEMENT

The Foley catheter is removed on the following morning, and the patient is allowed out of
bed intermittently throughout the day. The
dressing is removed on the second or third
day, and the patient applies povidone-iodine
ointment to the incision several times daily
for the first week. Unless some problem
arises, such as unusual edema or pain, he is
discharged on the third day. Antibiotics, consisting of tobramycin and carbenicillin, are
given prophylactically just before surgery and
for 2 to 3 days afterward, until discharge. Patients are seen several weeks after discharge
and are instructed that they may have coitus
after 1 month and must at first use a water-
based lubricant. Patients are seen for a final
check approximately 2 months after surgery
for evaluation of performance, satisfaction,
and healing (Fig. 21-6).

RESULTS

Over 250 implants have been emplaced since
March, 1976. The most frequent causes of
impotence have been peripheral vascular
disease, diabetes, CNS disease, and pelvic
surgery. If one uses the criteria used for some
other penile implants, that is, patients who
were discharged with a well-positioned, un-
infected implant, the success rate in this series is 98 percent. As is true with all current
double-rod, semirigid penile implants, all patients have been able to have coitus, and the
vast majority are quite satisfied. Satisfaction
seems to depend to a large extent on patient
expectations, and this, in turn, depends on
the care and time spent interviewing the patient before surgery.

Two patients, both diabetics, have developed a postoperative infection that necessitated removal of the prostheses. One of
these was reimplanted 6 months later with a
12-cm diameter Flexirod, although there was

considerable fibrosis; the other is awaiting reimplant.

The only long-term complication of semirigid implants, other than device failure, seems to be extrusion. Although in this series there have been no cases of extrusion through the skin, this can occur, especially in paraplegics. All patients are warned that extrusion may occur and that they should return promptly if the end of the implant bulges under the skin near the glans. An incipient extrusion through the skin may be prevented by removing an ellipse of tunica albuginea over the protruding end of the prosthesis and closing the defect. By this means, the glans is drawn back over the end of the prosthesis, and extrusion is prevented.

Two patients have extruded their implants through the urethra. One of these extrusions occurred in a patient who had a rather deep urethral meatotomy at the time of the penile implant. This patient had had a transurethral resection of the prostate three months before the implant and had developed a rather dense meatal stricture. From this experience, it would seem that meatal strictures should be corrected well in advance of implant surgery. A second patient extruded his implant 2 years after surgery, following an automobile accident in which he was thrown against the steering wheel. Once a semirigid implant breaches the skin or urethra, it should be removed at once. Surprisingly little sepsis and fibrosis occur after an extrusion, provided the prosthesis is promptly removed, and the corpora usually may be dilated easily at the time of reimplantation. If only one implant has breached the skin or mucosa, the opposite side usually need not be removed. After an extrusion, it is probably prudent to shorten the replacement by 0.5 cm.

Over a period of months, a young quadriplegic who was implanted to help maintain a condom sheath had his implant slowly migrate posteriorly through the crus into the perineal tissues. This seemed to be caused by his clothing and condom sheath pressing on the glans. The distal ends of the implant came to rest in the mid-penile shaft, and it was removed because it was no longer serving its intended purpose. This is the only patient in 250 implants who had his prosthesis permanently removed.

Early in this series, it was not uncommon for patients to have significant postoperative penile pain for several weeks. It was finally realized that in an effort to gain as much length as possible, too long an implant was being used. Since that time, an additional 0.5 cm has been removed, with a significant diminution in postoperative pain. During this earlier period, one man with persistent pain for 2 months had the implants removed through distal lateral penile incisions, shortened by 0.5 cm, and replaced. His discomfort subsided within 2 days. Prolonged pain in the glans is usually the result of an implant that is too long, whereas perineal and scrotal pain are due to pressure of the proximal implant on the pudendal nerves. This pain may take weeks to resolve.

PROBLEMS

The malpositioned implant sometimes can cause problems. In normal men, the corpora are very close to the same length. Quite often, when both sides are fitted separately and the prostheses are trimmed to different total lengths, one side ends up shorter than the other. This may not be a functional problem, but if it is, one or both prostheses may be removed by making a short incision lateral to the urethra near the coronal sulcus, extracting it, and inserting one of the proper length. The same implant may be trimmed and reinserted if only shortening is required.

Occasionally, when dilating the first corpus, one may pass through the septum into the contralateral corpus, either distally or into the crus. This may not be detected when the first implant is inserted, but it usually becomes quite evident when one tries to dilate the contralateral side. If difficulty in dilating the second crus or distal shaft is encountered, crossover should be suspected immediately. It may be overcome easily by removing the first prosthesis, inserting the second in its corpus, and then redilating the first side. With the contralateral corpus occupied by its prosthesis, the first side dilates easily, and insertion is not difficult.

Some men have very scarred crura from trauma, priapism, Peyronie's disease, or from a previously infected implant. It may be possible to dilate the penile shaft, but not the crus. In this case, if the crus can be dilated even for a short distance under the pubis, the Flexirod implant may be cut quite short, even into the soft hinge, to achieve the appropriate total length. When the crus is so fibrotic that dilation cannot be accomplished, it is firm enough to provide quite adequate support for coitus.

All current double-rod semirigid penile implants provide, in most cases, partner satisfaction, and they are the most popular type. Even if coitus is engaged in daily, as is quite unlikely for most patients, this still amounts to using the device for only a minute fraction of the total time it is implanted. The individual's day-to-day comfort and his ability to conceal the implant are most important, as is the fact that the failure rate of the Finney Flexirod device so far approaches zero.

REFERENCES

1. Barry, J. Clinical experience with hinged silicone penile implants for impotence. *J. Urol.* 123:178, 1980.
2. Barry, J., and Seifert, A. Penoscrotal approach for placement of paired penile implants for impotence. *J. Urol.* 122:325, 1979.
3. Finney, R. New hinged silicone penile implant. *J. Urol.* 118:585, 1977.
4. Finney, R., Sharpe, J., and Sadlowski, R. Finney hinged penile implant: Experience with 100 cases. *J. Urol.* 124:205, 1980.
5. Lash, H. Silicone implant for impotence. *J. Urol.* 100:709, 1968.
6. Melman, A. Experience with implantation of the Small-Carrion penile implant for organic impotence. *J. Urol.* 116:49, 1976.
7. Pearman, R. Insertion of a silastic penile prosthesis for the treatment of organic sexual impotence. *J. Urol.* 107:802, 1972.
8. Small, M., Carrion, H., and Gordon, J. Small-Carrion penile prosthesis: New implant for management of impotence. *Urology* 5:479, 1975.

22

The Small-Carrion Penile Implant

MICHAEL P. SMALL

In 1973, the Small-Carrion penile implant was introduced. The prostheses are made of a medical-grade silicone shell with a silicone sponge interior. The purpose of combining the two forms of silicone is to provide the implant with material that most closely simulates the erect penis. The consistency and durability of this prosthesis is excellent, and the surgical technique for its implantation relatively simple. These factors, together with the low complication rate both for the surgery and indefinite follow-up period, have helped make the Small-Carrion prosthesis the most frequently used penile implant and has done much to establish implantation as a treatment for erectile dysfunction.

Originally, the implants consisted of a medical-grade silicone shell with a silicone gel interior. The gel-filled prostheses were used in the first 10 patients to receive the Small-Carrion implant. Eventually, the gel was replaced by the silicone sponge because air tended to diffuse through the shell, causing the implant to become somewhat softer during its shelf life. Since modification of the silicone sponge in 1973, the implant has remained basically the same, except for the addition of sizes of 21-cm length and 1.3-cm diameter. The implants are now available in multiple sizes, starting at 12-cm length and 0.9-cm diameter through multiple intermediate lengths to a 1.1-cm diameter and to the 21-cm length in a 1.3-cm diameter.

It has been my experience that preoperative estimation of the size of the implant to be used is very unreliable. Because of this, I recommend that all sizes of the implant be available in the operating suite so the proper one can be selected at the time of surgery. A sizer set containing each size of prosthesis has been made available so that the sterile implants do not have to be opened for intraoperative measurements. The sizer set can easily be cleaned and sterilized and, of course, reused indefinitely. Not only is this a great convenience and time-saver, but it also provides an extra margin of safety from possible contamination and damage to the implants, because usually they are never opened until they are ready to be implanted.

The concept of implanting two semirigid silicone bodies intracorporally is quite simple.

The implants are secured by the normal intracorporal anatomy, and a normal erection is closely simulated. After the prostheses have been implanted and healing has taken place, a large percentage of patients will have sufficient blood circulating within the corpora to supplement the erection that was achieved by the surgery. It is interesting that with this additional blood flow, many partners are unaware that the patient has a penile implant.

In tissue response to the penile implant, a silicone capsule will develop around the implant, usually within 10 to 14 days. The inner aspect of the capsule reveals a glistening surface. On this inner side, the capsule is not attached to the implant. The outside of the capsule is attached to the inner aspect of the corpora and remaining cavernous tissue, and it is in this plane that additional blood circulates and provides the supplemental erection. We have followed the development of the silicone capsule microscopically, and it reveals formation of a fibrous cicatrix (pseudocapsule) that contains a few scattered eosinophils and histiocytes. There appears to be no difference in the pathologic findings in the pseudocapsule if a biopsy is taken either relatively soon after surgery or many months or years later.

The capsule that sometimes develops after a breast implant may cause contracture and, possibly, deformity and may therefore be undesirable. The capsule that forms after penile implant surgery, however, is beneficial, because it gives an additional layer of support. Should there ever be reason surgically to reexplore the patient's penis (possibly to insert a different-size implant), the capsule leaves a perfectly developed "channel" from which the existing prosthesis can be removed, and a new one inserted with great ease.

Table 22-1 summarizes the etiology of the impotence and the number of patients operated on in each category. The results and surgical success are tabulated.

SURGICAL TECHNIQUE
Preoperative, intraoperative, and postoperative prophylaxis against infection cannot be overemphasized. An aminoglycoside is given on call to the operating room in a dosage schedule such that the patient will get two-thirds of his daily dosage based on his body weight preoperatively. On the evening of surgery he will receive the remaining one-third of his daily dosage as an intravenous infusion. In the holding area, the patient receives 200 mg of doxycycline intravenously. The aminoglycoside is repeated on the first and second postoperative days in the same dosage schedule as given on the day of surgery. The afternoon or evening dosage is given intramuscularly after intravenous fluids have been discontinued.

For patients who have chronic renal failure, or for those who are on dialysis, the dosage of aminoglycoside is modified according to individual circumstances. In these patients, there have been no nephrotoxic or neurotoxic complications. The doxycycline is repeated on the first postoperative morning, and, starting on the second postoperative day, 100 mg is given orally every 12 hours. This is continued for an additional 5 days.

In addition to antibiotics administered directly to the patient, a solution of polymyxin B sulfate and neomycin is mixed in the operating room and used for several very important purposes. The sizer prostheses are soaked in this solution, and each layer of the wound is copiously irrigated with it at various points in the operative procedure. With this total antibiotic regimen and the povidone-iodine scrub before surgery, the incidence of post–penile implant infection has been decreased dramatically from the 15 percent reported in our first 20 patients.

My surgical technique has not changed from that I described in 1975 and again in 1978. I prefer the perineal approach because it leaves the patient with no penile scar and very little postoperative discomfort. There are many other approaches to the corpora, however, and the surgeon should be familiar with these so that alternative approaches will be available if indicated. The other approaches are the penoscrotal, ventral circumcision, and infrapubic. All have certain advantages and disadvantages. If the perineal incision is car-

Table 22-1. Diagnosis and surgical results in 610 patients (September, 1980)

Diagnosis	Number of patients	Results	Comments
After prostatectomy, cystectomy, abdominoperineal resection	87	Excellent (85) Poor (2)	Bilateral perforation at glans; 1 patient had radiation therapy
Aortobifemoral bypass	15	Excellent (15)	
After priapism	13	Excellent (11) Poor (2)	Unable to implant intracorporal prosthesis
Psychogenic	84	Excellent (83) Poor (1)	1 patient had prolonged discomfort in glans—gradually cleared; 1 patient never satisfied with size and underwent insertion of inflatable implant; 2 patients originally had inflatable penile implant
Pelvic fracture	26	Excellent (25) Good (1)	Lost one prosthesis secondary to infection; an occasional patient required a different length prosthesis on each side
Peyronie's disease	44	Excellent (40) Good (3) Poor (1)	Plaque incised (12); penis not straight (3); erosion of one implant in patient where plaque not incised
Arteriosclerotic or hypertensive vascular disease (and medications)	157	Excellent (154) Good (2) Poor (1)	One implant too small and replaced 6 weeks postoperative; erosion through glans with loss of one implant—2 patients; bilateral perforation at glanular-meatal junction with initial urinary retention; 1 patient originally had inflatable penile implant
Spinal cord injury	32	Excellent (32)	18 implanted solely for sexual dysfunction
After electrical burn	1	Excellent (1)	Required urethroplasty
After groin explosion	1	Poor (1)	Had 1 prosthesis but subsequently removed because of poor tissue healing
Diabetes mellitus	124	Excellent (120) Good (1) Poor (3)	Urinary retention (1); septicemia and loss of both implants (2); perforation of 1 implant, urethroplasty, and subsequent erosion of other implant (1)
Epispadias extrophy	1	Good (1)	Small phallus
Hypogonadism	3	Excellent (3)	1 patient had replacement of testicular implants
Scleroderma	1	Good (1)	Lost 1 implant secondary to surgical perforation at glans
Neurologic disease, i.e., multiple sclerosis	8	Excellent (8)	
Chronic renal disease	13	Excellent (12) Poor (1)	Because of persistent pain of unknown etiology both implants were removed from 1 patient
Total	610	Excellent (589) Good (9) Poor (12) Surgical success (excellent only) 96%	

ried too far forward into the base of the scrotum, the patient may develop temporary hypesthesia. With careful preoperative preparation and rectal coverage, the perineal approach is a clean and easy way to reach the corpus cavernosum or crus of the penis with very little risk of infection. It also makes it possible to have the urethra easily palpable or visible.

The patient is placed in the lithotomy position and receives a 15-minute povidone-iodine scrub. The operative field is then isolated from the rectum with an isolating adhesive drape. After the patient has been draped, a No. 16F Foley catheter is introduced into the bladder and will be used to help identify the urethra during surgery and to drain the bladder postoperatively. The catheter usually is removed on the first postoperative morning and is only left in this long because most patients who undergo penile implant have spinal anesthesia.

A vertical midline incision is made in the perineum, extending from the base of the scrotum toward the rectum. The posterior extent of the incision approximates the area of the deep bulbous urethra (Fig. 22-1), approximately 5 cm anterior to the anus. The incision is carried through the subcutaneous tissues until the bulbocavernosus muscle with its underlying corpus spongiosum, urethra, and urethral catheter can be identified. These structures are retracted laterally with a vein retractor to expose the ischiocavernosus muscle and crus of the penis or corpora cavernosa. If the skin incision is made long enough, the tunica albuginea of the corpora cavernosa will be visualized at the upper portion of the wound. At the middle and lower portion of the wound, laterally, the ischiocavernosus muscle will be overlying the crus of the penis (Fig. 22-2). There will be multiple small- to medium-size veins crossing this area. If necessary, the ischiocavernosus muscle may be dissected carefully from the crus and also where some of the fibers fan out onto the corpus cavernosum. The shiny tunica albuginea of the crus and/or corpora will then be visible. A vertical incision is made in this structure, carrying the incision into the cav-

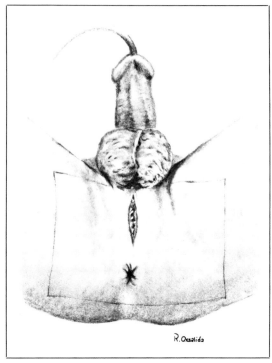

R. Oxsalida

Figure 22-1. A vertical midline incision used in perineal approach for prosthesis implantation is shown. Isolating adhesive surgical drape has been applied as outlined.

ernous tissue (Fig. 22-3). Proximal dilation is carefully performed by using the Hegar dilators, usually only a No. 7 or 8, because the prosthesis is thinner posteriorly (Fig. 22-4). If perforation of the crus does occur, closure should be accomplished with a figure-of-eight suture of 0 chromic catgut. Unless the damage is extensive, the operative procedure can go forward.

The Hegar dilator is then used to dilate the corpora distally, with dilation usually being carried out to a No. 12 or 13. If the 1.3-cm diameter implant is to be used, dilation will usually have to be continued to a No. 13 or 14. Care must be taken not to overdilate, or possibly tear, the corpora.

Extra care must be taken when dilating distally with the Hegar dilators, because there are a number of potential problems. The penis, and therefore the corpora, should be in the stretched position, so that the corpora do not "accordion" during dilation (Fig. 22-5). This could lead to unnecessary trauma and

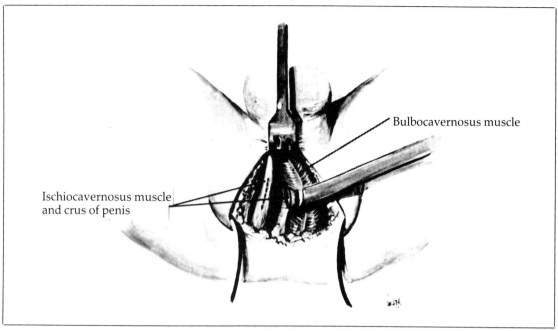

Figure 22-2. Ischiocavernosus muscle and penile crus are exposed by retracting the urethral bulb. (Reprinted from M. P. Small, H. M. Carrion, and J. A. Gordon, *Urology* 5:79, 1975. With permission.)

Figure 22-3. The corpus cavernosum has been incised, revealing spongy cavernous tissue within.

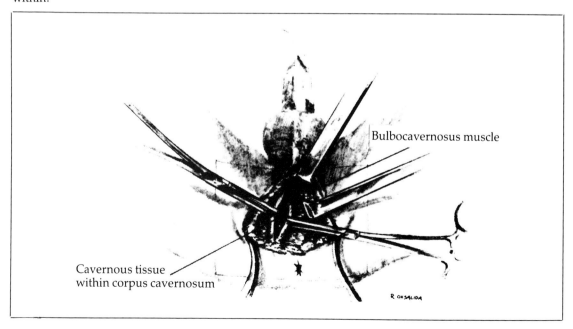

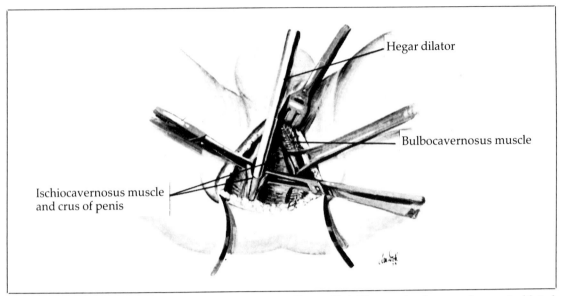

Hegar dilator

Bulbocavernosus muscle

Ischiocavernosus muscle
and crus of penis

Figure 22-4. The proximal corporal space is dilated with Hegar dilator. (Reprinted from M. P. Small, H. M. Carrion, and J. A. Gordon, *Urology* 5:79, 1975. With permission.)

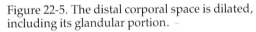

Figure 22-5. The distal corporal space is dilated, including its glandular portion.

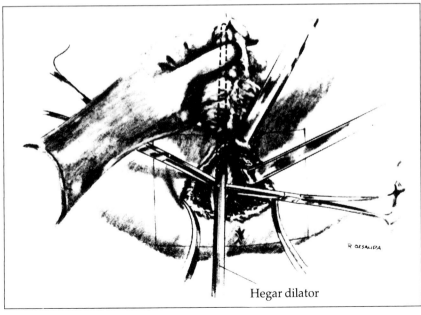

Hegar dilator

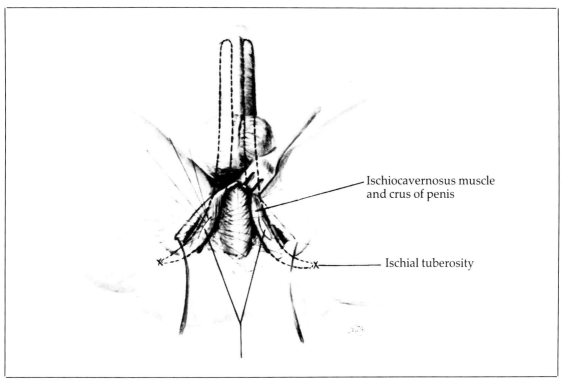

Figure 22-6. The dashed lines indicate prostheses placed within the corpora at completion of implantation. (Reprinted from M. P. Small, H. M. Carrion, and J. A. Gordon, *Urology* 5:79, 1975. With permission.)

possible perforation. It is imperative that the dilation extend to the end of the corpora and under the glans penis. The corpora are quite dense in this area and are embryologically separate from the glans penis. Perforation will not occur unless dilation has been too vigorous. However, disease processes such as priapism, scleroderma, or in some cases, Peyronie's disease may cause the corpora to become dense enough to require more vigorous dilation. In such cases extreme care must be taken to prevent perforation.

While dilating distally, it is extremely important to have the tip of the dilator turned laterally, rather than medially, to prevent perforation of the intracorporal septum. If perforation does occur, the implant will follow the same course and will cross over and be implanted in the contralateral corpus. Should this problem occur, it can be corrected by removing the implant and temporarily terminating the procedure on the ipsilateral side and proceeding to open, dilate, and irrigate the contralateral side. Once this has been accomplished and an implant of the proper size has been emplaced, it will be easier to implant into the original corpus. If necessary, further distal dilation can be accomplished before the proper size of implant is inserted. Figure 22-6 shows the implants fixed well under the glans penis distally and against the ischial tuberosities proximally. There should be no buckling of the prosthesis, because this would indicate excessive length and could result in eventual extrusion. There should also be no "drooping" of the glans penis, because this would suggest that the implant is too short.

The prostheses are easily implanted distally but may require an instrument to "flip" the tail into the crus posteriorly. To avert damage to the prosthesis, only smooth forceps should be used, because forceps with teeth may damage and weaken the implants.

After both implants have been positioned and the wound has been generously irrigated with the antibiotic solution, the corpora are closed with multiple interrupted sutures of 0

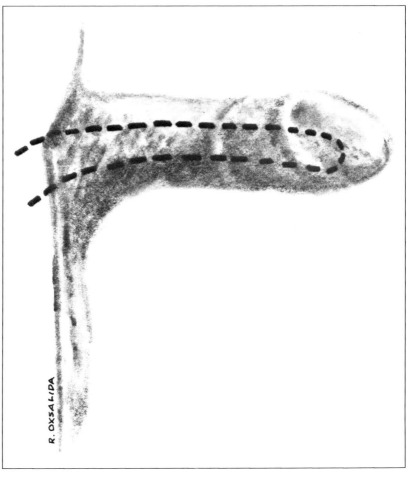

Figure 22-7. Lateral view of penile shaft showing intracorporal position of prosthesis (erect position).

chromic catgut. The wound is again copiously irrigated with the same solution, and the subcutaneous tissue is closed with multiple interrupted sutures of 3-0 plain catgut. The skin is closed with multiple interrupted sutures of 3-0 chromic catgut. Flexible colloidion is applied to the wound as a dressing. This wound covering works extremely well. Moreover, it is difficult to apply any other type of dressing to the perineal area, and the colloidion will remain in place for several days. It also acts as a barrier against contamination of the wound from the rectum.

Because all patients are evaluated routinely for any signs of prostatism or neurogenic bladder dysfunction before penile implant surgery, the incidence of difficulty in voiding, or frank urinary retention on removal of the Foley catheter on the first postoperative morning has been extremely rare. After the catheter has been removed, the patients may have some dysuria, but this gradually subsides with each voiding. The penis is kept in the position that is most comfortable for the patient, but he is cautioned to avoid excessive manipulation for approximately 2 weeks. This allows adequate time for the silicone capsule to develop around the implant.

The patient is usually discharged from the hospital on the afternoon of the second postoperative day, after he receives the last injection of aminoglycoside. Doxycycline, 100 mg every 12 hours, is prescribed for an additional 5 days, together with pain medication as indicated. The patient is instructed to start sitz baths immediately and to continue these for 20 minutes 4 or 5 times per day. These baths tend to diminish the need for postoperative

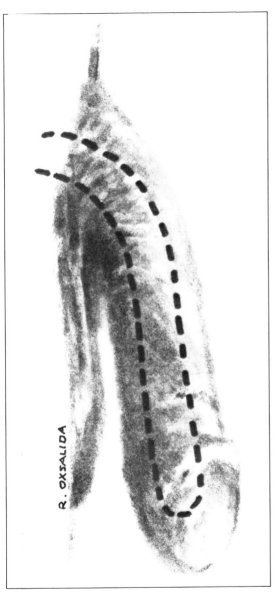

Figure 22-8. Lateral view of penile shaft showing intracorporal position of prosthesis (flaccid position).

pain medication and allow the patient to move the penis more easily. During this portion of the postoperative period, the patient is encouraged *gradually* to bend the penis downward, keeping it in the midline of the body. At the end of this time, most patients will be able to "wear" the penis in a downward position with minimal discomfort. Intercourse can be attempted safely at this time if there have been no complicating factors. Figures 22-7 and 22-8 show the penis postoperatively and

demonstrate its flexibility when implanted with the Small-Carrion prosthesis. After the discomfort of surgery has subsided, the penis will be relatively inconspicuous under the proper type of underclothing.

SPECIAL INTRAOPERATIVE
CONSIDERATIONS
Certain patients with Peyronie's disease may require more surgery than simple implantation of the Small-Carrion implant. Approximately 85 percent of patients with Peyronie's disease can be managed solely with the penile implant, because the implant makes the penis straight, or almost straight, and adequate for sexual intercourse. In the other 15 percent, even with the implant, the penis still has a chordee. It is in this group of patients that Raz and Kaufman [8] recommend incision of the Peyronie's plaque. I have found this to be most useful.

Once the prostheses have been implanted and the degree of chordee ascertained, a dorsal incision is made in the penis and carried down to the Peyronie's plaque, or band. Caution must be exercised to avoid damaging the midline neurovascular bundle. Multiple transverse incisions are then made into the plaques, or bands, in one or both corpora until the penis is straight. These incisions are carried down through the plaque, and the corpora so that the implant is exposed. Once the penis is straight, the tissue will granulate in, and therefore the opening in the corpora need not be closed.

Should a lateral distal chordee be present postoperatively, causing the glans to bend to one side and cover only one implant, excision of a wedge of corpora can correct the problem easily and effectively. An incision is made through the skin and subcutaneous tissue and is carried down to the Peyronie's plaque, if present, or down to the tunica albuginea of the corpora. An Allis clamp can be used to grasp the tunica. This will help determine how much tunica must be excised to bring the glans penis over the ipsilateral implant. Once the proper-size wedge of corpus and tunica has been excised, the wound is irrigated with the antibiotic solution and closed in a routine manner. This particular procedure also can be performed anytime in the postoperative period if it is noted that the glans penis bends to one side. This technique also may be used for patients with Peyronie's disease either at the time of implantation or anytime postoperatively.

Surgical perforation can occur, and if it occurs posteriorly in the crus, it can be closed with one or two figure-of-eight 0 chromic catgut sutures. The operative procedure can then proceed. If the surgical perforation is at the meatus or glans, however, that portion of the operative procedure would be terminated, and no implant will be placed in this side, because it will shortly erode through the opening even if an attempt is made to suture it. A contralateral implant can be inserted, and the patient can function satisfactorily until the perforated area has healed. This will usually take about 3 to 4 months; the other implant then can be inserted.

Paraphimosis is easily managed with a dorsal relaxing incision, because there usually is not enough skin to perform a circumcision after the implant has been inserted. After the relaxing incision has been made and allowed to heal, the scar is relatively inconspicuous.

In patients with severe vascular disease or in those who have had radiation therapy, implantation of the longest- and widest-diameter implant might not give them the best result and may even cause pressure necrosis. In this group of patients, I recommend implanting a prosthesis of a diameter that allows them to function sexually but not so wide that tissue necrosis might occur. The length of the implant must be sufficient to prevent the SST deformity, but again, oversizing should be avoided.

In patients who have severe fibrosis of the corpora it will be extremely difficult, or even impossible, to dilate. The use of instruments such as the Kohlman dilator, the Otis urethrotome, or even a scalpel blade may be necessary to cut this dense tissue. For this group of patients, I feel that the 0.9-cm diameter prosthesis is quite satisfactory and acceptable.

Although it is very rare not to be able to dilate the corpora at all, this is a distinct possibility in patients with severe fibrotic disease such as scleroderma or priapism. In this group of patients, I insert the Small-Carrion penile implant in the location that Lash [4] has recommended. In using the 12-cm prosthesis, the tip is placed under the glans. A certain amount usually will have to be cut off the prosthesis so that the proximal end will fit firmly against the symphysis pubis under the tunica albuginea. Obviously, this is less than ideal, but it does allow sexual functioning.

In patients who have not had erections for a long time, the corpora will develop some degree of atrophy. In these patients, I select the size implant that I consider proper for them at that time. As they start functioning normally, the penis will get longer and possibly even wider because of additional blood flow through the corpora. This additional blood flow expands the tissues that have been atrophic; in a small number of patients, replacement by a larger-size implant may be desirable. Should this be the case, I usually approach the surgery through the same perineal incision. The incision into the corpora is carried through the pseudocapsule. The interior, glistening surface of the pseudocapsule indicates that the proper plane has been reached. The implants are easily removed and replaced with the proper size, with or without further dilation.

The treatment of infection is varied, and if the infection is superficial and does not involve the corpora, the wound can be opened and treated like any other superficial infection. The implants do not have to be removed under these conditions. Rarely, one corpus may become infected, but this is usually late and secondary to a systemic infection. If this is the case, the implant should be removed from the infected side only, and the wound allowed to heal without primary closure. Extensive irrigation of the corpus usually will be required; this is done with a red rubber catheter that can be advanced gradually. The corpus that has not been involved should not be disturbed, because the pseudocapsule has protected that side. If both corpora are infected, as might occur in a diabetic patient, it is best to remove the implant as soon as the infection becomes obvious, and to irrigate copiously with an antibiotic solution through a deeply inserted red rubber catheter. Occasionally, a through-and-through incision and irrigation with the catheter must be carried out from one end of the corpus to the other for an extended period of time. In the latter group of patients, complete clearing of the infection and closing of the wound may take many months, especially if the diabetes is poorly controlled. In this group, it will be virtually impossible later to dilate the corpora sufficiently to implant a prosthesis. At this point one might consider placing the implant dorsally as Lash [4] and Pearman [6] have recommended and I have discussed under Peyronie's disease, above.

COMPLICATIONS

Table 22-2 lists complications in 590 patients undergoing implantation of the Small-Carrion penile prosthesis who received antibiotic therapy. The first 20 patients operated on are not included in this group, because antibiotics were not used routinely at that time. The incidence of infection was therefore much higher, approximating 15 percent. Since the use of the present antibiotic routine, the incidence of infection has decreased dramatically, and there have been only two serious infections in the subsequent 590 patients. Both of these infections occurred in diabetic patients and eventually required removal of the implants. Superficial wound infections have occurred in two patients, but these have been controlled easily and without sequelae. The implants were not affected.

Urinary retention has occurred in two patients, whose extruding implants were causing urethral pressure. One diabetic patient developed urinary retention secondary to neurogenic bladder dysfunction, and two patients required prostatectomy because of urinary retention secondary to benign prostatic hypertrophy. One patient was operated on with a retropubic prostatectomy, and postoperative drainage was by way of a suprapubic cystostomy. The other patient required transurethral resection through a perineal urethrostomy.

It has been suggested that patients who require frequent cystoscopies and/or transure-

Table 22-2. Complications in 590 patients receiving antibiotic therapy (September, 1980)

Complications	Number of patients
Urinary retention	
Diabetes	1
Perforation at meatus causing compression — unilateral or bilateral	2*
Benign prostatic hypertrophy	
Requiring TUR through perineal urethrostomy	1
Requiring retropubic prostatectomy	1
Perforation or erosion	
Surgical	
Scleroderma	1
Diabetic (required urethroplasty)	1
Postoperative — radical prostatectomy	1
Postoperative — radical prostatectomy and radiation therapy	1
Postoperative — penile implant (through glans or at glanular meatal junction)	3*
Perforation of crus (10 months postoperative and 2 years postoperative)	2
Postoperative — Peyronie's disease: Erosion of one implant where plaque was not incised	1
Inability to insert prothesis because of extensive scarring in corporum (post priapism)	1
Septicemia requiring removal of prosthesis, incision and drainage of perineum, and abscess of corporum (diabetes)	2
Paraphimosis — treated with dorsal relaxing incision	3
Inadequate size prothesis — subsequently had insertion of inflatable prosthesis	1
Superficial perineal wound infection without sequelae	2
Total patients	610
Complications	22
Complication rate	3.6%

*Same patients.

thral resections for problems such as recurrent bladder tumors should not be considered for Small-Carrion implant surgery. Indeed, it should be emphasized that transurethral resection should not be attempted through the urethra in a patient who has undergone implantation of any semirigid penile prosthesis. A perineal urethrostomy can easily be used to solve the original problem and still allow the use of the Small-Carrion implant. This procedure is quite simple and easy to perform and should prevent most postoperative urethral strictures, which are attributed to transurethral resection. An additional feature of the perineal urethrostomy is its low complication rate and the fact that the patients are so easily followed. It is therefore not necessary to rule out this category of patients as possible recipients of the Small-Carrion Implant.

Paraphimosis occurred in three patients and all have been treated adequately with a dorsal relaxing incision. Surgical perforation of the glans penis or the urethra is extremely rare, but excessive or difficult distal dilation can lead to this complication. I have had a surgical perforation occur in one patient with scleroderma in which the corpora were extremely fibrotic, as one sees in patients who have had priapism. Another surgical perforation occurred in a diabetic who had had three previous attempts at penile implant. (After one of the attempts, a urethrocorporal-cutaneous fistula developed.) Two patients had bilateral perforation at the glans. Both of these patients had undergone radical prostatectomy. One of these patients had also had radiation therapy for carcinoma of the prostate. Three prostheses eroded at the glandular-meatal junction, and two of these eroded only on one side; therefore only one implant was lost. One patient with Peyronie's disease had one implant eroded but was able to retain the other. This patient still had chordee after the penile implant, because the Peyronie's plaque was not incised. There was probably excessive pressure from the prosthesis in the one corpus, leading to the erosion.

In the two patients in whom the crura became perforated, neither was considered a postoperative complication, because they oc-

Table 22-3. Size of implant used in 610 patients (September, 1980)

Size prosthesis		Number of patients
Length (cm)	Diameter (cm)	
12.0	0.9	2
12.0	1.1	8
13.3	0.9	6
13.3	1.1	23
14.5	0.9	32
14.5	1.1	60
15.8	0.9	25
15.8	1.1	85
17.0	0.9	8
17.0	1.1	111
17.0	1.3	34
18.0	1.1	77
18.0	1.3	68
19.0	1.3	36
20.0	1.3	33
21.0	1.3	14

Note: Figures total more than 610 because a number of patients have returned for implantation of a larger prosthesis.

curred, respectively, 10 months and 2 years postoperatively. These were managed with surgical exploration and by suturing the perforation with a figure-of-eight chromic catgut suture, and reinsertion of the proper-size implant.

Table 22-3 shows the various lengths and diameters of implant that have been used in the 610 patients reported. One can see how essential it is that a broad selection of sizes be available in the operating suite to avert the problem of not having the size needed to provide optimum results. When one is sizing the patient, one must remember that there are certain patients who have a disparity in the length of the corpus and crus on one side as compared to the other. The etiology of this disparity of size may be congenital, inflammatory, or secondary to distortion of the pelvic bones after pelvic fracture. In this group of patients, the surgeon should be prepared to implant a different-size prosthesis on each side, so that both implants will rest evenly under the glans penis, even though there is no uniformity in the posterior location. It has been mentioned in the literature that the prosthesis can be trimmed and smoothed with fine sandpaper if the exact size of prosthesis is not available at the time of surgery. It has been my experience that this is adequate, but not desirable, because there may be some rough edges left on the implant that could lead to postoperative erosion. It is much more convenient, and certainly safer, to take the precaution of having an adequate size range available before surgery.

CONCLUSIONS

A normal state of erection can be achieved by bilateral intracorporal implantation of the Small-Carrion penile prosthesis. The implant gives adequate length and diameter to the penis so that normal intercourse can occur. Although the prosthesis is firm and considered semirigid, it has been adequately demonstrated that it is sufficiently flexible to allow the phallus to remain inconspicuous under the proper type of underclothing. In this reported series, there have been no patients who have requested that the implant be removed because they considered it too conspicuous. When discussing the surgery with the patient the fact that they will have a permanent erection has not appeared to be a deterrent or influencing factor in any case.

The goal of providing a penis with sufficient rigidity to allow intercourse has been achieved by a number of semirigid penile implants. If the operation is successful there is no need for reoperation, adjustment, repairs, or replacement. There are no mechanical parts to malfunction or hydraulic systems to become obstructed, leak, or otherwise fail in any way.

In my experience, the mechanical failure rate of the inflatable penile prosthesis has been underestimated in the literature. The success rates that are reported are usually achieved only after the patient has undergone as many as three operations after the initial surgery to correct a mechanical or hydraulic problem. With the Small-Carrion implant reoperation is rare and hospitalization is short.

For these reasons the cost is considerably lower and results more reliable than with the inflatable implant system. These are all important points that should be considered by both the physician and the patient in making a decision as to what type of prosthetic device to select for his use.

REFERENCES

1. Barry, J. M., and Seifert, A. Penoscrotal approach for placement of paired penile implants for impotence. *J. Urol.* 122:325, 1979.
2. Kramer, S. A., et al. Complications of Small-Carrion penile prosthesis. *Urology* 13:49, 1979.
3. Lange, P. H., and Smith, A. D. A comparison of the two types of penile prosthesis used in the surgical treatment of male impotence. *Sexual Disabil.* 1:307, 1978.
4. Lash, H. Silicone implant for impotence. *J. Urol.* 100:709, 1968.
5. Morales, P. A., et al. Penile implant for erectile impotence. *J. Urol.* 109:641, 1973.
6. Pearman, R. O. Treatment of organic impotence by implantation of a penile prosthesis. *J. Urol.* 97:716, 1967.
7. Raz, S., deKernion, J. B., and Kaufman, J. J. Surgical treatment of Peyronie's disease: A new approach. *J. Urol.* 117:598, 1977.
8. Raz, S., and Kaufman, J. J. Small-Carrion operation for impotence: Improved technique. *Urology* 6:68, 1976.
9. Scott, F. B., et al. Erectile impotence treated with an implantable, inflatable prosthesis: Five years of clinical experience. *J.A.M.A.* 241:2609, 1979.
10. Small, M. P., Carrion, H. M., and Gordon, J. A. Small-Carrion penile prosthesis: New implant for the management of impotence. *Urology* 5:79, 1975.
11. Small, M. P. The Small-Carrion penile prosthesis. *Urol. Clin. North Am.* 5:549, 1978.
12. Small, M. P. Small-Carrion penile prosthesis: A new implant for the management of impotence. *Mayo Clin. Proc.* 51:36, 1976.
13. Small, M. P. The Small-Carrion Penile Prosthesis: A Semirigid Penile Prosthetic for the Management of Erectile Dysfunction. In R. M. Ehrlich (ed.), *Modern Techniques in Surgery.* Mt. Kisco, N.Y.: Futura, 1980.
14. Sotile, W. M. The penile prosthesis: A review. *J. Sex. Marital Ther.* 5:90, 1979.
15. Wise, T. N. Sexuality in the aging and incapacitated. *Psych. Clin. North Am.* 1:173, 1980.

23

Silicone-Silver Penile Prosthesis

UDO JONAS

The criteria limiting the quality of a penile implant in treatment of erectile impotence are functional as well as cosmetic. An optimal solution would be a device that voluntarily allows a physiologic erection as well as a normal resting or shower position of the penis. This solution is achieved by the Scott inflatable prosthesis [2]. However, it requires a pumping maneuver before intercourse, and erection is effected by a complicated hydraulic system that has a high incidence of technical failures. The alternative consists of a non-inflatable prosthesis, e.g., that described by Small and Carrion [3]. This prosthesis has a simple design, much lower cost, and can be implanted with a simple surgical technique. However, there is the disadvantage of a more or less permanent erection.

To find a solution that has the advantages without the disadvantages, the silicone-silver penile prosthesis was developed.

DESCRIPTION OF PROSTHESIS

The prosthesis (Fig. 23-1) is made of silicone rubber. A silver inlay is imbedded inside the silicone rubber; it consists of twisted silver wires (999.7 fine silver). Thus, the penis can be directed into different positions and stabilized manually: erection for intercourse, downward for micturation as well as for resting.

The prosthesis is manufactured in two different diameters (Fig. 23-2) — 9.5-mm and 11-mm lengths and in lengths varying from 16 to 24 cm. The whole kit consists of 14 prostheses. At the distal end, which is implanted underneath the glans penis, the tip is significantly softer as protection against perforation (Fig. 23-3A). Individual adaptation can be done intraoperatively by cutting the proximal end (which is imbedded inside the crura) after selection of an appropriate size (Fig. 23-3B). However, a minimum of 3 mm of silicone rubber should be left beyond the silver inlay. For the length determination, a sizer, which has the shape of the prosthesis and a meter imbedded (Fig. 23-4), is included in the kit. Note that the calibration starts at each end for measurements of both the distal and the

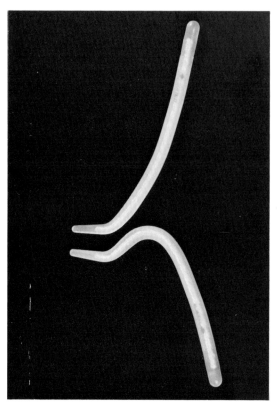

Figure 23-1. Silicone-silver penile prosthesis. A silver inlay embedded in the silicone rubber allows stabilization in different positions.

Figure 23-2. Full set consists of 14 prostheses: seven prostheses with a diameter of 9.5 mm (16- to 22-cm length) and seven pairs with a diameter of 11 mm (18- to 24-cm length).

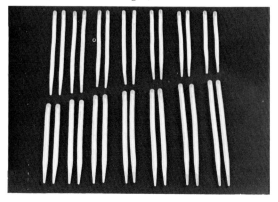

proximal distances from the incision site. The sum of the two measurements gives the exact prosthesis length required.

Stabilization in different positions is guaranteed by the silver inlay. Using a simulator (Fig. 23-5), bending maneuvers have been carried out to test the lifetime of the inlay. It became evident that there was no secondary hardening of the silver. However, breakage occurred in this very unphysiologic test (with double bendings 90 degrees upward and 90 degrees downward at a frequency of nine double bendings/minute) after 6000 bendings. This breakage, however, was never observed in the follow-up until 3½ years after implantation. However, two important facts were noted:

1. Even after breakage, the stability of the prosthesis was not at all jeopardized and the function was unchanged.
2. Even after more than 2 million bendings, the silver has never perforated through the silicone rubber. Thus, there does not appear to be any risk to the patient.

OPERATIVE APPROACH

The approach preferred in our institution utilizes a semicircular incision [1] at the dorsum penis in the sulcus coronarius (Fig. 23-6). After identification of Buck's fascia, the tunica albuginea is opened between two stay sutures. A dilation of the corpus is carried out down to the crura as well as distally underneath the glans (Fig. 23-7). Dilatation using Béniguet's probes starts at about No. 12F and is continued up to No. 30F. After exact length determination (Figs. 23-4 and 23-8), the prosthesis can be inserted easily (Fig. 23-9). As is seen in this schematic drawing, the use of an eyelid retractor eases the insertion distal to the sulcus coronarius. Closure of the tunica is accomplished using No. 0 Dexon sutures. The prosthesis should fit snugly into the straight corpus without tension (a prosthesis that is too long may lead to pain and possible perforation; a prosthesis that is too short may lead to kinking of the glans thus impeding

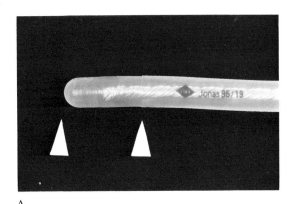 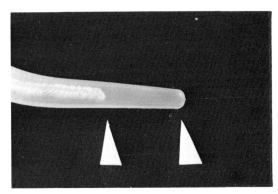

A
B

Figure 23-3. A. The tip of the prosthesis is of significantly softer material, to avert perforation. B. The proximal end (*arrows*) may be cut to an exact length.

Figure 23-4. A, B. Sizer for exact length determination which is included in the kit. Note the calibration starting at both ends for exact measurements.

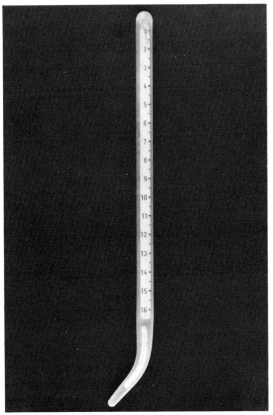 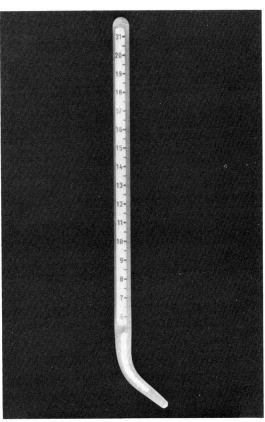

A
B

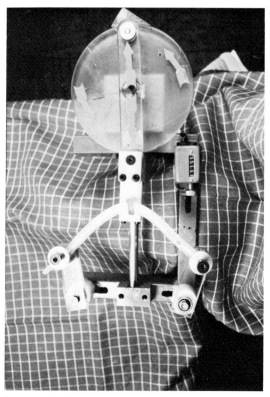

A

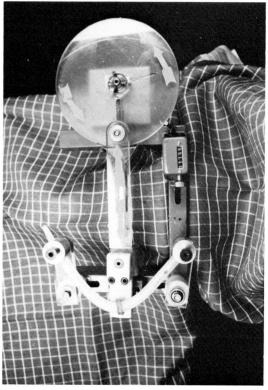

B

Figure 23-5. A, B. Simulator to test the lifetime of the silver inlay: double bending maneuvers 90 degrees upward and 90 degrees downward done through a piston. For further explanation see text.

intercourse). A mild compressive dressing is applied for 2 to 3 days (Fig. 23-10).

In patients with fibrosis of the corpora (e.g., status after priapism), an additional incision in the dorsum of the penis placed infrapubically is suggested to ease dilatation. A midshaft approach is also suggested in patients with spinal cord injury wearing a condom urinal.

Micturation is generally not inhibited, as is seen in Figure 23-11. There is no urethral compression either in the resting or in the erect position.

Figure 23-12 shows the postoperative appearance. Note the good cosmetic result with a stabilized erection in the upper half of the figure. Endoscopy is possible as long as the length of the prosthesis required does not exceed 21 cm. Above this length, the endoscope sheath is simply too short. However, special long endoscopes are commercially available (Storz). To gain some length for endoscopy, some torsion of the penis may be done. If this fails, a urethrotomy may be applied. Because

in our experience only 20 percent of the patients required a prosthesis longer than 21 cm, this does not seem to be a major problem.

RESULTS

Indication and diagnostic workup is not in the scope of this presentation. On results based on 55 implantations and a questionnaire regarding 350 implantations performed by 53 surgeons shows that this type of device produces excellent cosmetic and functional results. Complications included wound dehiscence (n = 3), which required secondary closure in two patients. On two occasions intraoperative perforation occurred requiring reimplantation. In our very first patient, postoperative bleeding requiring reoperation occurred. Since then the compressive dressing described has been applied and no further

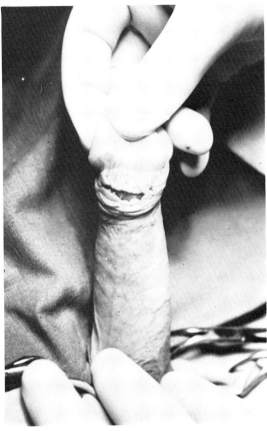

Figure 23-6. Operative approach: semicircular incision in the sulcus coronarius.

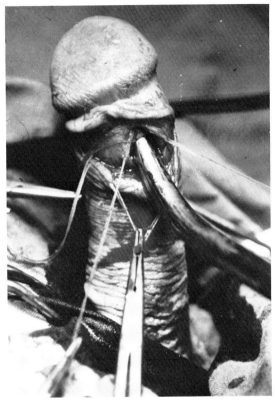

Figure 23-7. Dilatation distally and proximally from the incision site using Béniguet's probes.

bleeding problems have been noted. Two diabetic patients had the prosthesis removed due to infections. Another perforation occurred in a patient who underwent cast-bed treatment due to spondylolisthesis immediately following prosthesis implantation. In this case, the pressure from the cast against the crura had simply eroded the corpora.

Pain does not seem to be a big problem; it occurs in 14.6 percent of cases in the first 10 days postoperatively.

The success rate based on our results as well as on the results obtained via the questionnaire was 94 percent. About half of the physicians asked used the subcoronal incision described herein. Using this device with the operative technique described, improved treatment of erectile impotence has been achieved.

Figure 23-8. Length determination using the sizer seen in Fig. 23-4.

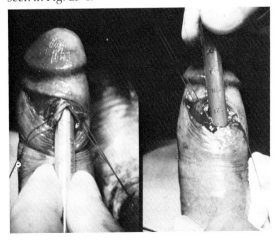

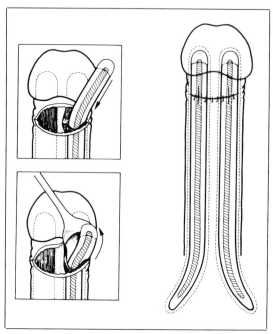

Figure 23-9. Insertion of the prosthesis: The eyelid retractor helps to implant the prothesis distally to the sulcus coronarius.

Figure 23-10. Postoperatively, a mild compressive dressing is applied for 2 to 3 days.

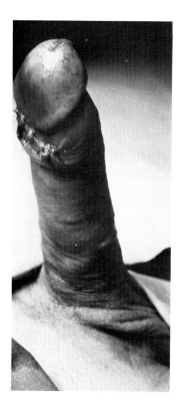
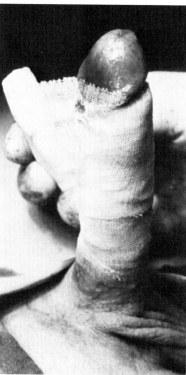
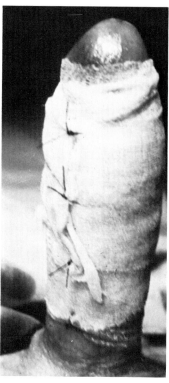

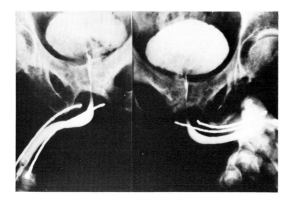

Figure 23-11. Postoperative x ray in the resting and erectile positions: the silver wires are easy to identify; note that there is no urethral compression.

Figure 23-12. Postoperative result in the erect (*above*) and the resting (*below*) position.

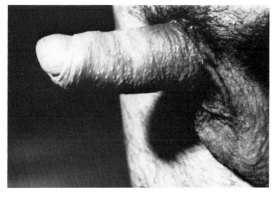

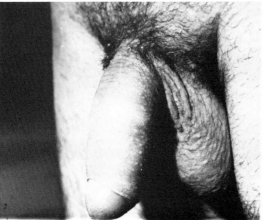

REFERENCES

1. Jonas, U., and Jacobi, G. H. Silicone-silver penile prosthesis: Description, operative approach, and results. *J. Urol.* 123:865, 1980.
2. Scott, F. B., Bradley, W. E., and Timm, G. W. Managements of erectile impotence. Use of implantable inflatable prosthesis. *Urology* 2:80, 1973.
3. Small, M. P., Carrion, H. M., and Gordon, J. A. Small-Carrion penile prosthesis: New implant for management of impotence. *Urology* 5:479, 1975.

24

Inflatable Penile Prosthesis

JERRY G. BLAIVAS

The inflatable penile prosthesis (IPP) was first developed and described by Scott, Bradley, and Timm [14] in 1973. The original prosthesis was constructed of Dacron-reinforced silicone rubber and consisted of four separate components: an "inflate" pump, a "deflate" pump, a fluid reservoir, and the paired penile cylinders. One pump was implanted into each side of the scrotum, the reservoir was placed in the prevesical space and the cylinders were placed beneath the tunica albuginea in each corpus cavernosum. All components were interconnected by silicone rubber tubing (Fig. 24-1). Subsequent design modifications have resulted in a less complicated, more reliable device, which consists of the two inflatable cylinders, a fluid reservoir, and a single inflate-deflate pump mechanism (Fig. 24-2).

The IPP is implanted completely within the body and can be inflated or deflated at will to mimic the natural cycle of erection and detumescence. Erection is produced by squeezing the pump mechanism in the scrotum. This transfers the fluid from the reservoir (located between the posterior rectus fascia and the rectus muscle) to the penile cylinders in the corpora. Detumescence is accomplished by pressing a release valve located on the edge of the pump mechanism. Varying degrees of tumescence and detumescence can be achieved by varying the amount of fluid transfer. Because the cylinders are expandable, they conform to each patient's corpora and produce an erection almost indistinguishable from a natural one.

INDICATIONS FOR SURGERY AND
PATIENT SELECTION

Candidates for implantation of an IPP must fulfill three broad criteria: They must have erectile impotence not amenable to conservative therapy; they must be psychologically and intellectually able to cope with the prosthesis; and they must be in general health good enough safely to undergo the surgical procedure. In addition, it is preferable that they have manual dexterity sufficient to operate the prosthesis by themselves. Occasionally, patients with Peyronie's disease in

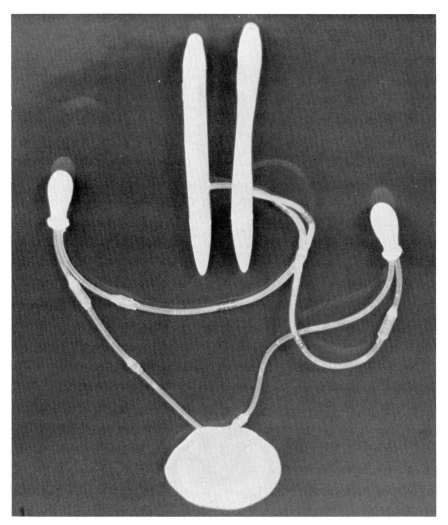

Figure 24-1. Original inflatable penile prosthesis. (Photograph courtesy of American Medical System.)

whom conservative treatment fails may also be candidates for IPP [11].

The decision as to whether impotence is amenable to nonsurgical treatment may be a difficult one. To this end, a careful medical evaluation seeking vascular, neurologic, psychiatric, endocrinologic, and anatomic abnormalities should be performed. A thorough review of the medication and drug history, including alcohol use, should be accomplished. Details of this extensive evaluation are found in Chapters 6 to 10.

Care should be taken not to confuse erectile impotence with premature ejaculation. *Erectile impotence* is defined as the inability to achieve or maintain an erection sufficient for vaginal penetration and intercourse. In most instances, the patient is able to achieve a partial erection that is insufficient for penetration, but he can achieve orgasm and ejaculation extravaginally [5, 17]. Some patients obtain full erections that simply detumesce before either orgasm or ejaculation has occurred. Patients with premature ejaculation usually achieve a full erection that is of adequate consistency for vaginal penetration, but ejaculation and orgasm occur either before or immediately after entry. Detumescence quickly follows, and further vaginal intercourse is impossible.

It should be determined preoperatively that

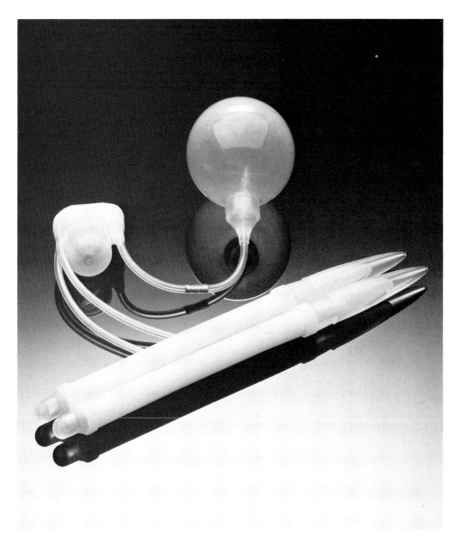

Figure 24-2. Current penile prosthesis. (Photograph courtesy of American Medical System.)

the patient can be expected to benefit from the procedure from a psychologic viewpoint. This requires that the patient, and, in many instances, his sexual partner have a clear understanding of the prosthesis. It should be emphasized that the prosthesis is only designed to *simulate* natural erection. If ejaculation and orgasm did not occur before implantation, they usually will not occur afterward; but if the patient was able to experience orgasm and ejaculation preoperatively, he should retain this capability. By itself, the prosthesis does not alter the relationship between a man and his partner. It does not increase his "manhood," nor does it necessarily make him more desirable. It only allows him to achieve an adequate erection, whereas that was formerly impossible. If partial erections were present preoperatively, it may be possible that this function will be retained, but only when the prosthesis is in the "deflate" position [5, 17]. When erection is accomplished by inflating the prosthetic device, no further erection is usually possible.

The requirement that the patient be a psychologically suitable candidate does not mean that he must have an organic etiology for his impotence, nor does it mean that he is psychologically normal. Certain patients with organic impotence are poor candidates for a penile prosthesis, whereas properly selected patients with a psychologic etiology may be excellent candidates. In the series of Furlow [3], Kessler [8], Malloy [9], and Scott [15], patients who underwent implantation of the prosthesis because of psychologic impotence fared just as well as those whose impotence was thought to be organically caused.

Once it has been determined that the patient is an acceptable candidate for a prosthesis, the decision to implant either an inflatable or a semirigid device must be made. Although it is ultimately the patient's decision, certain medical conditions favor one or the other prosthesis. All semirigid prostheses result in a permanently elongated penis. This often makes transurethral surgery impossible unless perineal urethrostomy is performed. Accordingly, patients who are likely to require repeated transurethral surgery (urothelial tumors, urethral stricture, neurogenic bladder) may fare better with an inflatable prosthesis, which generally does not interfere with cytoscopic procedures. It is my belief that the inflatable penile prosthesis may be a better choice for patients with absent or diminished penile sensation (especially due to spinal cord injury), because these patients are much more prone to erosion of semirigid devices [6, 10]. To date, there have not been any studies comparing inflatable and semirigid prostheses in spinal injury patients, but no erosions of the inflatable prosthesis have occurred in the absence of wound infection, whereas erosion of semirigid devices has occurred in up to 11 percent of patients [2, 6, 7, 10, 16, 17].

Insertion of the semirigid prosthesis is a simple operation that usually can be performed in 30 to 45 minutes with a minimum of postoperative complications [2, 7, 16]. Unless infection or erosion occurs, the likelihood of a secondary operation is remote. These considerations favor the use of a semirigid prosthesis for patients in borderline health in whom another operation might prove a hazard. Other advantages of the semirigid prosthesis include the fact that there are no mechanical parts to malfunction, hospitalization

is generally shorter, and the device is somewhat less expensive. The disadvantages of the semirigid prosthesis include the much higher incidence of erosion through the glans or urethra (0–11%) [2, 6, 8, 12, 16, 17] and the notion that permanent erection may prove embarrassing to the patient. In addition, the erection is usually less rigid than a natural one and sexual partners are more aware of the presence of the prosthesis than is the case with the inflatable type.

The main advantage of the inflatable prosthesis is that it effects a natural-appearing erection. The size of the penis can be varied, and, when flaccid, it appears perfectly normal. Transurethral surgery can be performed routinely without incident. The likelihood of erosion is remote. Major disadvantages include (1) there is a high mechanical failure rate (10–35%) [1, 4, 8, 9, 12, 13, 15, 17], even in the best of series; (2) it is more expensive; (3) the hospital stay is usually longer; and (4) the device requires a reasonable degree of manual and intellectual dexterity to operate.

Both types of prosthesis make it easier to apply and retain condom catheters. If the patient will ultimately require external sphincterotomy or transurethral surgery of the urethra, distal to its membranous portion, it is wise to perform that surgery first and wait at least several months before implanting the prosthesis. Failure to adhere to this principle may result in an inadvertent perforation of the corpora during surgery, exposing the prosthesis to a high likelihood of infection or extrusion.

SURGICAL TECHNIQUE

Because of the small caliber of the prosthetic tubing and valve mechanism, lint from surgical drapes or air bubbles that enter the system can cause device malfunction. Moreover, infection of the prosthesis site is a serious occurrence that requires complete removal of the device. For these reasons, special care must be taken by all members of the operating team to minimize such complications. Extraneous operating room traffic should be eliminated, and several authors recommend intermittent spraying of the wound with a broad-spectrum antibiotic solution [4, 15]. A separate Mayo stand or table should be prepared for handling the prosthesis in a lint-free environment before implantation. This table should have an uncovered metal tray on which the prosthesis can be stored and prepared for implantation. The operative site should be shaved immediately before surgery, to reduce the likelihood of wound infection. After routine prepping and scrubbing, the patient should be draped with lint-free drapes.

While the patient is being prepared, the surgeon should fill the reservoir and the inflate-deflate bulb according to the manufacturer's specifications. Because the device is constructed of semipermeable material, an isotonic solution must be used; otherwise there might be a net flow of fluid into or out of the system, resulting in possible device malfunction. The solution must be free of particulate matter that might clog the tubing or the inflate-deflate mechanism. Radiographic contrast medium is the solution preferred, to facilitate diagnostic evaluation should there be postoperative complications; but a history of allergy contraindicates its use, and normal saline may be substituted. Hypaque, 25%, diluted 1:1 or Cysto-Conray diluted 2:1 with sterile water are effective solutions. Higher concentrations of the contrast media should not be used; neither should Ringer's lactate solution be used as the diluent, because of the possibility of precipitation. After the reservoir and the inflate-deflate bulb are filled, they are submerged in a saline-filled basin until needed.

The operation may be performed through a midline or transverse suprapubic, or through a midline penoscrotal approach (Fig. 24-3). The penoscrotal approach should be used with caution in patients who have previously undergone retropubic surgery, because of the possibility of scarring and adhesions to bowel or bladder. A urethral catheter always should be inserted, to aid in the identification of the urethra before one incises the tunica albuginea. The catheter should be attached to a sterile drainage bag before passage, to avoid urinary contamination.

Suprapubic Approach

After the skin incision is made, the dissection is carried down just below the pubis, and the pale white, fibrous tissue characteristic of the tunica albuginea is identified; care is taken to avoid the midline neurovascular bundle. Stay sutures are placed, and incisions approximately 2 to 3 cm in length are made on the dorsolateral aspect of the tunica. Care must be taken to make this incision distal to the level of the pubis so that there will be no difficulty in introducing the distal part of the prosthesis (Fig. 24-4). By using a curved Metzenbaum scissors, a plane is identified just under the tunica on its dorsolateral surface. The urethra around the catheter is grasped with the left hand, and the urethra is pulled away from the corporal incision; a No. 7 Hegar dilator is introduced into the corpus. With lateral traction against the wall of the corpus and the urethra pulled away, the dilator is inserted distally into the glans, and then proximally to the crura. In this fashion, the corpus is dilated to a No. 11 or 12 Hegar, care being taken not to overdilate the glanular portion. Excessive traction on the stay sutures must be avoided, because this can weaken the wall of the tunica and may result in aneurysm formation postoperatively. If difficulty is encountered when one is dilating the distal corpora, the tip of the penis should be grasped by the surgeon, and downward traction exerted rather than pulling on the stay suture. Occasionally, the corpus may be so fibrosed that it is impossible to dilate with a blunt instrument. This is most commonly encountered after priapism or pelvic fracture. In these instances, it may be necessary to make several corporal incisions and incise the scarred area under direct vision.

There are several methods for determining the proper size of prosthesis. With the penis in the natural position, one should measure the distance from the midpoint of the corporal incision to the tip of corpora and then from the midpoint to the proximal end near the ischial tuberosity. A cylinder that is 0.5 cm shorter than the sum of the two measurements should be chosen. If the two sides vary in size, the smaller of the two sizes should be

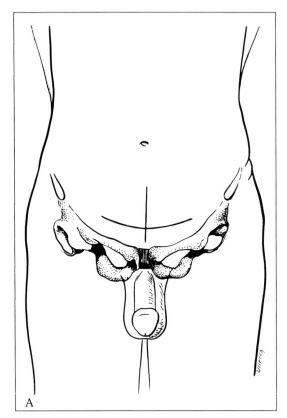

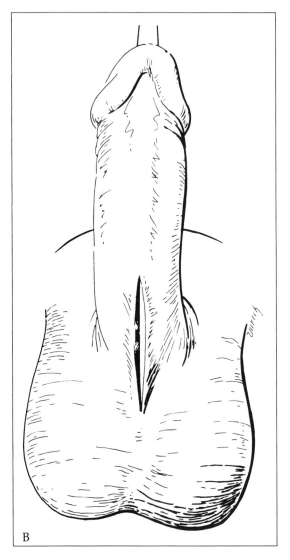

Figure 24-3. Incisions for inflatable penile prosthesis. A. Transverse and midline suprapubic incisions. B. Midline penoscrotal incision.

tried on both sides; but, occasionally, it may be necessary to use a different size for each side. A second method of sizing involves the use of the rear tip extenders (Fig. 24-5). This innovation permits the cylinder tubing to exit directly from the corporal incision at a right angle, without lying between the expandable portion of the prosthesis and the tunica, a position that may weaken the prosthesis. In addition, the surgeon can add 1 to 6 cm to the selected prosthesis to ensure an accurate fit for each side.

To select the proper size, the corporal incision should be made near the symphysis pubis. The distance from the midportion of the corporal incision to the distal end of the corpora is measured. That distance plus 4 cm is the size of the cylinder that should be implanted. To select the size of the rear tip extender that is needed, one should measure the distance from the midportion of the cor-

poral incision to the proximal extent of the corpus. One should subtract 4 cm from this measurement, and that is the distance that needs to be covered by the rear tip extender. The rear tip extenders come in 1-, 2-, and 3-cm lengths and can be added to one another to make up more distance. However, if the nonexpandable portion of the prosthesis can be palpated in the perineum, a larger-size cylinder should be substituted by using a smaller rear tip extender.

To prevent trauma to the prosthesis, it should be placed in the corpus with a Furlow inserter [3]. The Furlow inserter consists of a barrel and plunger. The barrel is placed into

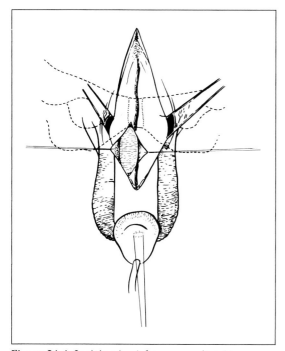

Figure 24-4. Incision in right corpus distal to symphysis pubis is demonstrated.

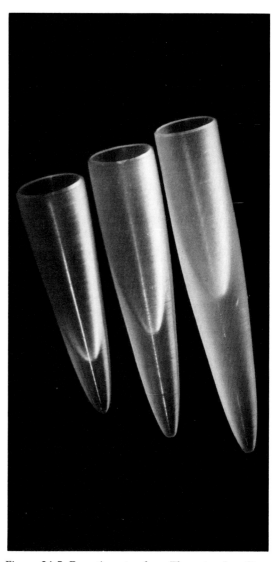

Figure 24-5. Rear tip extenders. The extenders fit onto the proximal end of the cylinder, increasing the length by 1-, 2-, or 3-cm intervals. (Photograph courtesy of AMS.)

the corpus, and the plunger is engaged to push a straight needle through the end of the corpus and out the glans. The penile cylinder is attached to the needle by a long suture. By grasping the suture, the prosthesis is pulled into position in the corpus (Fig. 24-6). The appropriate-size cylinder is selected and filled either with saline or radiographic contrast medium. The cylinder is filled with just enough fluid barely to distend the walls; care being taken not to overstretch it. With the obturator of the Furlow inserter in the retracted position, both ends of the suture attached to the tip of the prosthesis are passed through the eye of a 2- to 2½-in. Keith needle, and, with both ends of the suture folded back on themselves, the blunt end of the needle is pulled into the barrel of the inserter by placing the suture in the groove of the barrel and pulling until the tip of the needle is completely within the barrel. The inserter is then placed into the corpus in the same manner that the Hegar dilators were used. The tip of the inserter is palpated in an acceptable position in the glans, and the needle is pushed through the glans by inserting the obturator

fully into the inserter. After backing the inserter out of the corpora, while the suture is being held, the cylinder is pulled into position by gentle traction on the suture. Care must be taken to ensure that the tip of the cylinder is in good position in the glans and that the tubing is aligned with the incision in the tunica. Further traction on the suture usually allows easy placement of the proximal end of the cylinder in the corpus. Before cutting the suture and removing it from the tip of

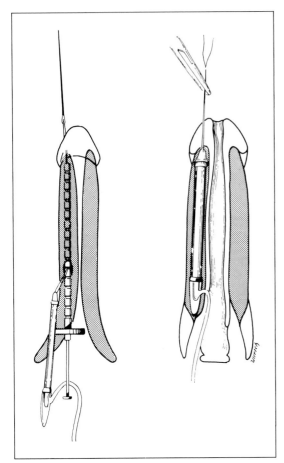

Figure 24-6. Insertion of penile cylinder into corpora using Furlow inserter. Furlow inserter with plunger in forward position and needle protruding through the glans is shown (left). Traction on the suture gently pulls the cylinder into position in the corpus (right) (see text).

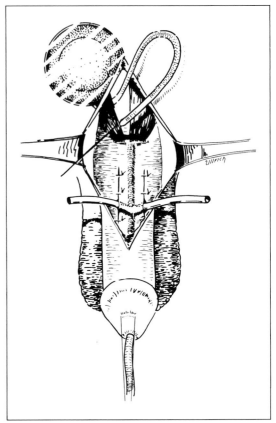

Figure 24-7. The reservoir is placed beneath the rectus fascia. The tubing is passed through the rectus muscle and fascia by attaching it to a specially designed needle.

the cylinder, one should check the size and position of the prosthesis by completely inflating it. In most instances, it is possible to place the tip of both cylinders well into the glans penis, but satisfactory results can be attained as long as at least one cylinder is in that position.

The coporal incisions are closed with a running or interrupted 000 monofilament nonabsorbable suture. Because of the superficial position of the corporal incisions, the knots may be palpable postoperatively and may cause discomfort. A single suture, beginning at the proximal edge of the wound just adjacent to the cylinder tubing, may be stitched in

a running fashion to the distal edge of the wound and then back again and tied to itself. This results in a single knot, next to the exit tubing, which is usually no more obvious than the tubing itself. The corporal incisions should be closed under direct vision, with care taken to avoid injuring any part of the prosthesis with the needle.

For placement of the reservoir, an incision is made in the rectus fascia, and the rectus muscle is split in the midline. With blunt dissection, a space is created between the rectus muscle and the posterior rectus sheath, and the reservoir is placed there. The tubing is brought out through a separate opening in the rectus fascia made by attaching the tubing to a specially designed needle, which is then pulled through the fascia (Fig. 24-7).

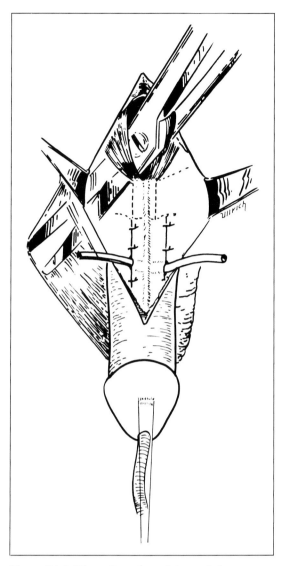

Figure 24-8. Dissection of scrotal pouch for placement of inflate-deflate mechanism is performed with scissors.

The inflate-deflate bulb is positioned beneath the dartos layer in the right hemiscrotum after a pouch is created by blunt dissection with a Metzenbaum scissors (Fig. 24-8). A large Hegar dilator may be used to enlarge the pouch to the proper size. The bulb should be placed as far distally as possible in the scrotum so that tubing will not be stretched when the patient operates the device.

The tubing from the two cylinders, the reservoir, and the inflate-deflate bulb are connected just distally to the external inguinal ring, in a plane just superficial to the fascial layers. Care should be taken to keep the ends of the tubing free of blood, lint, or air bubbles when the connections are made. To facilitate this, the open end of the tubing is irrigated with normal saline each time a connection is made. The appropriate length of tubing is selected by grasping the inflate-deflate bulb and pulling it into the most distal position in the scrotum. The tubing from the cylinders and the reservoir is then placed in a gentle arc so that it meets the tubing from the inflate-deflate bulb just distally to the external inguinal ring. After being occluded at the appropriate site with a silicone-shod hemostat, the tubing is transected with a clean, sharp scissors. The ends of the tubing are irrigated with normal saline by inserting the end of a blunt-tipped 21-gauge needle into the cut end of the tubing. Being careful to eliminate debris, lint, and air bubbles from the tubing, one makes the connections with 00 monofilament nonabsorbable sutures. Care should be taken not to pull too tightly on the suture, because this may cut through the tubing. Once all connections have been made, one fully inflates and deflates the prosthesis and carefully checks the position of all components. The wound is closed in layers with 000 nonabsorbable monofilament suture, care being taken to test the prosthesis after each layer is closed. At the end of the procedure, the prosthesis is left partially inflated.

The Foley catheter is removed the morning after surgery. The catheter is taped either to the thigh or the abdomen, in such a way as to ensure that it exits from the penis without exerting pressure on the side wall of the meatus or the glans. As soon as the patient can tolerate operation of the prosthesis, it should be inflated and deflated daily and he should be taught how to operate it himself. This is usually accomplished within the first 1 to 2 weeks postoperatively. It should be cautioned that failure fully to deflate the prosthesis can result in the formation of a constricting tissue capsule around the reservoir. Once formed, this capsule prevents full deflation, and the penis then continually remains in a partially erect state.

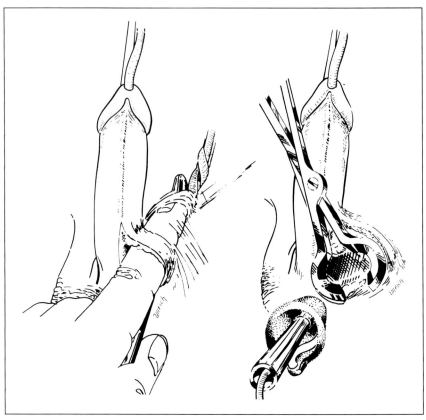

Figure 24-9. Creation of retropubic space for reservoir (left). Reservoir and reservoir carrier about to be placed into the retropubic space through the inguinal ring (right).

Scrotal Approach

A midline penoscotal incision is made and the tunica albuginea is identified (Fig. 24-3B). Care being taken to avoid the urethra, corporal incisions are made on the ventrolateral surface, and the cylinders are inserted just as in the suprapubic approach. After testing the position and function of the cylinders, one inserts the reservoir in the following fashion: The pubic tubercle is palpated through the scrotal wound, with the left index finger just lateral to the base of the penis. The finger is passed directly into the inguinal canal through the external inguinal ring. The floor of the inguinal canal (transversalis fascia) is palpated and a Metzenbaum scissors is placed adjacent to the index finger and the fascia is bluntly perforated. The retropubic space thus entered, blunt finger dissection widens the space in which the reservoir will lie. Retraction is accomplished through use of an extra long speculum or small right-angle retractors. The reservoir is placed beside the index finger

and it is gently advanced into place, care being taken to avoid formation of kinks or twists in the tubing. A specially designed carrier is available to facilitate placement of the reservoir (Fig. 24-9). Immediately after positioning the reservoir, one inflates it to its 65-ml capacity. The junction of the tubing and the reservoir should be palpated to ensure that there are no kinks.

With blunt dissection, a scrotal pouch is made for the inflate-deflate bulb, just as in the suprapubic approach. The tubing from the cylinder on the side opposite the inflate-deflate bulb is attached to the needle and brought across the scrotal septum to the other side. The tubing connections are made, and the wound is closed in layers. Postoperative care is the same as for the scrotal approach.

RESULTS OF SURGERY

The overall success rate of implantation of the inflatable penile prosthesis has been most encouraging. All recent large series have reported that between 91 and 96 percent of patients are able to use the prosthesis to their satisfaction with a minimal follow-up of 6 months. These excellent results, however, are at the expense of a reoperation rate of 6 percent to 42 percent [4, 8, 9, 11–13, 15, 17]. With continued improvement in prosthetic design and surgical technique, the surgical complication rate has steadily declined while the rate of success has accelerated. In Scott's original series [14], five of the first 12 patients were unable to use the device to their satisfaction and five required reoperation. In contrast, only 13 of the last 78 patients (17%) required reoperation and all have had a satisfactory outcome [15]. Similarly, in Furlow's latest series [4], the device malfunction rate has been decreased from 27 percent initially to 6 percent in the last 72 patients.

In a retrospective questionnaire study [5] of 61 patients (in a series of 180), 45 patients (74%) were satisfied with the prosthesis and 44 of their 59 sexual partners were satisfied (75%). Of the 13 patients who were clearly dissatisfied, eight had mechanical complications, and, after surgical replacement or repair, all reportedly were satisfied with the prosthesis. The other 5 complained of pain [2] or loss of sensation [1].

In Smith's series [17], 10 patients experienced partial erections prior to implantation and they all retained this capability postoperatively, but only when the prosthesis was deflated. When inflated, no further erection was possible. In Gerstenberger's series [5], 58 percent of the patients who were capable of partial erections preoperatively lost that ability after implantation.

COMPLICATIONS

Complications of emplacing the inflatable penile prosthesis may be categorized as either mechanical or pathologic (Table 24-1). Mechanical failure, such as cylinder or reservoir rupture, pump malfunction, or fluid leaks may be due either to faulty surgical technique or to prosthetic design problems (Table 24-2). In Scott's initial prosthesis, there were two pumps and four valves that could malfunction, whereas in the current design, there is a single pump and valve. In the original prosthesis, the reservoir had a seam that was frequently the site of fluid leaks; in the current one, the reservoir is seamless and the incidence of rupture or leak has been reduced dramatically. The problem of cylinder rupture also has been reduced. This is probably due as much to the introduction of the Furlow inserter for placing the cylinders into the corpora as to design improvements in the cylinder itself.

The major surgical complications include (1) infection of the prosthesis site (0–3%), which requires complete removal; (2) scrotal erosion of the pump (0–3%); (3) phimosis (1%); and (4) scrotal hematoma (0–2%) [1, 4, 8, 9, 12, 13, 15, 17]. It is important to note that erosion of the prosthesis itself, seen in up to 10 percent of semirigid prostheses [2, 6, 7, 10, 16], was only reported in 1 of 1243 implantations of the inflatable prosthesis.*

In order to determine the etiology of mechanical complications, a careful history is necessary. The patient usually complains of the inability either to inflate or deflate the prosthesis. The most common symptom is a gradual decrease in the size of the erection produced by fully inflating the prosthesis, which progresses to the inability to inflate the prosthesis at all, signifying a fluid leak. This may be confirmed by obtaining an x ray of the prosthesis that reveals little or no remaining contrast (Fig. 24-10B). On examination, the penis is flaccid and the bulbous portion of the pump mechanism may feel empty. If a small amount of fluid remains in the bulb, it does not refill after being squeezed. A sudden deflation of the prosthesis may signify rupture of the reservoir or a cylinder.

Although the diagnosis of fluid leak is usually apparent from the history and physical

*"Inflatable Penile Prosthesis Clinical Experience (1973–1979)." Compiled by American Medical Systems, Inc., 3312 Gorham Avenue, Minneapolis, Minnesota 55426, 1979.

Table 24-1. Surgical results of the inflatable penile prosthesis

| Author | Number of patients | Complications (%) | | Reopera-tions (%) | Success (%) |
		Mechanical (%)	Patho-logic (%)		
Scott, et al. [15]	245	42		42	96
Furlow [3]	175	21	7	29	96
Malloy, et al. [9]	105	23	5	31	93
Kessler [8]	50	14	6	14	96
Smith, et al. [17]	17	24		6	94
Montague, et al. [12]	17	12	6	12	94
Schreiter, et al. [13]	14	29	7	21	92
Fallon, et al. [1]	12	25	8	25	93

Table 24-2. Mechanical failures of the inflatable penile prosthesis

Author	Number of patients	Fluid loss	Cylinder rupture	Reservoir rupture	Pump malfunction	Tubing kink	Cylinder aneurysm	Buckling of cylinder
Furlow [4]	175	7	3	0	3	8	9	5
Malloy, et al. [9]	105		17	5	4	2		
Kessler [8]	50	4			2	1		
Smith, et al. [17]	17	2					2	
Montague, et al. [12]	17	1	1			1		
Fallon, et al. [1]	12	2				1		
Schreiter, et al. [13]	14	2	2				2	

examination, the site of the leak may be difficult to pinpoint. If there is still some fluid left in the prosthesis, physical examination and x ray may disclose that one cylinder is empty while the other is not, indicating a leak in the empty cylinder or its tubing. More often than not, the diagnosis is not as straightforward. Schreiter and co-workers [13] recommend re-inflating the prosthesis with radiographic contrast medium and obtaining serial x rays to demonstrate the site of the leak. Because of the minute size of most leaks, this technique is generally unsuccessful. Scott recommends utilizing an electrical continuity test* to demonstrate the site of a fluid leak but this generally has been unsuccessful in our hands.

*Available from American Medical Systems, Inc.

When the patient complains of the inability to deflate the prosthesis completely, there may be a tubing kink, a valve malfunction, or a constricting tissue capsule surrounding the reservoir. This latter condition is caused by one's not deflating the prosthesis completely during the postoperative period. If the cylinders are not fully deflated, some of the fluid remains in them and the reservoir never attains its full size. During healing, the tissue capsule that forms around the reservoir is too small to accommodate all of the fluid from the cylinders. Hence, even though the pump and valve mechanism operate normally, it is impossible to deflate the prosthesis fully.

A tubing kink often can be visualized radiographically, but oblique and lateral exposures must be obtained for one to be certain. On

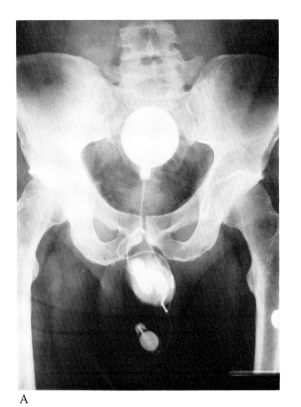

A

examination, the bulb of the pump can be deflated once, but it does not refill until the deflate mechanism is activated.

Other mechanical complications include improper sizing and placement of the prosthesis. If the tip of at least one cylinder does not extend distally to the corona of the penis, the glans may buckle during intercourse and cause pain. Placement of the pump mechanism too high in the scrotum may make manipulation of the device difficult or painful. If the tip of the cylinder is placed too far distally in the glans, pain or, in rare instances, erosion may occur.

Once an accurate diagnosis has been made, corrective surgery is usually simple and straightforward. The prosthesis is surrounded by a well-defined tissue capsule. If the dissection is performed with electrocautery, the proper plane is easily established, because the cautery will not damage the silastic components of the prosthesis. When a fluid leak has been localized, the damaged component should be replaced, and the sys-

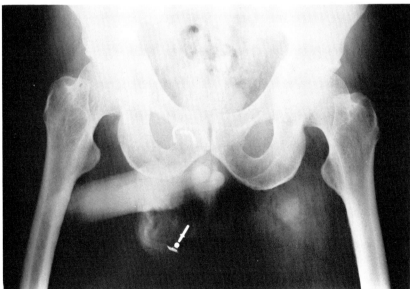

B

Figure 24-10. A. Normal x ray of prosthesis. The reservoir, tubing, cylinders, and inflate-deflate mechanism all contain radiographic contrast medium. B. X ray demonstrating loss of fluid with only faint visualization of the prosthesis (see text).

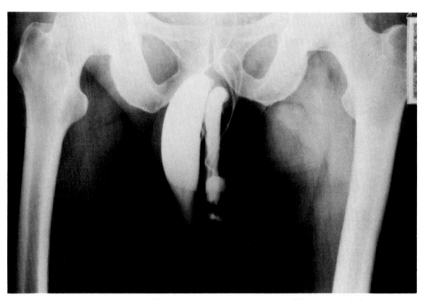

Figure 24-11. Aneurysmal dilatation of the right corpus is seen on radiograph.

tem retested for additional leaks; but if the site of the leakage cannot be determined accurately, it is preferable to replace the entire prosthesis. When a tubing kink or pump malfunction is diagnosed, the entire prosthesis must be carefully tested after repair to be certain that there are no other problems.

Aneurysmal dilatation of the corpora may manifest itself as an asymptomatic bulge when the prosthesis is inflated or it may be associated with pain (Fig. 24-11). It is not known whether the etiology is an inherent weakness of the tunica albuginea, an acquired defect due to excessive traction on the corporal stay sutures, or poor healing of the corporal wound. It is well documented, however, that once an elastic substance is stretched beyond its normal limits, it will subsequently bulge at that location when stretched again. Since both the silastic cylinders and the tunica albuginea are elastic substances, excessive stretching of either will result in a permanent defect.

In most instances, aneurysmal dilatation of the corpora causes only a minor cosmetic problem and requires no treatment. However, when the condition is painful and interferes with intercourse, surgical repair is indicated. The cylinder on the affected side must be removed, and the thinned out aneurysmal dilatation of the tunica albuginea must be

completely excised until normal tunica tissue is exposed. The resulting defect may be repaired with a patch of prosthetic vascular graft material such as Dacron mesh. The graft should be sutured to the tunica with interrupted monofilament nonabsorbable suture material. The prosthesis should be left in the "deflate" position for 6 to 8 weeks. At the end of that period, it should be inflated and deflated each day, with gradual increasing of the amount of inflation until a full erection is achieved after 1 week.

Infection of the prosthesis is, by far, the most serious of the pathologic complications. It necessitates its complete removal, because the entire device is contained within a single tissue capsule. When the patient has the classic signs of infection — fever, local erythema, tenderness, and leukocytosis — the diagnosis is straightforward. In many instances, the however, the only symptom is persistent pain in the penis, scrotum, groin, or suprapubic area. Constitutional signs and symptoms may be absent, and the correct diagnosis is appreciated only after overt signs of purulent wound drainage or abscess formation are apparent. These conditions call for prompt removal of the entire prosthesis, thorough irrigation of the wound with a broad-spectrum antibiotic solution, and maintenance of specific antibiotic treatment for 2 weeks because it is impossible to obtain adequate surgical drainage of all parts of the wound.

REFERENCES

1. Fallon, B., Milleman, L. A., and Culp, D. A. The use of an inflatable penile prosthesis for treatment of impotent men. *J. Iowa Med. Soc.* 12:444, 1978.
2. Finney, R. P. New hinged silicone penile implant. *J. Urol.* 118:585, 1977.
3. Furlow, W. L. Inflatable penile prosthesis: New device for cylinder insertion. *Urology* 12:447, 1978.
4. Furlow, W. L. Inflatable penile prosthesis: Mayo Clinic experience with 175 patients. *Urology* 13:166, 1979.
5. Gerstenberger, D. L., Osborne, D., and Furlow, W. L. Inflatable penile prosthesis: Follow-up study of patient-partner satisfaction. *Urology* 14:583, 1979.
6. Golji, H. Experience with penile prosthesis in spinal cord injury patients. *J. Urol.* 121:288, 1979.
7. Jonas, U., and Jacobi, G. H. Silicone-silver penile prosthesis. *J. Urol.* 123:865, 1980.
8. Kessler, R. Surgical experience with the inflatable penile prosthesis. *J. Urol.* 124:611, 1980.
9. Malloy, T. R., Wein, A. J., and Carpiniello, V. L. Further experience with the inflatable penile prosthesis. *J. Urol.* 122:478, 1979.
10. Malloy, T. R., Wein, A. J., and Carpiniello, V. L. Comparison of the inflatable penile and small-Carrion prosthesis in the surgical treatment of erectile impotence. *J. Urol.* 123:678, 1980.
11. Malloy, T. R., Wein, A. J., and Carpiniello, V. L. Advanced Peyronie's disease treated with the inflatable penile prosthesis. *J. Urol.* 125:327, 1981.
12. Montague, D. K., Hewitt, C. B., and Stewart, B. H. Treatment of impotence with an inflatable penile prosthesis. *Ohio State Med. J.* 75:9, 1979.
13. Schreiter, F., Skoluda, D., and Bressel, M. The surgical treatment of erectile impotence with the AMS penis prosthesis. *Urologe Ausg.* 15:276, 1976.
14. Scott, F. B., Bradley, W. E., and Timm, G. Management of erectile impotence: Use of implantable inflatable prosthesis. *Urology* 2:80, 1973.
15. Scott, F. B., et al. Erectile impotence treated with an implantable inflatable prosthesis. *J.A.M.A.* 241:2609, 1979.
16. Small, M. P. Small-Carrion prosthesis: Report on 160 cases and review of the literature. *J. Urol.* 119:365, 1978.
17. Smith, A. D., Lange, P. H., and Fraley, E. E. A comparison of the Small-Carrion and Scott-Bradley penile prostheses. *J. Urol.* 121:609, 1979.

Vascular Surgery for the Treatment of the Impotent Male

IBRAHIM S. HAWATMEH
ERIK HOUTTUIN
JOHN G. GREGORY
MICHAELA H. PURCELL

HISTORY

Successful penile erection requires that blood flow normally to and from the penis in response to nervous stimuli. Since the beginning of this century, much work has been done to enrich our understanding of the vascular components of erection. In 1902, Wooten [27] described a disorder that he termed *atonic impotence*. He reported that this condition resulted from loss of tissue tonicity and from relaxation and dilatation of veins and sinuses of the penis. The condition was treated by attempting to occlude venous outflow by ligation of the dorsal vein and thereby restore tumescence.

In 1908, Lydston, another pioneer, published the results of 100 cases in which he too employed "resection of the vena dorsalis penis" in the treatment of vasculogenic impotence. He attributed his success to the fact that both the superficial and deep dorsal veins of the penis were ligated. Lydston believed that this procedure resulted in two favorable situations that contributed to the success of the surgery. First, mechanical obstruction to venous outflow caused transient enlargement of the penis postoperatively, and, second, in his words, "the larger the penis following the operation the more the patient is impressed, and he feels that the results are successful, and his confidence is built, and permanent results often ensue" [5, 20]. Given what we know about the synchronous relationship that must exist between blood inflow and outflow for successful erection to occur, it is clear that simple obstruction of venous outflow does not solve the problem of vascular impotence [14].

In 1936, Lowsley and Bray [19] reported results of an operation for the relief of impotence in which the bulbocavernosus muscle was shortened and the ischiocavernosus muscle was plicated in addition to ligation of the deep dorsal vein of the penis. Of 51 patients reported, results were excellent in 31. The best results were in those who were made impotent by trauma to the perineum or urethra.

Attention turned toward the arterial components of erection in 1923, when Leriche described a specific syndrome that predominantly affected males between 40 and 60 years of age. This syndrome was characterized by pain in the thighs, hips, and/or buttocks; claudication; and inability to obtain or maintain a stable erection. The pathophysiologic aspects of this disorder involved gradual obliteration of the terminal aorta by atherosclerosis with superimposed thrombosis [10, 15]. In 1940, Leriche further explained the etiology of vasculogenic impotency by his observation that impaired blood flow to the pelvic viscera, specifically to the penis, resulted in decreased tumescence. It was noted that isolated lesions in the aortic tree, as well as vascular spasms, could cause erectile failure [16, 17]. It is interesting that reconstruction of the arterial tree has now been shown to improve erection in many patients [4].

Despite the steady growth of knowledge in the area of vascular surgery in general, the hemodynamics of erection received little further surgical consideration until 1972, when Michal described revascularization of the corpora cavernosa. Through his work, Michal has made dramatic contributions to the field of vascular impotence. He and Ginestié, in 1976, were the first to publish the results of revascularization of the corpora in which they employed microsurgical techniques and anticoagulation [7, 24]. Since that time, many centers in the United States and Europe have explored the vascular components of erectile failure. For example, we recently have been able to produce impotence in dogs by ligating the penile arteries, and then have been able to restore erectile function by revascularizing the penile bulb by direct implantation of the femoral artery [13].

Vasculogenic impotence has been clearly demonstrated to be an existing pathologic phenomenon. However, successful management by selection of appropriate surgical intervention depends on accurate delineation of the disorder. Our experience has led us to the development of a specific protocol of diagnosis and a set of criteria of operative management.

DIAGNOSIS

The first task undertaken in the evaluation of the impotent male is to differentiate between those who are impotent as a result of psychologic trauma and those who are physiologically impotent (Table 25-1). Once the possibility of psychogenic impotence has been excluded (or if extended psychotherapy has proved unsuccessful), surgical management is considered. Initially, we identify those with vascular abnormalities by detailed physical examination. The penile and peripheral pulses are palpated, and the abdomen is auscultated for the presence of bruits. Penile blood flow is measured by an infant blood-pressure cuff. An instrument that has been useful to us in screening potentially impotent patients after renal transplant is the Doppler ultrasound, which has assisted us in obtaining a gross evaluation of vessel patency [1]. However, the most important tool employed in the evaluation of penile vascular insufficiency is the midstream flush and selective bilateral internal pudendal arteriogram [8] (Fig. 25-1). By this technique, not only the extent, but also the precise location, of vascular obstruction can be identified. In addition, very useful information about the functional efficiency of the penile neurovasculature also can be obtained by transrectal electrical stimulation of the nervi erigentes. For this to be done, the patient is put under general anesthesia. A 19-gauge needle is placed into one corpus for the purpose of recording intracorporal pressures. A second needle, through which a solution of saline and/or contrast medium is to be injected, is placed in the other corpus; and a third needle is placed into the femoral artery to provide direct means of monitoring the patient's blood pressure during electrical stimulation. The rectal probe is then introduced, and stimulation to the nervi erigentes is given at 26 cycles per second. If erection occurs, it is concluded that peripheral neurovascular functions are intact. If erection does not occur, however, the corpora are infused with fluid at a constant rate of 50 ml/min, and the patient is again stimulated. One may conclude that vascular insufficiency does exist if erection occurs, and occurs only, during combined stimulation and infusion [12].

Finally, if revascularization is considered,

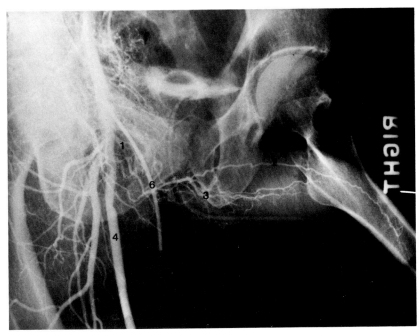

Figure 25-1. Left selective internal pudendal arteriogram showing (1) internal pudendal artery, (2) dorsal penile artery, (3) bulbar artery with its branches, (4) femoral artery, (5) Foley catheter, (6) angiography catheter.

one must investigate the competence of penile venous outflow in order to avoid postoperative priapism, a condition that is a particular risk after direct revascularization procedures. To do this, a cavernosogram is done, in which flat films of the penis are taken during detumescence after the injection of contrast medium and saline [11].

SURGICAL TECHNIQUES

The protocol outlined above assists the physician in obtaining an accurate diagnosis of vasculogenic impotence. Depending on the specific lesion identified, many surgical techniques are applicable in the restoration of normal penile blood flow. Procedures such as aortic reconstruction, endarterectomy, and thrombectomy have been used with varying degrees of success [4]. Moreover, several techniques employing revascularization of the penis have been described. Direct techniques provide arterial flow directly to the corpora, whereas indirect techniques employ arterial

shunting to the penile vasculature. Both types of procedures are presented below.

Direct Revascularization

FEMORAL CORPORAL SHUNT USING SAPHENOUS VEIN GRAFT. In this procedure, arterial blood is shunted from the femoral artery to the corpora cavernosa by using a saphenous vein graft (Fig. 25-2). To harvest the saphenous vein, a subinguinal incision is made lateral over the femoral pulse. Another similar incision is made distal to this at a distance determined by the length of the saphenous graft needed. The vein is exposed. Alternatively, one may make a transverse incision anterior to the tip of the medial malleolus. This will expose the trifurcated origin of the saphenous vein. Once the vein graft is harvested, it should be irrigated with heparinized solution and distended, so that any small break in the wall that might have occurred during harvesting may be recognized and closed. With the vein graft prepared, a tunnel is made by blunt dissection between the femoral artery and the base of the penis or the lateral aspect of the penis. It is important to remember during dissection that the graft when in place should pass beneath the spermatic cord structure. Because of the presence of valves, the vein graft must be reversed before anas-

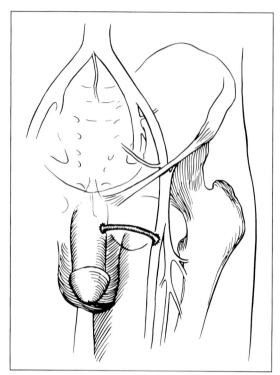

Figure 25-2. Femoral corporal shunt using saphenous vein graft.

function, gradually, over a 12-month period, all again became impotent [2, 11, 18].

EPIGASTRIC CORPORAL SHUNT. In this procedure, arterial blood is directed to the penis by direct anastomosis of the epigastric artery to the corpora (Fig. 25-3A). A paramedial incision extending to the base of the penis is made. The epigastric artery and vein are exposed and dissected free to the umbilicus, where the artery is ligated and divided (Fig. 25-3B). A tunnel is made under the inguinal ligament, and the inferior epigastric artery is swung down to the base of the penis and sutured end-to-side to the corpus cavernosa by using microsurgical techniques. With the epigastric corporal shunt, there is less flow directly to the corpora cavernosa as compared to the previous technique described. Therefore, there is a decreased incidence of postoperative priapism. Another advantage of this procedure is that the femoral artery need not be clamped. Success with this procedure is reported to be 70 percent [6, 23, 28].

EPIGASTRIC CORPORAL SHUNT USING SAPHENOUS VEIN GRAFT. In this procedure, arterial blood is directed to the penis from the epigastric artery to the corpora by interposing a saphenous vein graft between the inferior epigastric artery and the corpora cavernosa (Fig. 25-4). When compared to a simple epigastric corporal shunt, this procedure is associated with a greater incidence of vessel occlusion [28].

Indirect Revascularization

EPIGASTRIC DORSAL ARTERY BYPASS. By using the technique described in the direct epigastric corporal shunt, the inferior epigastric artery is swung down to the dorsal artery of the penis, and an end-to-side anastomosis is then made by using microsurgical techniques (Fig. 25-5). The patient must receive anticoagulant therapy in the postoperative period. Michal and Ginestié [6, 23] report successful results in 60 percent of their patients who have been revascularized by using this technique. However, in patients who have severe vascular disease, it may be difficult to find a patent dorsal artery of the penis, as this artery is

tomosis, to ensure optimal blood flow to the corpora. With noncrushing clamps in place, the femoral artery should be irrigated with a heparinized solution. An end-to-side anastomosis is made between the artery and the saphenous vein. A lateral incision is made at the base or lateral aspect of the penis, and an end-to-side anastomosis between the corpora and saphenous vein is made. This anastomosis is more difficult due to the hard, fibrous character of the tunica albuginea. A button can be taken from the corpus cavernosa to improve the anastomosis. Before the clamps are opened, the graft should be irrigated, and air completely evacuated from the system. Tumescence will occur after the clamps are opened, but this will subside within the first few postoperative days. Short-term results with this technique have been favorable, but long-term results are discouraging. In our series, over a 6-month period, five patients underwent revascularization through use of this technique. Although all patients initially enjoyed return of erectile

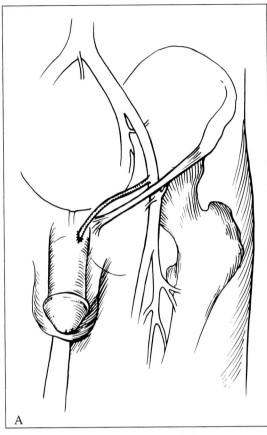

Figure 25-3. A. Epigastric corporal shunt.
B. Exposure of epigastric artery using paramedian incision.

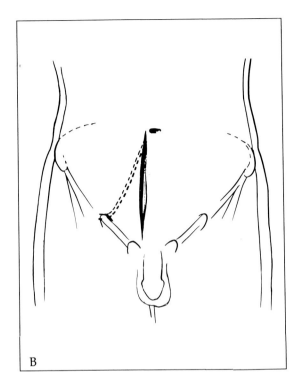

Figure 25-4. Epigastric corporal shunt using saphenous vein graft.

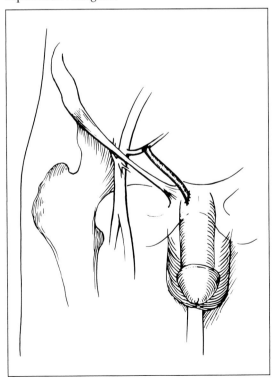

often found to be small and friable.

FEMORAL PUDENDAL BYPASS USING SAPHENOUS VEIN GRAFT. In this procedure, arterial blood from the femoral artery is shunted indirectly to the corpora cavernosa (Fig. 25-6). An incision is made on the perineum from the anal opening to the ischiotuberosity. The pudendal artery is isolated, and using a microsurgical technique, an end-to-side anastomosis is made between the pudendal artery and a prepared segment of saphenous vein graft. Next, the lower extremities are extended, and the common femoral artery on the right side is exposed anteriorly through an inguinal incision. The bypass is brought through a subcutaneous tunnel in the scrotal region and the femoral genital line in such a manner as to avoid the sharp edge of the pubic ramus of

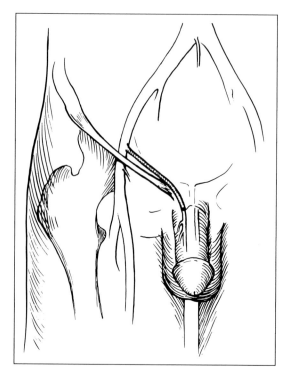

Figure 25-5. Epigastric dorsal artery bypass.

the ischial bone. The proximal anastomosis is made on the medial side of the common femoral artery, just below the inguinal ligament. Michal [22] performed this procedure on a 34-year-old patient who had previously undergone bilateral ligation of the hypogastric artery in an attempt to halt excessive bleeding consequent to pelvic trauma. After revascularization, this patient was potent for 12 months, but erections subsequently ceased.

SINGLE TO QUADRUPLE FEMORAL DORSAL BULBAR BYPASS. In this procedure, the saphenous vein is harvested with its tributaries (Fig. 25-7). An end-to-side anastomosis is made between the femoral artery and one to four of the dorsal and/or bulbar arteries; this results in a single, double, triple, or quadruple bypass, respectively. The bulbar artery is exposed by opening the corpus anteriorly with a long incision. Using a right angle clamp the corpus is gently probed until the bulbar artery is exposed. Preliminary reports of this operation are encouraging. Success is reported to be over 60 percent at 12 months' follow-up [3].

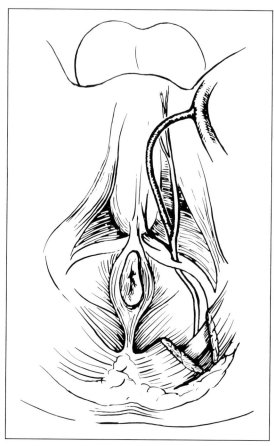

Figure 25-6. Femoral pudendal bypass using saphenous vein graft.

ARTERIALIZATION OF THE PENILE VENOUS SYSTEM (FEMORAL DORSAL VEIN BYPASS). This procedure is accomplished by using techniques described in the direct femoral corporal shunt (Fig. 25-8). However, the saphenous vein is interposed between the femoral artery and the dorsal vein of the penis by using microsurgical techniques. This directly arterializes the dorsal vein, and thus, indirectly, the corpora cavernosa. In some cases an opening is made between the arterialized dorsal vein and the corpora cavernosa, thus improving blood flow to the corpora. Verag [25, 26] reports 75 percent success at 6 months' followup using this technique.

DISCUSSION
Although great strides have been made in the treatment of vasculogenic impotence, much

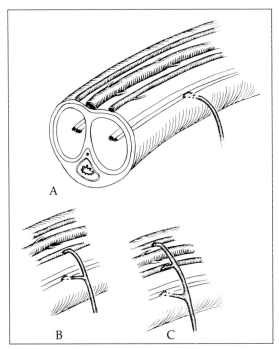

Figure 25-7. Femoral dorsal-bulbar bypass. A. Single bypass (femoral bulbar). B. Double bypass (femoral, bulbar dorsal). C. Triple bypass (femoral, bulbar, dorsal dorsal).

Table 25-1. Protocol employed in the evaluation of erectile failure

Psychogenic versus organic etiology
  History and physical examination
  Nocturnal penile tumescence meter
  Minnesota Multiphasic Personality Inventory
    Test (MMPI)
  Rorschach test
  Psychiatric evaluation if indicated
Neurogenic versus vascular etiology
  Glucose tolerance test and serum
    hormone levels
  Detailed neurological examination
  Cystometrogram (CMG) and sphincter
    electromyography (EMG)
Penile blood supply evaluation
  Palpation for penile pulse
  Penile blood pressure measurement by means
    of the Doppler ultrasound
  Selective bilateral internal pudendal
    arteriograms
  Corpus cavernosogram
  Intraoperative electrical transrectal stimulation
    of the nervi ergentes with infusion of the
    corpora cavernosa
  Miscellaneous: thermographic-penile scan

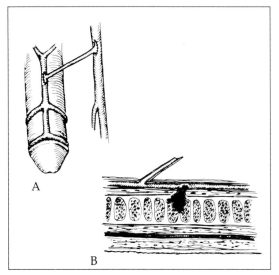

Figure 25-8. Arterialization of the penile venous system. A. Femoral dorsal vein bypass. B. Dorsal corporal shunt.

still needs to be learned about diagnosis and surgical management. Long-term follow-up, when available, reveals that surgical revascularization yields promising, but less than fully acceptable, results. In addition, the methods of diagnosis and the interpretation of the diagnostic findings are as yet unrefined. For instance, the Doppler ultrasound, though useful, provides no more than screening information. This technique can assess grossly the presence or absence of blood flow, but it cannot differentiate among the various vessels in the penile bodies.

The arteriogram is by far the most useful method of localization of vascular abnormalities, but results disclosed are often confusing. We have seen patients who are impotent with only unilateral vascular insufficiency. On the other hand, we have also seen patients regain potency after extensive trauma to the pelvic area with bilateral pudendal artery occlusion. Moreover, we have noted that some patients with bilateral renal transplants in which both hypogastric arteries were used regained potency after a time, even though both pudendal arteries had been ligated. It appears that some patients with severe vascular occlusion develop collateral circulation that is sufficient for erection, whereas others remain impotent with only minor vascular insufficiency. In addition to the above inconsistencies, the arteriogram is invasive and usually requires general anesthesia. Finally, much is yet to be learned about transrectal electrical stimulation. Although important information about the neurovasculature of the penis often is obtained, this procedure should be considered experimental. It is invasive, and we have found it to be associated with such complications as increase in blood pressure and burning of the rectal mucosa in dogs.

It is apparent from numerous reports that there is still no guarantee of success in the impotent male through use of any surgical technique, including the prosthetic implants [9]. For this reason, we feel the field of male erectile failure is open to the development of new methods of treatment. Although improvement is needed, firm foundations have been laid in the area of vascular correction of impotence. The use of anticoagulant therapy and of microsurgical techniques has furthered success in this area and has advanced urologic surgery into a new, exciting era.

EDITORS' NOTE

Indirect revascularization of the penis by the different techniques mentioned in this chapter offers several theoretical advantages over direct corporal body revascularization. With an anastomosis to the terminal penile vessels instead of the tunica albuginea, arterial blood flow is always proximal to the vasomotor control area of the corporal erectile tissue. Moreover, with a penile arterial anastomosis, systemic systolic blood pressure is not directed in a sustained fashion into the corporal spaces. It is not surprising, then, that the complications of direct corporal revascularization such as priapism and corporal fibrosis have not been seen with indirect penile revascularization.

There are essentially two options for redirecting arterial blood flow to the penile vessels. A saphenous vein bypass graft can be interposed between the femoral artery and the terminal penile vessels or the inferior epigastric artery can be anastomosed directly to the terminal penile vessels. As resting penile blood flow is low (10 ml/minute) the saphenous vein graft [3] may be in chronic danger of occlusion and thrombosis. It appears that the end-to-side microsurgical anastomosis between the inferior epigastric artery and the dorsal penile artery (the Michal II procedure) may well provide the best combination of achieving both physiologic regulation of corporal blood flow and adequate prolonged patency of the donor vessel. As previously stated, Michal quotes a 60 percent restoration of potency response.

Several modifications of the Michal II procedure have already developed. MacGregor and Konnack reported on the successful restoration of erectile potency using the inferior epigastric artery end-to-side to the corporal artery [21]. We have successfully performed revascularization in selected cases of vasculogenic impotence using the inferior epigastric artery end-to-end to the proximal dorsal penile artery. Indirect microsurgical revascularization using the inferior epigastric artery to any of the terminal penile vessels may provide the consistent, long-term successes that have not been realized during direct corporal revascularization.

REFERENCES

1. Burns, J. R., et al. Vascular induced erectile impotence in renal transplant recipients. *J. Urol.* 121:721, 1979.
2. Casey, W. C. Revascularization of corpus cavernosum for erectile failure. *Urology* 14:135, 1979.
3. Crespo, E., and Zorgoniotti, A. Personal communication, May, 1981.
4. DePalma, R. G., Levine, S. B., and Feldman, S. Preservation of erectile function after aortoiliac reconstruction. *Arch. Surg.* 113:958, 1978.
5. Gee, W. F. A history of surgical treatment of impotence. *Urology* 5:401, 1975.
6. Ginestié, J. Results of the Revascularization of the Corpus Cavernosum. In A. W. Zorgoniotti and G. Rossi (eds.), *Vasculogenic Impotence: Proceedings of First International Conference on Corpus Cavernosum Revascularization.* Springfield, Ill.: Thomas, 1980. Pp. 235–237.
7. Ginestié, J. F., and Romieu, A. Traitement d'impuissance d'origine vasculaire: La revascularisation des corps caverneux. *J. Urol Nephrol. (Paris)* 10:853, 1976.
8. Ginestié, J. F., and Romieu, A. *Radiologic Ex-*

ploration of Impotence. Amsterdam: Martinus Nijhoff, 1978.

9. Gerstenberger, D. L., Osborne, D., and Furlow, W. Inflatable penile prosthesis: Follow-up study of patient-partner satisfaction. *Urology* 14:538, 1979.

10. Hassan, P. W., and Busuttil, R. W. Leriche syndrome. *Surg. Rounds* 9:39, 1979.

11. Hawatmeh, I. S., et al. The diagnosis and surgical management of vasculogenic impotency. *J. Urol.* 127:5, 1982.

12. Houttuin, E., Hawatmeh, I. S., and Gregory, J. G. Clinical Differentiation Between Neurogenic and Vasculogenic Impotence Using Transrectal Electrical Stimulation. In A. W. Zorgoniotti and G. Rossi (eds.), *Vasculogenic Impotence. Proceedings of First International Conference on Corpus Cavernosum Revascularization.* Springfield, Ill: Thomas, 1980. Pp. 67–71.

13. Houttuin, E., et al. Surgical correction of erectile impotence due to vascular insufficiency in the dog. *Clin. Res.* 26:93a, 1978.

14. Krane, R.J., and Siroky, M. B. Neurophysiology of erection. *Urol. Clin North Am.* 8:91, 1981.

15. Leriche, R. Des oblitérations artérielles hautes comme cause d'insuffisance circulatoire des membres inférieures. *Bull. Soc. Chir.* Paris 49:1404, 1923.

16. Leriche, R., Beaconsfield, P., and Boely, C. Aortography, its interpretation and value—report of 200 cases. *Surg. Gynecol. Obstet.* 94:83, 1952.

17. Leriche, R., and Morel, A. The syndrome of thrombotic obliteration of aortic bifurcation.

Ann. Surg. 127:193, 1948.

18. LeVeen, H. H. Vein graft for vascular impotence. *Medical World News,* April 3:73, 1978.

19. Lowsley, O. S., and Bray, J. C. The surgical relief of impotence. *J. A. M. A.* 107:2029, 1936.

20. Lydston, G. F. The surgical treatment of impotence. *Am. J. Clin. Med.* 15:1571, 1908.

21. MacGregor, R. J., and Konnack, J. W. Treatment of Vasculogenic erectile dysfunction by direct anastomosis of inferior epigastric artery to central artery to corpus cavernosum. *J. Urol.* 127:136, 1982.

22. Michal, V., Kramar, R., and Bartak, V. Femoral pudendal bypass in the treatment of sexual impotence. *J. Cardiovasc. Surg.* 15:356, 1974.

23. Michal, V., Kramar, R., and Hejhal, L. Revascularization Procedure of the Cavernous Bodies. In A. W. Zorgoniotti and G. Rossi (eds.), *Vasculogenic Impotence. Proceedings of First International Conference on Corpus Cavernosum Revascularization.* Springfield, Ill.: Thomas, 1980. Pp. 239–257.

24. Michal, V., et al. Direct arterial anastomosis on corpora cavernosa penis in the therapy of erective impotence. *Rozhl. Chir.* 52:587, 1973.

25. Verag, R. Personal communication, 1980.

26. Verag, R., et al. L'impuissance vasscularie. *Actualités d'Angeologie* 1:13, 1980.

27. Wooten, J. S. Ligation of the dorsal vein of the penis as a cure for atonic impotence. *Tex. Med. J.* 18:325, 1902–1903.

28. Zorgoniotti, A. W., et al. Diagnosis and therapy of vasculogenic impotency. *J. Urol.* 123:674, 1980.

Index